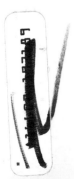

Beyond Cholesterol

Peter O. Kwiterovich, Jr., M.D.

Director, Lipid Research Clinic
The Johns Hopkins University School of Medicine

Beyond Cholesterol

The Johns Hopkins Complete Guide for Avoiding Heart Disease

The Johns Hopkins University Press
Baltimore and London   1989

IMPORTANT NOTE TO THE READER

Diets, exercise programs, and the use of medications are all matters that of their very nature vary from individual to individual. You should speak with your own doctor about your individual needs before initiating any diet or exercise program. It is especially important to discuss the use of any medication with your physician. These precautionary notes are most important of all if you are already under medical care for an illness or if the use of diet or medication is being considered for your child.

The Johns Hopkins University Press, 701 West 40th Street, Baltimore, Maryland 21211
The Johns Hopkins Press Ltd., London

The paper used in this publication meets the minimum requirements of American National Standard for Information Sciences—Permanence of Paper for Printed Library Materials, ANSI Z39.48-1984.

Library of Congress Cataloging-in-Publication Data

Kwiterovich, Peter.
　　Beyond cholesterol.

　　Includes index.
　　1. Coronary heart disease—Prevention—Popular works.
2. Cholesterol—Health aspects. I. Title.
RC685.C6K86　1989　　　616.1′205　　　89-2548
ISBN 0-8018-3828-2 (alk. paper)

This book is dedicated to my patients in the Lipid Clinic and to the participants in the Lipid Research Clinics Coronary Primary Prevention Trial and other research endeavors, who have given so much of themselves in the hope that they and future generations will be free from coronary heart disease.

Contents

Acknowledgments

I wish to express my deepest thanks to each of the following individuals for their contributions to this book.

First, I thank my wife Kathy and our three children, Kris, Peter, and Karen for their patience, devotion, and unqualified support while this book was being written. Anders Richter, Senior Editor at the Johns Hopkins Press, provided invaluable help and guidance, particularly during the formative stages of the manuscript. Jess Bell has my admiration and gratitude for the speed and authority of his complete editing of the manuscript. I am indebted to Joyce Kachergis for her excellent work with the figures and for designing the book cover.

I am indebted to all my patients, past, present, and future, who continue to teach and challenge me in the clinical practice of lipidology. Further, I wish to thank in particular those patients who contributed their favorite recipes, and who allowed me to use their personal vignettes as teaching examples for the reader.

I am greatly indebted to the staff of the Johns Hopkins University Lipid Research–Atherosclerosis Unit and Lipid Research Clinic, who have supported my efforts in both clinical and laboratory investigation and have become true friends as well as co-workers. In particular, the outstanding efforts of my secretary of ten years, Carol McGeeney, and her most able successor, Pauline Divel, in the typing and editing of numerous drafts of the manuscript are acknowledged.

Ginny Hartmuller, R.D., M.S., currently the chief nutritionist in the Lipid Research Clinic, and her predecessor, Katherine Boyd, R.D., M.S., both contributed in a most significant way to the chapters dealing with nutrition and the preparation of the two-week menu plan and recipes. Judith Chiostri, R.D., M.S., prepared the food tables in Appendix B and also contributed to Part III, Diet and Cholesterol. I thank Katie Hanna, a predoctoral student, for her help with the analysis of the nutritional content of the recipes. Thomas Weber, Clinic Manager, and Ann Schmidt, Clinic Co-ordinator, provided valuable assistance with the patient vignettes, and Noreen Porell helped immensely with the references. I thank Hazel Smith for her help and devotion to the families of Tracey Bechard and Barbara Allen and other patients who have serious lipid problems.

The following members of the Lipid Research Clinic staff reviewed various parts of the book: Paul S. Bachorik, Ph.D., Stephanie D. Kafonek, M.D., and Michael Miller, M.D. Others who provided valuable reviews of certain parts of the book were: Peter Wood, D.Sc., Ph.D., Bonnie Weiner, M.D., Kerry Stewart, Ph.D., Bernard Wolfe, FRCPC, Kenneth Carroll, Ph.D., Diane Becker, D.Sc., Thomas Pearson, M.D., Ph.D., Donald Hunninghake, M.D., Ph.D., Ronald Lauer, M.D., Frank Franklin, M.D., Ph.D., Reg Murphy, Don Graham, and my sisters Pamela Skwish and Deborah Kwiterovich-Hoover.

I wish particularly to thank Mary Pugh of Ally and Gargano, Inc. for her many astute suggestions for making the manuscript suitable for the layman. Vera Belsky of Merck Health Information Services, Merck, Sharp & Dohme, also provided useful suggestions in this regard, and I am grateful for the support of her department for the artwork for the book. Morton Levinstein read the entire manuscript and had many pertinent comments. Finally, I thank Jeanne Moody for preparing the indexes in such a professional way.

It's More Than Just Cholesterol

Cholesterol. You have heard or read the word a hundred times on television, on radio, and in the newspaper. Just about every magazine has featured articles about cholesterol, and several books have been written about how to cure it or control it. Despite all this fanfare, many Americans are still not sure what cholesterol is, or what they should be doing about it. Just a few short years ago the National Heart, Lung, and Blood Institute and the Food and Drug Administration found that although 46 percent of the respondents reported having had their blood cholesterol measured, only 7 percent actually knew what their cholesterol level was. In the same survey it was found that only 23 percent of Americans had attempted dietary changes to lower their blood cholesterol levels.

It's no wonder there is so much confusion about cholesterol. Even the truth can be misleading. A product says "No cholesterol" but is bad for you anyway because it is high in saturated fat. Another product states "Only vegetable shortening used," but the vegetable oil has been hardened by a process that increases its content of saturated fat. Just several years ago, didn't you read that olives weren't good for you? Now, all of a sudden, people are saying that olive oil is wonderful. A woman in the supermarket says, "This product has coconut oil; I'm not going to buy it, it's too high in cholesterol." She is right not to buy it, but for the wrong reason! A man says, "Why does this recipe call for egg whites, don't they know that eggs are high in cholesterol?" Eggs are; egg whites aren't.

And if it isn't confusing enough about what you should eat to help you have a healthy heart, along comes all the complicated jargon about cholesterol in your blood. You have probably heard about "good cholesterol" and "bad cholesterol," but isn't this a contradiction in terms? Could someone please explain in simple terms what the difference is and why it matters?

Your next-door neighbor's husband had a heart attack. Why? His cholesterol level was perfectly normal, he wasn't overweight, and he had eaten a healthy diet for years. How can this happen? Does research on cholesterol have fundamental flaws? You might ask, "If cholesterol isn't the answer, what is? What can I do to help avoid heart disease?"

Or a doctor tells you that your child's cholesterol level is too high. You are terrified. You may wonder, "Is my child going to have a heart attack? How can that be?"

Perhaps you or your child is on the pudgy side, and you think maybe exercise would help, but then why did Jim Fixx, the health writer and marathon runner, die suddenly and unexpectedly from heart disease? Good heavens, you say, are there no absolutes? Are there no straightforward answers?

Perhaps you have already tried a diet low in cholesterol and saturated fat. Or you have jumped on the recent oat bran bandwagon to get more fiber in your diet, or the fish oil bandwagon to increase your omega-3 intake. But your cholesterol is still too high. Should you take some new wonder drug that lowers blood cholesterol and cleans it out of the body, or take any drug at all? What should you do?

You may be one of hundreds of thousands of Americans who have had coronary artery bypass surgery or coronary balloon angioplasty. You still have a lot to live for. But to understand what you can do to decrease the chance of future blockages, you need to understand the basic reasons why you developed the problem in the first place.

I have written this book because I believe it is time that an expert in cholesterol answered questions of this sort in a clear, simple manner. The American public does not need to be misled or misinformed, let alone to live in fear of food. If you read this book, you will be able to assess more completely and confidently your risk of heart disease, and you will understand better what you and your doctor can do to help you prevent it.

Nothing takes the place of experience and knowledge. Over the past seventeen years, I have worked with many adults and children who have problems with cholesterol and other fats in their bodies. I have learned firsthand what their concerns are and what needs to be done to help them increase their chances of living longer and better lives. I have taken these lessons and used them as examples to help you understand the basic points made in this book. Finally, my patients have even provided their very own favorite recipes for you.

Cholesterol is the central problem, but not the whole story. As this book's title, *Beyond Cholesterol*, implies, there are other factors that either make things worse or make things better. On the bad side, these include saturated fats, low levels of "good cholesterol," and triglyceride problems; on the good side, weight control, exercise, and the judicious use of drugs when all else fails. This book tells you, in the simplest possible language, what is known about the causes of heart disease and what you can do to avoid it, both for yourself and for those you love.

PART ONE

Coronary Heart Disease and Cholesterol

CHAPTER I

Introduction

I walked along the beach. I couldn't believe both Tracey and Barbara were gone. Only fifteen years old, they had died from complications of the most severe kind of cholesterol problem; despite a decade of work with these children, I had failed to save them. But perhaps they will not have died in vain if only people can be made to realize how important cholesterol can be. At that moment, I resolved to write this book.

There is only one chance in a million that your child has the same cholesterol problem as Tracey and Barbara. But there is one chance in four that your child's blood cholesterol level is too high, and one chance in two that your own blood cholesterol level is higher than 200 mg/dl (milligrams per deciliter), now considered at the top of the desirable range. In fact, the odds are one in four that your blood cholesterol level is above 240 mg/dl, placing you at a significantly higher risk of coronary heart disease.

Why are the odds so great that your blood cholesterol level may be too high? It could be that your diet contains too much total fat, saturated fat, cholesterol, and simple sugars, and is lacking in fiber and complex sugars. If so, you're not alone. Americans are brought up to eat plenty of meat, whole milk, cheese, ice cream, butter, and fancy desserts. It's not just your diet; other factors such as physical inactivity, obesity, diabetes, and inherited genetic conditions may be involved. In summary, both nature and nurture, both genes and diet, are important factors that can influence your blood cholesterol level and lead you to develop coronary heart disease.

Are your children at risk? This too depends both on what genes they have inherited and on the lives they lead. A heart-healthy lifestyle for your children starts with learning good nutrition and forming proper eating habits. Good habits of exercise are essential and are easier to form in childhood. Understanding about foods high in calories and fat will help them from becoming obese. Knowing the dangers of smoking can help keep your teenagers away from cigarettes.

In the past twenty years, exceptional progress has been made in understanding the role of cholesterol in the development of coronary heart disease. It is now established not only that an elevated blood cholesterol level is a strong risk factor for the development of coronary heart disease, but also that lowering elevated blood cholesterol levels *decreases* deaths and heart attacks from coronary heart disease. Further, doctors now better understand the fundamental processes involved in the body's handling of cholesterol. This has led both to better diagnosis of people who have inherited types of cholesterol problems, and to more specific and effective treatment with diet and drugs.

The theme of this book is preventing coronary heart disease by recognizing and modifying risk factors, particularly the blood cholesterol level. Do you know your blood cholesterol level? If it is high, do you know why? Finally, do you know what you and your doctor can do to reduce your risk of coronary heart disease? Although it is now possible to prevent coronary heart disease by controlling cholesterol, only one in ten Americans knows his or her blood cholesterol level and what can be done to lower it. People are much more knowledgeable these days about high blood pressure and cigarette smoking, also risk factors for coronary heart disease, but few know as much about cholesterol.

Deaths from coronary heart disease in the United States have decreased over 30 percent since 1967, but in 1987 an estimated 514,000 Americans were killed by this disease (Figure 1-1) and over 700,000 others were admitted to hospitals because of heart attacks. In the same year, some 332,000 open heart operations, called coronary artery bypass grafts, were performed on patients with coronary heart disease.

More recently, a newer procedure that does not require open heart surgery, called coronary artery balloon angioplasty, has been used to treat blocked coronary arteries. Using a flexible artery-thin tube, an uninflated balloon is inserted into the artery underneath the blockage, and the balloon is then inflated to "squash down" the blockage. Coronary angioplasty procedures jumped from 6,000 in 1980 to 184,000 in 1987, and continued growth can be expected.

In all, almost five million Americans know they have coronary heart disease. They know because the blockages in their coronary

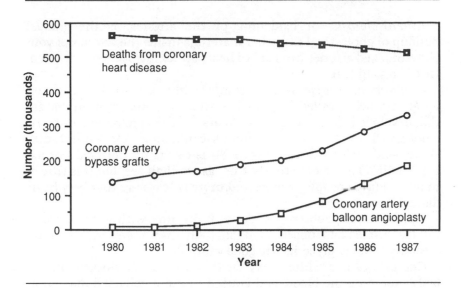

Fig 1-1. Coronary heart disease in America, 1980–1987.
Data from National Center for Health Statistics: Hospital Discharge Survey (August 1988).

arteries are so advanced that they have suffered a heart attack or other heart-related problems. Many more millions of people have "hidden" coronary artery disease. One or more of their coronary arteries have accumulated enough cholesterol to cause at least 50 percent blockages, but the blockage has not yet caused any signs of coronary heart disease such as chest pain or a heart attack.

Is it worthwhile to prevent coronary heart disease? The answer is plainly yes in personal terms; it is better to be alive than dead, better to be healthy than sick. But the answer is also yes in terms of national policy. In 1984, 1 percent of the gross national product went for coronary artery bypass operations alone, and coronary heart disease cost this country over $50 billion.

This book will give you the tools to work with your doctor to reduce your risk of coronary heart disease and avoid becoming another coronary disease statistic. In the following chapters I will translate the results of years of research into practical recommendations for you and your family, recommendations based on my own experiences with patients. Certain words and phrases that may be unfamiliar are defined in the text, and a Glossary is also provided at the end of the book. Let me begin by defining some of the common words and phrases used throughout the book.

Atherosclerosis, or hardening of the arteries, is the gradual buildup of cholesterol and other materials inside the arteries of your body. Blocked arteries can lead to heart attack, stroke, or poor circulation in your legs.

Coronary heart disease is the result of atherosclerosis in the arteries of your heart, called the coronary arteries. Coronary heart disease that develops before the age of 55 years is called premature (or early) coronary heart disease. The famous cardiologist Dr. Paul Dudley White said, "Heart disease before 80 is our fault, not God's or nature's will." This is not strictly true, as we shall see, but it is true of more and more people as more and more is learned about how heart disease occurs.

Lipids are fats, substances that will not mix with water. Cholesterol, saturated fats, unsaturated fats (polyunsaturated and monounsaturated), and triglyceride are good examples.

Cholesterol is a white, waxy fat found naturally throughout the body including the blood, and is used to build cells and make hormones. The liver and other organs can manufacture all the cholesterol your body needs. However, cholesterol also comes from the animal foods you eat, such as eggs, meats, butter, and whole milk. Cholesterol is not found in plant foods.

Saturated fats are white, oily substances that are solid at room temperature. They are the main component of the white marbling in meats, the visible fat around meat, meat drippings that become solid after cooling, and butter and cheese. In addition to their presence in animal products such as red meats, whole milk, cheese, and ice cream, saturated fats are also plentiful in coconut oil and palm oil, two plant oils widely used in commercially processed foods.

Unsaturated fats are clear, oily substances that are liquid at room temperature. They are the main component of oils that come from plants. *Monounsaturated fats* are found in olive oil and canola oil. *Polyunsaturated fats* are found in corn oil, sunflower seed oil, and safflower oil.

Triglyceride is a fat that contains three fatty acids (*tri* means three). It is found in the food you eat and in your body, including your bloodstream. The fatty acids may be saturated, monounsaturated, or polyunsaturated. The type of fatty acid that predominates determines whether the triglyceride is a saturated fat, a monounsaturated fat, or a polyunsaturated fat.

Lipoproteins. Just as "oil and water do not mix," cholesterol and triglyceride cannot dissolve in your blood unless they are mixed

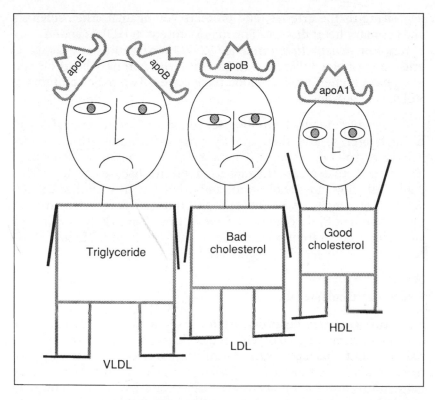

Fig. 1-2. Schema depicting the three major lipoproteins in blood from fasting patients: VLDL (very-low-density lipoprotein), LDL (low-density lipoprotein), and HDL (high-density lipoprotein). VLDL and LDL increase the risk of coronary heart disease; HDL appears to protect against it.

with proteins. Lipids travel in your blood in packages of fat and protein called lipoproteins.

✶ *Low-density lipoprotein (or LDL)* carries most of the cholesterol in your blood (Figure 1-2). LDL is often called the "bad" cholesterol because high levels of LDL lead to the buildup of cholesterol in your arteries. The major protein in LDL is apoB (*apo* here refers to the ability of the protein to associate with lipid).

✶ *High-density lipoprotein (or HDL)* carries less of your blood's cholesterol (Figure 1-2). HDL is often called the "good" cholesterol because it appears to carry cholesterol from the lining of the arteries back to the liver for disposal. HDL thus prevents cholesterol from depositing in the arteries, and protects you against atherosclerosis and coronary heart disease. The major protein in HDL is apoAı.

Very-low-density lipoprotein (or VLDL) carries most of the triglyceride in your blood (Figure 1-2). Patients with coronary heart disease often have higher levels of blood triglyceride. Two major proteins in VLDL are apoB and apoE.

To prevent coronary heart disease, you must identify your risk profile (Chapter 5) and then modify your risk factors through diet (Chapters 10–14), exercise (Chapter 15), and possibly medication (Chapter 16) to decrease the rate at which the disease develops. This book will show how cholesterol and other fats in your diet can adversely influence the nature and amount of lipoproteins in your blood. You will find a comprehensive Action Plan to help you change your blood lipoprotein profile from a bad one (high LDL, low HDL) to a good one (lower LDL, higher HDL).

Genes and Cholesterol

Premature coronary heart disease most often runs in families: thus a man whose father died of a heart attack at age 50 may himself be at risk at about that age. Other families appear to be relatively protected from it. A thorough knowledge of your family history may help you to avoid coronary heart disease and live longer, and may also help you determine whether your own children are at risk. In Chapter 5 you will learn how to assess this risk by drawing up a family tree.

In the second part of the book, "Genes and Cholesterol," you will read about people who have inherited different kinds of blood lipid problems and how these problems are also present in their relatives (Chapters 7, 8, and 9). If you or a member of your family has one of these problems, this part of the book may help you to understand the basic problem and what can be done about it.

For example, there is the common genetic condition called familial hypercholesterolemia, where LDL and cholesterol are removed too slowly from the blood owing to a deficiency of special proteins on the surface of cells called LDL receptors (Chapter 7). In some families with premature coronary heart disease, triglyceride levels may be too high; you will find out whether you have a blood triglyceride problem that may place you at risk (Chapter 8). You will also learn how to determine if you are at risk for coronary heart disease *even if your blood cholesterol is normal* (Chapter 9).

Any of these genetic conditions will be worsened by the burden of a diet high in cholesterol and saturated fats, or by the presence of other risk factors such as high blood pressure, cigarette smoking, and obesity. Another risk factor, unfair as it may seem, is simply being male. Men have approximately three times as many heart attacks, bypass operations, and the like as women.

Diet and Cholesterol

In Chapters 2 and 10, you will learn how cholesterol and saturated fat in your diet increase your blood cholesterol level, and how polyunsaturated and monounsaturated fats lower it. Your diet can therefore either increase or decrease your blood cholesterol level and your risk of coronary heart disease. However, you will also learn that diet is not the only answer. If you eat a standard American diet, *two-thirds of the cholesterol in your body is manufactured by your cells; only the remaining one-third is derived from your diet.* An elevated blood cholesterol level may in fact be due to a diet rich in cholesterol and saturated fat; but another possibility is that your liver is manufacturing too much cholesterol and triglyceride (Chapter 8), or that LDL and its cholesterol are being removed too slowly (Chapter 7).

You will learn how atherosclerosis causes blockage of the coronary arteries, and how it produces signs of coronary heart disease. You will see that lowering blood cholesterol reduces the risk of heart disease (Chapter 3). And you will learn how HDL, the "good" cholesterol, affects your risk of developing coronary heart disease, and what factors can increase or decrease the level of HDL cholesterol in your blood (Chapter 4).

In Chapter 5, "Your Risk Profile," you can review your diet to determine if it contains too much cholesterol or saturated fat. You will also find the normal values for total cholesterol, HDL cholesterol, and LDL cholesterol; helpful guidelines for determining whether you have high blood pressure and how much you should weigh; and an explanation of the importance of other risk factors for coronary heart disease such as cigarette smoking, lack of exercise, obesity, diabetes, and stress.

In the third part of the book there are five chapters related to diet. You will learn *how much lowering* of blood cholesterol you might expect by modifying the cholesterol, saturated fat, and unsaturated fat in your diet (Chapter 10). You will find the latest information on the use of monounsaturated fat, particularly olive oil and canola oil, to replace saturated fats in the diet. In Chapter 12, you will learn the difference between water-insoluble and water-soluble fibers, and how water-soluble fibers such as oat bran, guar gum, and pectin help to lower cholesterol levels. Chapter 13 discusses whether fish oils have a role in preventing coronary heart disease. Finally, are shellfish good or bad for you? On this score we know more than we did only a few years ago (see Chapter 11).

Eating is one of the great pleasures of life. To help you eat wisely and well, a cholesterol-lowering Action Plan is presented in Chapter 11. Have you often wondered whether a particular food was good or bad for you? Have you struggled to read the labels on foods? Guides to help you read labels are found in Chapter 11, and the saturated fat and cholesterol content of most commonly eaten foods is summarized in the Food Tables at the back of the book. Since about one-third of American's meals are eaten in restaurants, special sections on eating out and fast food guidelines are provided.

Also at the back of the book you'll find nearly a hundred quick and easy recipes for delicious low-fat hors d'oeuvres, soups, salads, entrees, and desserts, most of them provided by my patients. Cholesterol, saturated fat, and calorie content are listed for each recipe. These recipes have been used in Chapter 14 to prepare two weeks' worth of quick, easy menus.

To help children establish healthy habits early (Chapter 6), the National Institutes of Health Consensus Conference on Lowering Blood Cholesterol to Prevent Heart Disease recommended that healthy American children over two years of age follow a prudent diet low in cholesterol and saturated fat. It is hoped that by starting proper nutrition early in life we can lower the blood cholesterol levels of our children and slow the development of the early lesions of atherosclerosis. Whether this prudent diet will promote optimal growth and development in our children is an important issue that I discuss in Chapter 6.

Exercise, Drugs, and Cholesterol

The fourth part of the book deals with how exercise and drugs can help reduce your risk of coronary heart disease. The relationship between physical inactivity and the development of coronary heart disease is impressive (Chapter 15). Aerobic exercise can have a positive effect on your weight, your general well-being, and your blood levels of LDL cholesterol, HDL cholesterol, and triglyceride. Guidelines are provided to help you to decide what kind of exercise you should be doing, and whether you are doing enough exercise to help prevent coronary heart disease and control your weight.

If diet and exercise do not lower your blood cholesterol or triglyceride levels sufficiently, it may be necessary to add medication to your treatment program. In Chapter 16 you will learn about the latest medications that are available, how they work in the body, and what side effects you might expect from taking these medications.

CHAPTER 2

Do You Understand the Risk?

$\mathbf{T}$his chapter describes coronary heart disease and its causes, and presents evidence linking intake of dietary cholesterol and fat with levels of blood cholesterol and rates of coronary heart disease.

How Is Coronary Heart Disease Detected?

Unfortunately, in one-third of all cases the first sign of coronary heart disease is sudden, unexpected death. The victims are completely unaware of the blockages in their coronary arteries until it is too late.

In the rest of the cases, coronary heart disease first appears as chest pain or even a heart attack. Chest pain due to coronary heart disease is usually brought on by physical exertion. Physical activity increases the demand of the heart muscle for oxygen; if significant blockage is present in a coronary artery, the demand cannot be met. This produces pain, usually in the middle of the chest behind the breastbone. The pain is often pressing or constrictive. Some people describe it by clenching their fist over their chest. The pain may radiate up into the throat or jaw.

You may have heard the phrase *angina pectoris* used to describe such pain (*angina* from the Latin for throat, *pectoris* from the Latin for chest). The pain of angina pectoris may also radiate up into the left shoulder and down the left arm. When triggered by exercise or exertion, angina pectoris is usually relieved by rest. Occasionally, angina is brought on by tension or emotions; or it may occur after eating a meal, or even at night when sleeping. Angina that occurs at rest is an indicator of even more serious atherosclerosis, because the heart is not getting enough oxygen even when it is not working hard.

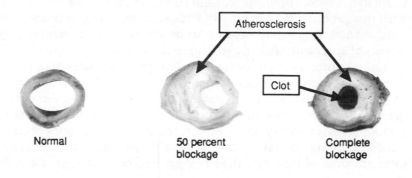

Fig. 2-1. Cross section of three coronary arteries. (A) A normal coronary artery with a completely open lumen. (B) An abnormal coronary artery whose lumen is blocked over 50 percent by atherosclerosis. (C) An abnormal coronary artery whose lumen became completely blocked when a clot formed on top of the atherosclerotic plaque, leading to a heart attack and death. The coronary arteries are enlarged three to four times to present detail.

Angina pectoris may be the first signal that you have underlying coronary heart disease.

A heart attack develops when a clot forms on top of the blockage in a coronary artery (Figure 2-1). This completely prevents blood from flowing through the artery, and deprives the tissue beyond the blockage of needed oxygen and nutrients. The cells in the heart muscle (*myocardium*) then die, producing what is commonly referred to as a heart attack (*myocardial infarction*).

Often the first sign of a heart attack is the development of pressing chest pain. When a heart attack is taking place, the chest pain is often not relieved by rest. This persistent chest pain is often also accompanied by weakness, fainting, profuse sweating, nausea, and vomiting. Emergency medical attention is needed, and hospitalization is required. When a heart attack occurs, the part of the heart muscle that is injured is left with a scar.

Is your heart being deprived of oxygen without symptoms? If you have significant blockages in your coronary arteries, you may be having "silent" episodes in which your heart muscle is not receiving enough oxygen (ischemia). Such episodes are transient, lasting only several minutes at a time, and are termed "silent myocardial ischemia" by heart doctors (cardiologists). As reported by Dr. Peter

Cohn in his book *Silent Myocardial Ischemia and Infarction*, people with this problem may be totally without symptoms, may have suffered a heart attack but gone on to be symptom-free, or may have attacks of angina alternating with episodes of silent ischemia.

How common is silent ischemia? Dr. Cohn estimates that two to three out of every 100 healthy men have silent ischemia during exercise; that survivors of heart attacks have one chance in ten of having silent ischemia; and that of the four million patients with angina pectoris in this country, about 80 percent also have episodes of silent ischemia. If you are having angina attacks, you probably are having more episodes of ischemia than is suggested by your angina attacks alone.

How is ischemia detected? Your doctor can use several different tests.

Resting electrocardiogram. The electrocardiogram (or EKG) is the best-known test for heart disease. The muscle cells of your heart contract in response to electrical impulses from the nerves. Electrodes attached to your body detect these impulses as they travel through the various parts of your heart. The recording or tracing that results is the EKG. If part of your heart muscle has been damaged by a heart attack, the electrical impulses do not travel through it properly, producing an abnormal EKG. A resting EKG (one taken while you are at rest) can also detect abnormalities (arrhythmias) in the rhythm of your heart.

The resting EKG has its limitations. For example, about three out of four patients with angina pectoris have normal resting EKGs. Many patients with significant blockages of their coronary arteries have normal EKGs. Having a normal resting EKG does not mean that you do not have any blockages in your coronary arteries, nor does it mean that you can ignore risk factors you may have for coronary heart disease.

Stress exercise electrocardiogram (stress test). If you have a positive family history of premature (before age 55) coronary heart disease, and one or more other risk factors for coronary artery disease, such as high blood cholesterol, high blood pressure, or cigarette smoking, your doctor may recommend that you have a stress exercise electrocardiogram (stress test).

A stress EKG is obtained while you exercise. Electrodes are hooked up to your arms, legs, and chest, and you begin by walking on a treadmill, whose speed and incline are gradually increased so that you are running in place as if you were running up hills of increasing steepness. During your stress test, the work that your heart must do rapidly increases, and the amount of blood that your heart needs increases. A significant blockage in one or more of your coronary arteries may then be detected as an abnormality in the EKG tracing. This abnormality reflects the decreased delivery of oxygen to the muscle cells of the heart during the stress of exercise.

The stress EKG can help your doctor determine if you have hidden blockages in your coronary arteries, but it is not a perfect test. Some people with significant blockages have perfectly normal stress EKGs. Such false negative tests may be due to small vessels called "collaterals" that develop to compensate for blockages in the coronary arteries.

On the other hand, some patients who do not have blockages in their coronary arteries have false positive stress tests. False positive tests can occur, for example, in patients who take the heart medicine digitalis, patients with rheumatic heart disease, those with a rapid pulse (tachycardia), and women at menopause.

Stress thallium exercise electrocardiogram (stress thallium test). If your stress test is positive and there is no apparent explanation for the result, your doctor may order a more sensitive test called a stress thallium test. Such a test is particularly indicated if you have a positive family history of premature coronary heart disease or other risk factors. A small amount of radioactive thallium is injected into the vein in your arm. The blood passes through the coronary arteries, delivering the thallium to your heart. The distribution of the thallium throughout your heart is determined, using a special kind of X-ray. If a certain area of your heart does not receive a normal amount of blood during exercise, less thallium accumulates in that part of the heart. Most of your heart will be lit up with the radioactive thallium, but areas with less thallium will show up as holes or spots of darkness.

If your first stress EKG is normal, should the test be repeated in the future? *Yes.* In the Lipid Research Clinics Coronary Primary Prevention Trial, conducted over a ten-year period (1973–83) in twelve medical centers in the United States and Canada, stress EKGs were performed at regular intervals for up to ten years in middle-aged men at high risk for coronary heart disease because of high blood cholesterol levels. The stress EKGs were done to check for abnormalities indicating that blockages in the coronary arteries had gotten bigger. Men whose performance on stress tests changed from negative to positive went on to develop more coronary heart disease than those whose tests remained negative. If you are at high risk for coronary heart disease, you and your doctor should probably plan on repeating your stress test every two or three years. If your test changes from negative to positive, further evaluation by a cardiologist may be indicated.

Holter EKG monitoring. In this test, you are connected to a small, battery-operated device that provides a continual EKG tracing over a period of 24 hours or more. You continue all your regular activities during the period of monitoring. The Holter EKG will determine whether you are having irregular heartbeats (arrythmias) or ischemic episodes. The frequency and duration of any ischemic episodes, their relationship to activity, and whether they are silent or accompanied by angina pectoris can all be determined by sensitive Holter EKG monitoring.

Coronary angiography. Since the three major coronary arteries in the heart cannot be seen in standard chest X-rays, a more sophisticated test, called coronary angiography, is required to view blockages. This test may be administered to patients with known coronary heart disease, to determine if they are candidates for a coronary artery bypass or balloon angioplasty, or to those in whom coronary heart disease is suspected but cannot be proved by any other tests.

In coronary angiography, a hollow plastic tube (catheter) is inserted in the large femoral artery in the groin. The catheter is threaded through the femoral artery, into the aorta, and up to the aortic valve, which separates the aorta from the main pumping part of the heart, the left ventricle. This test is also sometimes referred to as "cardiac catheterization."

The catheter is placed very precisely in the openings of the right or left coronary arteries (Figure 2-2), which begin just above the aortic valve, and a small amount of dye is injected. The appearance of the dye in the arteries is photographed using a special procedure that enables the cardiologist to watch the heart on a TV monitor. The dye shows up easily, allowing the cardiologist to determine how much dye is present in each of the coronary arteries.

The coronary arteries are those whose branches supply blood to your heart (Figure 2-2). There are three major ones: the right coronary artery, the left anterior descending coronary artery, and the left circumflex coronary artery. The right coronary artery is fairly long and gives rise to the posterior descending coronary artery. The left main coronary artery is usually very short (about an inch in length) and divides into the left anterior descending and left circumflex coronary arteries. These arteries supply blood to different parts of the heart. There are also many connections (anastomoses) between the

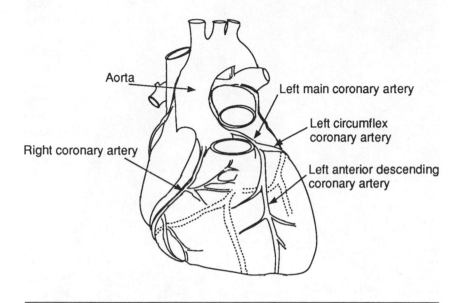

Fig. 2-2. Diagram of the major coronary arteries of the heart. The right coronary artery and the left main coronary artery both originate from openings in the aorta. The left main coronary immediately gives rise to the left anterior descending coronary artery and to the left circumflex coronary artery. The dotted lines indicate those vessels that are not seen from the front of the heart.

branches of the coronary arteries, resulting in a network of blood vessels that facilitates the delivery of blood to the muscle cells of the heart.

Blockages of the coronary arteries show up as narrowed areas in coronary angiography (Figure 2-3). The diameter of the narrowed sections of the coronary artery is measured to determine the amount of blockage. Blockages of 50 percent or more are significant. The greater the blockage, the less blood will flow through that segment of the artery and reach the parts of the heart beyond the blockage. Blockages can occur in one, two, or all three of the major coronary arteries; these conditions are referred to as "single-vessel," "two-vessel," and "three-vessel" disease.

Let's take an example. John Covington was first seen in our Lipid Clinic at the age of 34, when he was referred by his son's pediatrician. He looked well and had a perfectly normal physical examina-

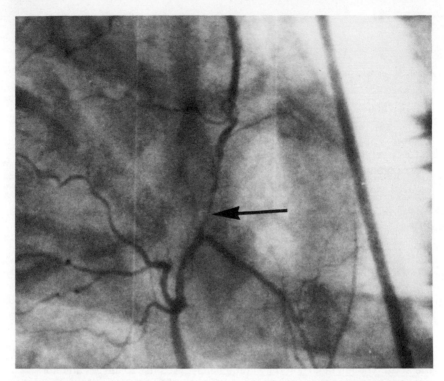

Fig. 2-3. Coronary angiogram of the right coronary artery. The portion of the artery that is almost completely narrowed by atherosclerosis is indicated by an arrow.

tion. But his blood cholesterol was 313 mg/dl, and a large amount of it was in LDL (252 mg/dl) and too little in HDL (30 mg/dl). His older brother had had a heart attack at 35, and his father had died from coronary heart disease in his early fifties.

Because of John's markedly abnormal blood lipid profile and positive family history for premature coronary heart disease, I recommended a stress test, which revealed ischemia. He next had a coronary angiogram, which showed a complete blockage of his right coronary artery (Figure 2-3) and many other areas of less severe atherosclerosis. Without his cholesterol testing and the subsequent tests, he still would be walking around totally unaware of his problem—if he was walking around at all. His blood cholesterol level has now been reduced to 176 mg/dl by changes in his diet and by drug treatment with a bile acid binding agent and niacin.

Coronary Heart Disease and Atherosclerosis

Although testing can be valuable in detecting existing blockages in your coronary arteries before sudden death, angina pectoris, or a heart attack occurs, ideally you should try to prevent blockages from forming in the first place. This is why it is important for you to understand how atherosclerosis develops, and what factors accelerate it. Even if you already have coronary heart disease and have had coronary artery bypass surgery, you will want to decrease the chance that the blockages will return.

Coronary heart disease results from the gradual development of atherosclerosis in the coronary arteries. The term atherosclerosis comes from the Greek *atheroma,* meaning porridge, and *skleros,* meaning hard. At birth our coronary arteries are completely open, no blockages are present, and blood flow is unimpaired. Between the ages of 10 and 20, small deposits of lipid, called "fatty streaks," begin to appear in the lining of the coronary arteries. Over time, some fatty streaks change gradually into larger deposits, called "fibrous plaques." As the fibrous plaque forms, it protrudes into the opening (lumen) of the coronary artery.

These early stages of atherosclerosis progress slowly through the teen-age years and through the twenties and thirties, but by age 45 or 50 many people in our society have more advanced atherosclerosis that may lead to coronary heart disease. If you have risk factors (discussed in Chapter 5) or have inherited a genetic problem in processing fat in your body (discussed in Chapters 7–9), you are much more likely to have atherosclerosis. The same factors may accelerate the early deposits of fatty streaks in the coronary arteries of your children.

Atherosclerosis has afflicted many populations throughout the history of mankind—for example, it has been found in Egyptian mummies—but not all mammals are susceptible to this disease. Rats and dogs are quite resistant, at least partly because most of their blood cholesterol is in high-density lipoproteins (HDL), the "good" cholesterol. In contrast, humans carry most of their blood cholesterol in low-density lipoproteins (LDL), which promote atherosclerosis. When animals consume diets rich in cholesterol or saturated fat, those that are susceptible, such as some nonhuman primates and rabbits, develop atherosclerosis; those that are resistant, such as dogs and rats, do not.

The relationship between cholesterol in the diet and atheroscle-

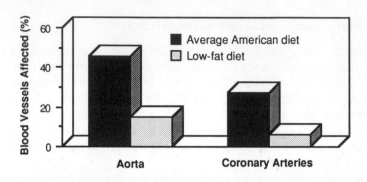

Fig. 2-4. Proportion of blood vessels affected with atherosclerosis in monkeys fed an average American diet and a low-fat diet. (Blood cholesterol: average diet, 383 mg/dl; low-fat diet, 199 mg/dl.)
From data provided by R. W. Wissler in E. Braunwald, ed., *The Myocardium: Failure and Infarction* (New York: HP Publishing Co., 1974), pp. 155–166.

rosis was first observed in rabbits in 1908 by a Russian pathologist named Ignatowsky. Later studies of nonhuman primates demonstrated the direct relationship between cholesterol and saturated fat in the diet, cholesterol level in the blood, and the development of atherosclerosis. The results of one such study are summarized in Figure 2-4. Dr. Robert Wissler and his co-workers fed one group of monkeys a "typical American diet" high in total fat, saturated fat, and cholesterol, and fed another group a "prudent diet" lower in fat. The animals on the typical American diet had significantly higher levels of blood cholesterol and much more atherosclerosis in their coronary arteries than those on the prudent diet.

But can the process of atherosclerosis be reversed? The answer is yes. Studies have shown that when the level of cholesterol in the blood of nonhuman primates is lowered by diet or drugs, the deposits of atherosclerosis in their coronary arteries become smaller. A study discussed in Chapter 3 has also reported this result in humans.

In the 1960s, medical researchers established that not all countries had the same amount of atherosclerosis in their populations. The International Atherosclerosis Project studied people in fourteen different countries. Arteries from 22,509 people who died between the ages of 10 and 69 years were examined under the microscope. In his book *Geographic Pathology of Atherosclerosis*, Dr. Henry McGill ranked twelve of the fourteen populations according to fat intake, blood cholesterol level, and atherosclerosis. He found a direct and highly significant relationship between these factors; locations with the greatest amount of atherosclerosis, such as the United States and Norway, had significantly higher average blood cholesterol levels and a significantly greater fat consumption.

Population Studies

A number of major studies have documented the link between blood levels of cholesterol and risk of coronary heart disease in humans.

The Multiple Risk Factor Intervention Trial (MRFIT), the latest and largest of these studies (1986), found the strong relationship between death from coronary heart disease and blood cholesterol levels shown in Figure 2-5. For six years the study followed 356,222 American men aged 35 to 57 years with no history of heart attack. It was found that the risk of death from coronary heart disease begins to increase gradually at blood cholesterol levels of 180 mg/dl, accelerates at about 200 mg/dl, doubles at about 220 mg/dl (in comparison to 180 mg/dl and below), and triples at about 245 mg/dl. The find-

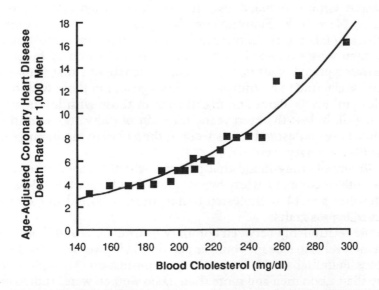

Fig. 2-5. Relationship between blood cholesterol level and death from coronary heart disease in men aged 35–57 studied over six years.

Data from the Multiple Risk Factor Intervention Trial (MRFIT) Study, as reported by J. Stamler, D. Wentworth, and J. D. Neaton in *Journal of the American Medical Association* 256 (1986): 2823–2828.

Table 2-1. Blood Cholesterol Level and
Chance of Developing Coronary Heart
Disease in Middle-Aged American Men

Blood cholesterol level (mg/dl)	Percent developing coronary heart disease over nine years
Below 194	4%
194–218	6
218–240	9
240–268	11
Above 268	15

Source: The Pooling Project Research Group,
Journal of Chronic Diseases 31 (1978): 201–
306.

ings were adjusted for the ages of the men, and persisted after other risk factors such as high blood pressure and cigarette smoking were considered.

How well does your blood cholesterol level predict the likelihood that you will develop coronary heart disease? The Pooling Project Research Group included two studies in Chicago and others in Albany, New York; Framingham, Massachusetts; and Tecumseh, Michigan (Table 2-1). Cholesterol values from over 8,000 middle-aged men were examined with regard to risk of coronary heart disease over a period of almost nine years. The rate of a first "coronary event" was found to be almost four times greater in those with blood cholesterol levels above 268 mg/dl than in those with levels below 194 mg/dl. In less than ten years, nine out of every 100 men in the study whose cholesterol levels were in the 218–240 mg/dl range had their first coronary event.

A Montreal study found that patients who developed atherosclerosis in their coronary artery bypass grafts had higher blood levels of cholesterol and LDL cholesterol than those who did not develop blocked bypass grafts.

Is the relationship between coronary heart disease and blood cholesterol level also true for younger people and for women? Yes. In the famous Framingham Heart Study in Framingham, Massachusetts, more than 2,000 men and more than 2,000 women were studied over fourteen years. For both younger men and women (ages 30 to 49 years) the risk of coronary heart disease increased appreciably at a blood cholesterol level of *about 200 mg/dl*. However, the rates of coronary heart disease were lower for the women. For the older group (ages 50–82 years), risk did not increase noticeably below a blood cholesterol level of about 240 mg/dl in men and 260 mg/dl in women. Thus blood cholesterol level appears to be even more important in younger adults than in older ones, and is relevant for women as well as men. As we shall see in Chapter 4, the level of HDL cholesterol provides insight into risk in older people, and also into why women have less coronary heart disease than men.

Coronary Heart Disease, Dietary Cholesterol, and Blood Cholesterol

A number of studies have demonstrated a link between the amount of cholesterol and saturated fat in the diet, the levels of total and LDL cholesterol in the blood, and coronary heart disease.

In the Coronary Heart Disease Study in Seven Countries, performed in the 1960s and published in 1970, a strong relationship was found between the percentage of calories eaten as saturated fat and the average blood cholesterol level (Figure 2-6). People in the four locations where more than 15 percent of calories were consumed as saturated fat had average cholesterol levels of 230 mg/dl or higher and the highest rates of coronary heart disease. People who consumed about 10 percent or less of their calories as saturated fat had average cholesterol levels, no higher than about 200 mg/dl, and lower rates of coronary heart disease.

Several studies were made in the 1970s of people who had moved from their native country to another country. One compared Japanese in Japan with Japanese who had moved to Hawaii and San Francisco. The average dietary intake of total fat, saturated fat, polyunsaturated fat, and cholesterol in the emigrant groups changed from typically Japanese to typically American (Figure 2-7); so did their blood cholesterol levels and their rates of death from coronary heart disease. Since all the people studied had similar genetic backgrounds, it seems clear that environmental differences, especially diet, led to the significant differences in their blood cholesterol levels and their rates of coronary heart disease.

Studies within a single population, such as the Framingham study, were more problematic because it is harder to detect small differences in dietary intake between people who are eating similar foods. Moreover, some people have large changes in their blood cholesterol levels when they change the content of cholesterol in their diet, others much smaller changes. Nevertheless, scientists now believe

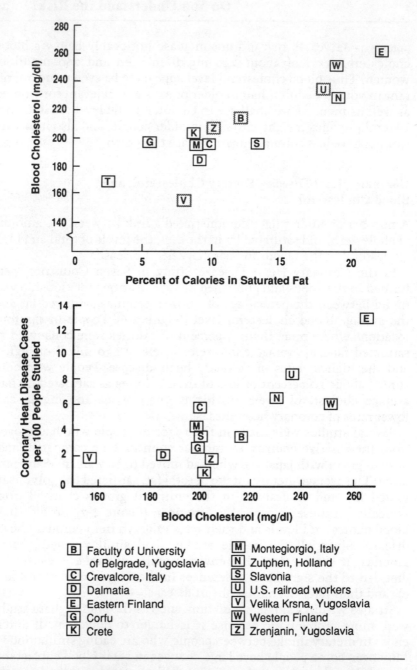

Fig. 2-6. Blood cholesterol level, dietary saturated fat, and coronary heart disease. The correlations (0.89 and 0.81, respectively) rate as highly significant. Broken lines indicate values determined from dietary records rather than from direct chemical analysis.

From the Coronary Heart Disease Study in Seven Countries, *Circulation,* 41 (1970): 162–185, Supplement 1, by permission of the American Heart Association, Inc.

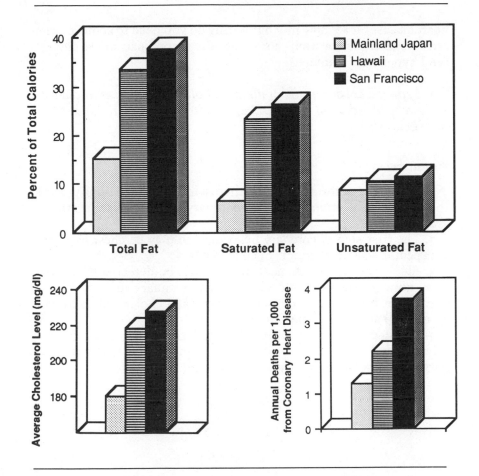

Fig. 2-7. Dietary fat intake, blood cholesterol levels, and comparative death rates from coronary heart disease in three Japanese populations.
Data from "Conference on the Health Effects of Blood Lipids: Optimal Distributions for Populations," *Preventive Medicine* 8 (1979): 628.

there is sufficient evidence to prove the first part of the cholesterol hypothesis:

1. *Increased consumption of dietary cholesterol and saturated fats → elevates blood total and LDL cholesterol levels → increases coronary heart disease.*

In the next chapter, you will learn that lowering your dietary content of cholesterol and saturated fat can lower your blood cholesterol level. But will lowering your blood cholesterol level prevent coronary heart disease? If so, how much lowering do you need to achieve? The answers to these questions constitute the second part of the cholesterol hypothesis, namely:

 2. *Reduced consumption of dietary cholesterol and saturated fats → lowers blood total and LDL cholesterol levels → reduces coronary heart disease.*

Summary

1. Hardening of the arteries, or atherosclerosis, is a lifelong process that starts early, often leading to coronary heart disease in middle age and later.

2. The first sign of coronary heart disease may be chest pain (angina pectoris), a heart attack, or sudden death.

3. Blockages of the coronary arteries can be detected by special tests, notably stress electrocardiogram and coronary angiography.

4. A diet high in total fat, saturated fat, and cholesterol increases blood total and LDL cholesterol levels.

5. Elevated levels of total and LDL cholesterol help cause atherosclerosis and coronary heart disease, and increase the risk of coronary heart disease for men and women of all ages.

CHAPTER 3

How Much Can You Reduce the Risk?

This chapter will review evidence showing that you can reduce your risk of coronary heart disease. It is shown first that treatment with diet and drugs can lower your blood cholesterol level, and second that such lowering actually reduces your risk of coronary heart disease. You will learn that the second part of the "cholesterol hypothesis" has been proved: namely, that reducing elevated blood total and LDL cholesterol levels decreases the number of heart attacks and deaths due to coronary heart disease.

The National Diet-Heart Study

In the 1960s, the National Institutes of Health sponsored the Diet-Heart Feasibility Study to determine if it was possible to lower the blood cholesterol levels of Americans eating at home by changing the kind and amount of fat in their diet. About a thousand men aged 45–54 in five cities, all healthy volunteers, were assigned to one of the three diets summarized in Table 3-1. Diets 1 and 2 were low in cholesterol and saturated fats but high in polyunsaturated fats; that is, they had a higher ratio of polyunsaturated to saturated fats, or P/S ratio. Diet 2 differed from Diet 1 in that it contained more polyunsaturated fat and monounsaturated fat. The "control" diet (Diet 3) was similar to a typical American diet, that is, high in cholesterol, total fat, and saturated fat but with a low P/S ratio.

The men picked up all their food at special distribution centers. The food containers did not list the ingredients, and neither the participants nor the doctors who conducted the study knew who was assigned to which diet. This research design, called "double-blind," is designed to reduce unintentional bias on the part of either the

Table 3-1. Diets Used in the National Diet-Heart Study

Type of diet	Amount of cholesterol (mg/day)	Total fat in diet (% of daily calories)	Saturated fat in diet (% of daily calories)	Balance of polyunsaturated to saturated fat (P/S ratio)
Low-cholesterol, low-saturated-fat				
Diet 1	350–450	30%	Below 9%	1.5
Diet 2	350–450	40	Below 9	2.0
Typical American				
Diet 3	650–750	40	16–18	0.4

study subjects or the medical scientists, since neither knows who is in what program until the end of the study.

After one year on the assigned diets, the blood cholesterol levels fell between 11 percent and 12 percent in the men on Diets 1 and 2 (Figure 3-1). The average cholesterol level in the group on the typical American diet (Diet 3) fell only 3 percent.

The next question was "Will lowering blood cholesterol by diet in healthy Americans decrease the rate of coronary heart disease?" There were several problems in trying to answer this question. First, the symptoms of coronary heart disease usually take four or more decades to manifest themselves. Second, although coronary heart disease is the major cause of death and disability in this country, the actual rate of *new* cases per year in middle-aged people is relatively low, about five to ten new cases per 1,000 middle-aged male adults. Third, what control group might such a study use?

Ideally, neither the participants nor the staff conducting the study should know which participants are in the treatment group and which are in the untreated control group. Diets that are high or low in animal fat and cholesterol are clearly different, and unless unlabeled foods were given out at a commissary, everyone would realize whether he was assigned to a diet low or high in cholesterol and saturated fat. Because 100,000 men were needed for a definitive diet-heart study, it was not feasible to have a blind control group of the necessary size.

The Lipid Research Clinics Coronary Primary Prevention Trial

Because of these difficulties and a prospective price tag of about $1 billion (in 1971 dollars), another approach was taken. First, only patients with very high blood cholesterol levels were selected; second, a drug treatment was chosen that lowers the blood cholesterol level to a greater extent than diet alone. This approach reduces the number of participants needed to a manageable level. A drug trial can replace a diet trial, provided that the drug has a specific effect on lowering blood cholesterol (and LDL cholesterol). This permits a direct test of the hypothesis that a decrease in the blood cholesterol level reduces coronary heart disease. Further, a drug trial allows medical scientists to develop a suitable "inactive medication" or placebo that will not lower the blood cholesterol level, thus permitting the study to be double-blind.

In the 1970s the Lipid Research Clinics Coronary Primary Prevention Trial study was initiated with support from the National Heart, Lung, and Blood Institute. About 4,000 healthy middle-aged men with high levels of blood total and LDL cholesterol were assigned by a flip of a coin either to a treatment group, which received an active medication called cholestyramine, or to a control group that received a placebo. Cholestyramine was known to produce a significant decrease (10–20 percent) in the level of total and LDL cholesterol in the blood.

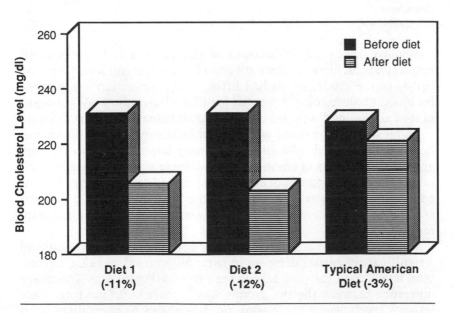

Fig. 3-1. National Diet-Heart Study results.
Data from the National Diet-Heart Study Final Report, *Circulation* 37 (1968): 181–223, Supplement 1.

Both the treatment and control groups were put on the same diet, moderately reduced from standard American fare in total fat, saturated fat, and cholesterol. Neither the participants nor the medical staff knew to which of the two groups a participant was assigned. The men's blood cholesterol levels were checked every other month during the seven years of the study, but were kept confidential. The two groups did not differ on other risk factors for coronary heart disease, such as smoking and high blood pressure. In addition, these factors were not intervened on or subjected to treatment, thus providing a true test of the cholesterol (LDL) hypothesis.

Let's take two examples of participants from the Johns Hopkins Clinic. Charles Maddox, then 50, was assigned to the active drug; Marshall Fields, then 56, was assigned to the placebo. Neither man knew which of the two preparations he was taking, but each took six packets per day every day for over seven years. Let's compare the results (figures are blood levels in mg/dl):

	C.M. (active drug)		M.F. (inactive drug)	
	Beginning of study	End of study	Beginning of study	End of study
Cholesterol	281	189	273	274
LDL cholesterol	199	118	196	191

Maddox had average reductions of 25.7 percent and 39.2 percent, respectively, in blood cholesterol and LDL cholesterol levels over the period of the study; Fields had little average reduction (0.6 percent for blood cholesterol; 3.7 percent for LDL cholesterol). Most important of all, Fields developed coronary heart disease; Maddox did not.

The results of the study were judged by comparing the number of heart attacks and deaths due to coronary heart disease in the two groups. Other signs of coronary heart disease were also assessed, including the development of chest pain (angina pectoris), the need for coronary artery bypass surgery, and the development of a positive stress electrocardiogram. These tests were reviewed for you in Chapter 2.

The men taking cholestyramine, the active study medication, had a significantly greater decrease in their blood total and LDL cholesterol levels than the men taking the placebo (Figure 3-2). The major difference between the two groups was in their LDL (and total) cholesterol levels, since there were no differences in their diets or in other risk factors such as high blood pressure, cigarette smoking, or obesity. In this study there was also a small increase in the level of

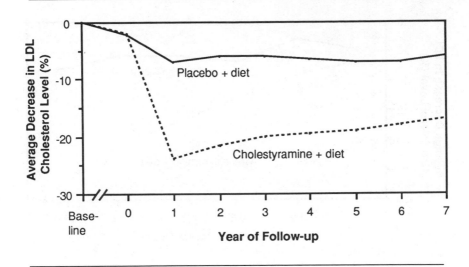

Fig. 3-2. Results for LDL cholesterol lowering of the Lipid Research Clinics Coronary Primary Prevention Trial.
Redrawn from the press release of the Lipid Metabolism Branch, National Heart, Lung, and Blood Institute, National Institutes of Health, January 1984.

the "good" high-density lipoprotein (HDL) cholesterol in the choles-tyramine group, an effect that was of some benefit in reducing coronary heart disease.

Did the significant average differences of about 10 percent in blood cholesterol and LDL cholesterol levels between these two groups result in different rates of coronary heart disease? Yes. Coronary heart disease deaths and heart attacks were reduced almost 20 percent in those on cholestyramine compared with those on placebo. *For each 1 percent reduction in blood cholesterol (and LDL cholesterol), there was a 2 percent reduction in coronary heart disease.* There were also significant differences of a similar magnitude between the two groups for angina pectoris, a positive stress electrocardiogram, and coronary artery bypass surgery.

Those men who took all their cholestyramine faithfully had a significantly greater fall in their LDL (and total) cholesterol levels than those who took little or none of their medication (Figure 3-3). Did they also have less coronary heart disease than those who did not take their medicine? Indeed they did. The greater the lowering of the LDL cholesterol, the greater the reduction in the risk of coronary heart disease (Figure 3-4).

It is of interest that about one-third of the participants in the Cor-

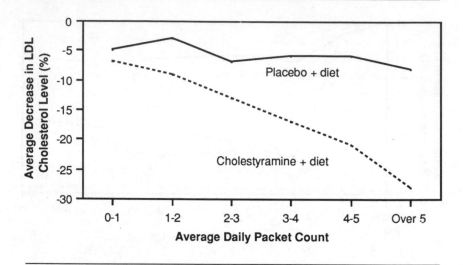

Fig. 3-3. Relation between number of doses of cholestyramine taken and the lowering of the LDL cholesterol level in the Lipid Research Clinics Coronary Primary Prevention Trial.
Redrawn from the press release of the Lipid Metabolism Branch, National Heart, Lung, and Blood Institute, National Institutes of Health, January 1984.

onary Primary Prevention Trial were not taking any study medication at all. For those on the placebo this was unimportant, but for those assumed to be taking six packets a day of cholestyramine, the fact that they did not take their medication unquestionably affected the results of the study. Their noncompliance made the drug appear less effective than it actually was when conscientiously taken by the other participants. This shows how difficult it is to prove a hypothesis for humans. Even so, however, the results shown in Figures 3-2 through 3-4 conclusively proved the cholesterol hypothesis.

The Coronary Drug Project

The results of the Coronary Drug Project were reported in the early and middle 1970s. Four medications were initially used: nicotinic acid, clofibrate (Atromid-S®), dextrothyroxine, and estrogen. Two of the medicines, dextrothyroxine and estrogen, had to be discontinued because of their side effects. Dextrothyroxine is very similar to the natural thyroid hormone (levothyroxine) made by your thyroid gland; it can lower the blood cholesterol level, but can also actually increase angina pectoris, abnormal heartbeats (arrhythmias), and heart attacks because of its adverse effect on the functioning of the heart. Estrogen, a female hormone, produced undesirable side effects such as breast enlargement in the men.

The effects of the two remaining drugs, nicotinic acid and clofibrate, are of considerable interest. Small amounts of nicotinic acid, also called niacin, are present in your food as part of one of the B vitamins, vitamin B_3. When nicotinic acid is given in high doses, it lowers the total cholesterol (and also triglyceride) in blood. Clofibrate (Atromid-S®), made in the laboratory and related to a compound called fibric acid, can not only lower your total cholesterol level but dramatically lower your triglyceride level.

The Coronary Drug Project asked the question, "If men who have suffered coronary heart disease are treated with an appropriate drug, will they be less likely to have their heart disease recur than other men with the same history who are treated with a placebo?" Since the men had already developed coronary heart disease, this type of study is called a "secondary prevention trial."

The participants were assigned by a random procedure similar to flipping a coin to either the nicotinic acid group (1,119 men), the

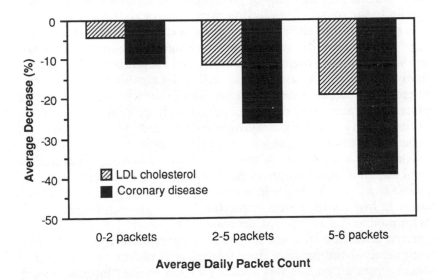

Fig. 3-4. Relation between reduction in LDL cholesterol and reduction in coronary heart disease risk.
Data from the Lipid Research Clinics Coronary Primary Prevention Trial, *Journal of the American Medical Association* 251 (1984): 365–374.

clofibrate group (1,103 men), or the placebo group (2,789 men). Neither the men nor the investigators knew whether they were taking the medication or the placebo. The men were followed for five years, and the numbers of new heart attacks and deaths due to coronary heart disease were documented for each of the groups.

What were the results of the study? The average blood cholesterol levels in the men in the three groups during the study were: nicotinic acid, 226 mg/dl; clofibrate, 235 mg/dl; and placebo, 251 mg/dl. There were fewer cases of recurrent coronary heart disease in the nicotinic acid group (287 cases) and the clofibrate group (309 cases) than in the placebo group (839 cases). In comparison to the placebo group the incidence of coronary heart disease was 19.8 percent less in the nicotinic acid group and 9.5 percent less in the clofibrate group. *Even in these men, who had already had a prior heart attack, you can see that for each 1 percent decrease in blood cholesterol there was about a 2 percent decrease in recurrence of coronary heart disease.*

If you already have coronary heart disease, both these results and those reviewed below indicate that you and your doctor should seriously consider trying to lower your blood cholesterol level, even if it is only in the so-called borderline-high range of 200 to 239 mg/dl.

Is nicotinic acid clearly more effective than clofibrate in preventing coronary heart disease, as the above figures suggest? Apparently so. After the study, the men were followed for ten years. Those originally treated with nicotinic acid still had a significantly lower rate of recurrent coronary heart disease than those who were taking the placebo, and this beneficial effect persisted despite the fact that most of the men were no longer taking nicotinic acid. No such long-term benefit was found in those who had taken clofibrate.

Nicotinic acid is not only more effective in lowering blood cholesterol and preventing coronary heart disease than clofibrate, but appears safer than clofibrate. In the World Health Organization (WHO) study of healthy men with borderline-high cholesterol levels, clofibrate produced a 10 percent decrease in blood cholesterol and a 20 percent reduction in coronary heart disease, compared with those who received the inactive drug (placebo). However, the number of *deaths from all causes* was actually higher in the clofibrate group. These excess deaths were due to diseases affecting the liver and the gall bladder, and to tumors of the intestines. Consequently, clofibrate (Atromid-S®) is no longer prescribed for most patients with high blood cholesterol.

The Helsinki Heart Study

Late in 1987, the results of the Helsinki Heart Study were published in the *New England Journal of Medicine*. The drug tested in this study was gemfibrozil (Lopid®), a cousin of clofibrate and also a derivative of fibric acid. Gemfibrozil significantly lowers both VLDL cholesterol and triglyceride levels, and usually increases the "good" HDL cholesterol level. A moderate decrease in the total of LDL cholesterol levels also often occurs.

In this five-year trial, healthy Finnish middle-aged men without heart disease but with high blood levels of LDL cholesterol and VLDL cholesterol were assigned to either gemfibrozil (2,051 men) or an inactive placebo (2,030 men) by a flip of a coin. The rates of heart attacks and death due to coronary heart disease in the treatment and placebo groups were compared throughout the five years.

What were the results? In the gemfibrozil group, both the average blood total cholesterol and the combined "bad" LDL plus VLDL cholesterol levels fell about 8 percent. The total triglyceride level decreased about 35 percent, and there was a significant increase of about 10 percent in the "good" HDL cholesterol level. The balance in the blood between "good" and "bad" cholesterol was thus markedly shifted for the better. In contrast, those in the placebo group had only minimal changes in their total, LDL, VLDL, and HDL cholesterol and triglyceride levels.

There were fewer new cases of coronary events in the gemfibrozil group (56 cases) than in the placebo group (84 cases); this overall difference of 34 percent was highly significant. Once again a study showed that lowering LDL cholesterol helps prevent coronary heart disease; once again it was estimated that for each 1 percent decrease in LDL there was about a 2 percent decrease in the risk of coronary heart disease. The results of the study suggest further that increasing HDL cholesterol decreases the risk of coronary heart disease, a new and important finding. The importance of HDL cholesterol in decreasing your risk for coronary heart disease is reviewed for you in greater detail in the next chapter. Finally, the use of gemfibrozil in this study was found to be safe and without the significant adverse effects reported for clofibrate.

Of the eleven other major clinical trials dealing with the cholesterol hypothesis, all but two found a significant reduction (range 9.5 to 43.8 percent) in the incidence of coronary heart disease after treatment of elevated blood cholesterol levels either with diet alone or with drugs. Three of the four diet trials were successful. The only drug trial that failed to show a treatment effect was the dextrothyroxine trial in the Coronary Drug Project discussed earlier in this chapter.

Can Lowering the Blood Cholesterol Level Reverse Blockages in the Coronary Arteries?

So far, you've learned that your risk of coronary heart disease can be decreased by lowering your blood total and LDL cholesterol levels. But what if, like so many others, you have existing cholesterol deposits or blockages in your coronary arteries? Will lowering your blood cholesterol levels diminish or remove those deposits?

There appear to be four possibilities (Figure 3-5):

1. *No change in progression.* Atherosclerosis may continue to progress with time despite treatment.

2. *Decreased progression.* After treatment starts, the process may be slowed but not stopped completely.

3. *No progression.* The process may be halted completely with treatment, so that no additional blockages develop but those that were present in the arteries remain.

4. *Regression.* The blockages in the coronary arteries may decrease in size, or even go away completely.

The National Heart, Lung, and Blood Institute Type II Coronary Intervention Study

This study was conducted in Bethesda, Maryland, at the National Heart, Lung, and Blood Institute. The phrase "type II" is shorthand for the kind of blood cholesterol problem that the participants had, namely, very high levels of LDL cholesterol in the blood. In addition, at least half had the inherited cholesterol problem called familial hypercholesterolemia, which is discussed in Chapter 7.

The question the study asked was, "Will lowering blood total and LDL cholesterol levels affect blockages in the coronary arteries?" The participants were 115 men and 28 women with type II cholesterol problems and coronary atherosclerosis. By a flip of the coin, half the participants were given cholestyramine to lower their blood total and LDL cholesterol levels, and the other half were given a placebo.

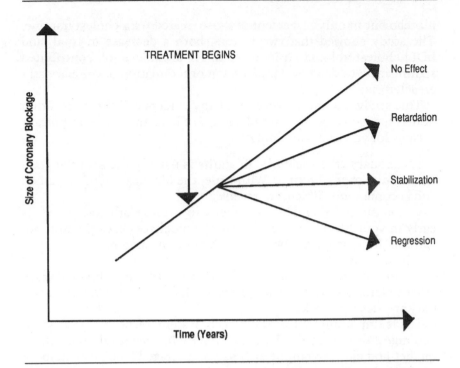

Fig. 3-5. Possible effects of lowering blood cholesterol on blockages in coronary arteries.

To measure the amount of blockages in the coronary arteries, coronary angiograms were performed at the beginning and end of the five-year study. At the end of the study, a panel of three doctors examined the repeat coronary angiogram to determine if any new blockages had started, and whether the old blockages had grown in size, remained the same, or become smaller.

It was found that the average levels of total and LDL cholesterol were significantly lower in the cholestyramine group (256 mg/dl and 178 mg/dl) than in the placebo group (289 mg/dl and 219 mg/dl). The average HDL cholesterol level was 41 mg/dl in those taking cholestyramine and 39 mg/dl in those on placebo.

The blockages in the coronary arteries had worsened in 49 percent (28 of 57) of the placebo-treated patients, but in only 32 percent (19 of 59) of the cholestyramine-treated patients. Of the patients whose coronary arteries were blocked by 50 percent or more at the beginning of the study, the disease got worse in 33 percent of those on placebo but in only 12 percent of those treated with cholestyramine. The study showed that two factors, both a decrease in total (and LDL) cholesterol and an increase in HDL cholesterol, contributed significantly to decreased progression or retardation of coronary atherosclerosis.

This study did not, however, find any evidence of the diminution or disappearance of coronary blockages. There are several important lessons for you from this study:

1. Coronary atherosclerosis in adults is usually the result of gradual buildup over a lifetime. With time, the blockages tend to harden and become more difficult to reverse.

2. You should therefore take steps to prevent atherosclerosis as early in your life as possible, before the blockages become more advanced. (It is also important to teach your children proper habits of nutrition early in life.)

3. Most doctors believe, as I do, that treatment *before* coronary atherosclerosis develops will be more effective than *after* the coronary arteries are blocked.

4. It is important that your blood cholesterol level be kept down to 200 mg/dl or less. In the Type II Coronary Intervention Study, those on diet and cholestyramine still had an average blood cholesterol of 267 mg/dl, a value still in the high-risk category for coronary heart disease. The ideal cholesterol level is not known, but the average adult cholesterol level in societies with little if any coronary atherosclerosis is about 150 mg/dl. Some researchers have accordingly argued that if there is any hope of reducing blockages in the coronary arteries by lowering cholesterol, the target level should be 150 mg/dl.

The Cholesterol-Lowering Atherosclerosis Study (CLAS)

In 1987, the Cholesterol-Lowering Atherosclerosis Study (CLAS) was reported in the *Journal of the American Medical Association* by Dr. David Blankenhorn and collaborators. This study also addressed the question of whether treatment with lipid-lowering drugs could affect blockages in the arteries.

The participants were 188 middle-aged men who had had coronary artery bypass grafts because of coronary atherosclerosis. The men were assigned by a flip of a coin to one of two groups: a treatment group that received the drugs colestipol and nicotinic acid, or a control group that received placebos. Colestipol acts the same way as cholestyramine and produces a significant fall in total and LDL cholesterol levels. Nicotinic acid, as we have seen, reduces both the total cholesterol and total triglyceride levels and raises the HDL cholesterol level. The treatment group was given a very strict diet (22 percent of calories as total fat and less than 125 mg of cholesterol per day). The placebo group was also given a fairly strict diet (26 percent of calories as total fat, less than 250 mg of cholesterol per day).

After two years of treatment, coronary angiograms were repeated and blockages in both the coronary arteries and the bypass grafts themselves were measured to determine what differences there were between the two groups.

When the 188 men entered this study, they had average total and LDL cholesterol levels of about 245 mg/dl and 170 mg/dl, respectively. After two years of drug treatment there was a marked fall of 26 percent in total cholesterol and of 43 percent in LDL cholesterol. In addition, the HDL cholesterol level increased 37 percent, and the total triglyceride level fell 22 percent. The new coronary angiograms showed that for 16.2 percent of the drug treatment group blockages of their coronary arteries had became smaller, compared with only 2.4 percent of the placebo group. Also those that became larger did so at a significantly slower rate in the treatment group. Finally, only 10 percent of the treatment group developed new coronary artery lesions, compared with 22 percent in the placebo group.

In the coronary artery bypass grafts the treatment group again did much better than the placebo group: only 24 percent experienced adverse changes in their bypass grafts, compared with 39 percent in the placebo group. And only 18 percent of the treatment group developed new lesions of atherosclerosis in their bypass grafts, a significantly lower rate than the 30 percent in the placebo group.

In conclusion, you have seen that drug therapy can both decrease LDL cholesterol and increase HDL cholesterol, thus markedly improving the balance of "bad" and "good" cholesterol. You have seen further that atherosclerosis in the coronary arteries of humans appears reversible by such therapy, as previous studies had shown for nonhuman primates. This does not mean that coronary artery bypass procedures are no longer worthwhile, because some operations are necessary in life-threatening circumstances. Though all those recent studies add up to good news, the final word must be one of caution: *if you already have coronary heart disease, a low-cholesterol, low-saturated-fat diet is important but may not by itself be sufficient.*

Summary

1. There is now overwhelming evidence that lowering blood total and LDL cholesterol by diet or drugs produces a reduction in coronary heart disease.

2. Two distinguished panels of medical experts, the Consensus Conference on Lowering Blood Cholesterol to Prevent Heart Disease (1983) and the Adult Treatment Panel (1988), both sponsored by the National Institutes of Health, have considered the available evidence and agreed as follows:

Is the relationship between blood cholesterol levels and coronary heart disease causal? *Yes.*

Will reduction of blood cholesterol levels help prevent coronary heart disease? *Yes.*

Should an attempt be made to reduce the blood cholesterol levels of the general population? *Yes.*

In the remaining chapters of this book, you will learn what you can do to take advantage of these latest scientific advances.

CHAPTER 4

HDL Cholesterol:
How Important Is It?

In the past ten years, no other lipoprotein in blood has generated more interest in lay and medical circles than high-density lipoprotein, or HDL. Much of the literature makes the point that if your level of HDL cholesterol is low, you are at increased risk of coronary heart disease. You will be pleased to learn, however, that if your HDL cholesterol is *high*, you are at *decreased* risk for coronary heart disease. In fact, you may be heading for longevity. Thus, although most of the cholesterol in your blood is carried on LDL (low-density lipoprotein), the lesser amount carried on HDL is still important for you.

It is important to have your blood level of HDL cholesterol measured by your doctor, particularly if you have a positive family history of premature coronary heart disease or have already suffered from a heart attack, angina pectoris, stroke, or poor circulation.

In this chapter, the effect of adverse factors that can decrease your HDL cholesterol level, such as obesity, physical inactivity, and cigarette smoking, will also be reviewed for you. You will learn that weight reduction, aerobic exercise, and stopping smoking may raise your HDL cholesterol level. You will be encouraged to take advantage of this "good" factor in your blood, HDL cholesterol, which may protect you against the development of coronary atherosclerosis.

HDL Cholesterol and Your Risk of Coronary Heart Disease

Over thirty years ago, Doctors Barr, Russ, and Eder observed that the level of HDL cholesterol was lower in patients with coronary heart disease. In 1966, Gofman and his associates published the results of a ten-year study of 1,961 men in Livermore, California. HDL and two subfamilies of lipoproteins within HDL, called HDL_2 and HDL_3, were lower in the 38 men who developed coronary heart disease than in men of the same age who did not. These two studies, and several others, were largely ignored until the 1970s. For example, HDL cholesterol levels were not determined in several of the major population studies reviewed in Chapter 2.

The famous Framingham Heart Study was begun in Framingham, Massachusetts, in 1949. The HDL cholesterol level was not measured until twenty years later, by which time many of the people in the study were middle-aged or older. HDL cholesterol levels were measured in this older group of 2,815 men and women, aged 49 to 82 years. In four short years, 79 of the 1,025 men and 63 of the 1,445 women who were previously free of coronary heart disease developed it. As you can see in Table 4-1, there was a steady decrease in the rate of coronary heart disease as the HDL cholesterol level increased from about 25 mg/dl to 75 mg/dl. This relationship was true for both men and women.

This striking effect of HDL on the risk of coronary heart disease was not explained by the presence of other risk factors such as high levels of blood total cholesterol, high blood pressure, or cigarette smoking. For example, in Figure 4-1 you can see that the risk of coronary heart disease increases as the HDL cholesterol level decreases at three different levels of the "bad" LDL cholesterol and systolic blood pressure. This finding was again true for both men and women. Of all the major risk factors, HDL cholesterol was the best

Table 4-1. HDL Cholesterol Level and Chance of Developing Coronary Heart Disease

HDL cholesterol level (mg/dl)	Percent of men developing heart disease	Percent of women developing heart disease
Below 25	18%	a
25–34	10	16%
35–44	10	5
45–54	5	5
55–64	6	4
65–74	3	1
Above 75	0	2

Source: Data derived from Framingham Heart Study, Exam 11, reported by T. Gordon et al. in *American Journal of Medicine* 62 (1977): 707–714.
aOnly four women were in this category; none developed coronary heart disease.

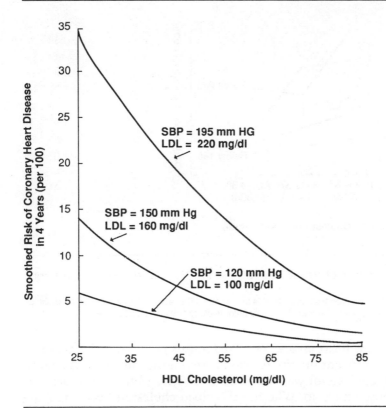

Fig. 4-1. Risk of coronary heart disease in four years for men aged 55 according to HDL cholesterol level. (SBP = systolic blood pressure.)
From the Framingham Heart Study, reproduced, with permission, from W. B. Kannel et al. in *Annals of Internal Medicine* 90 (1979): 85–91.

predictor of coronary heart disease in this older population.

In another program, people who were already participating in a study of cardiovascular disease in Albany, Framingham, Honolulu, San Francisco, and Evans County, Georgia, had their levels of HDL cholesterol measured. The findings of this study, called the Co-operative Lipoprotein Phenotyping Study, were consistent with those from the Framingham Study. A total of 6,859 men and women had a blood sample taken; all but 467 (6.8 percent) were 50 or older. For each of the five populations, HDL cholesterol was strongly and inversely related to the rate of coronary heart disease.

In the Israeli Ischemic Heart Disease Study, started in 1963, HDL cholesterol levels were measured in 6,562 men who were 40 or older.

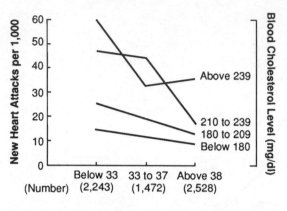

Initial HDL Cholesterol Level (mg/dl)

Fig. 4-2. Incidence of clinical heart attacks in 1963–1968 by HDL cholesterol level in 1963.
Redrawn with permission from the Israeli Ischemic Heart Disease Study, as reported by U. Goldbourt and J. Medalie in *American Journal of Epidemiology* 109 (1979): 296–308.

Over 150 new heart attacks occurred in this group over the next five years. A significant inverse relation between the rate of heart attacks and HDL cholesterol was found in those who were 50 or older, but not in those under 50. Whether the blood cholesterol was high, average, or below average (Figure 4-2), this relationship between a low HDL cholesterol and a higher rate of new heart attacks persisted.

Although the results of the three studies reviewed above were consistent with each other, the information from them was largely confined to men and women older than 50. What about younger people? In the Tromso Heart Study in Norway, Dr. N. E. Miller and colleagues examined the relation between the development of coronary heart disease and blood HDL cholesterol level in 6,595 men aged 20–49 years over a two-year period. In the seventeen men who suffered a coronary event, the average HDL cholesterol level was very low, only 26 mg/ml, compared with 39 mg/dl in 31 controls of the same age. The average LDL cholesterol level (222 mg/dl) in the coronary event cases was significantly higher than that (190 mg/dl) in the controls.

In regard to other variables such as blood total cholesterol, blood pressure, weight, and cigarette smoking, the group with coronary heart disease was similar to the control group. In fact, of the eight different risk factors for coronary heart disease determined in the Tromso study, HDL cholesterol was *the most important predictor* of future coronary heart disease in this group of younger men. Finally, you can see that a low HDL cholesterol level *preceded* the onset of coronary heart disease, and did not merely follow it as a consequence of subsequent changes in living habits.

Does Your HDL Cholesterol Level Predict How Much Blockage You May Have in Your Coronary Arteries?

Over a dozen studies have examined the relationship between HDL cholesterol and the degree of blockage due to coronary atherosclerosis. The blockages in the coronary arteries were determined by coronary angiography, a test reviewed for you in Chapter 2. In one such study of 483 men and women at Johns Hopkins, we found that the severity of the blockages was the greatest in those with the lowest HDL cholesterol levels. This relationship held for both men and women, and for both younger people (under 50) and older people (over 50).

Recently, when this study was expanded to 1,000 patients undergoing coronary arteriography, Dr. Michael Miller, our colleagues, and I found that more than one-third had a blood cholesterol level of 200 mg/dl or less. Of this normal cholesterol group, two out of three men and four out of five women with significant blockages in their coronary arteries had low HDL cholesterol levels. This emphasizes the importance of a low HDL cholesterol level, even if the blood cholesterol level is not significantly elevated.

What If a Low or a High HDL Cholesterol Level Runs in a Family?

Some families have a genetic condition in which HDL cholesterol levels are very low, and people in such families often develop premature coronary heart disease even when their blood total cholesterol level is less than 200 mg/dl. If you have a positive family history of premature coronary heart disease, or if you already have coronary heart disease, you should ask your doctor to determine your HDL cholesterol level. A level less than 35 mg/dl is definitely too low. Such families are discussed in more detail in Chapter 9.

In some families, the levels of HDL cholesterol are very high, as high as 80, 90, or 100 mg/dl. Dr. Charles Glueck and co-workers found that people from such families have a low rate of coronary heart disease. In fact, it is not unusual to find octogenarians in such families. Is there someone in your family who lived to be 80 years old? Have your HDL cholesterol level checked and see if you have inherited the "longevity factor."

Coronary Heart Disease and HDL Cholesterol: Can You Change the Inverse Risk?

After reviewing the above studies, you may be asking, "If I increase my HDL cholesterol level, will I decrease my risk of coronary disease?"

It has not been proved conclusively that increasing your HDL cholesterol level decreases your risk of coronary heart disease. But the results from three clinical trials, the Lipid Research Clinics Coronary Primary Prevention Trial, the NHLBI Type II Coronary Trial, and the Cholesterol-Lowering Atherosclerosis Study (Chapter 3), all point that way. These studies showed that the increased HDL cholesterol levels that occurred in the treatment group contributed to the decrease both in coronary heart disease events and in coronary atherosclerosis. Although these clinical trials were not designed to test directly an HDL cholesterol hypothesis, each found that an increase in HDL cholesterol produced a reduction in coronary heart disease in addition to the beneficial effect of lowering the LDL cholesterol level.

In the Helsinki Heart Study discussed in Chapter 3, doctors tested the effect of a drug called gemfibrozil (Lopid®) in men with combined high blood levels of LDL cholesterol and VLDL cholesterol. The major effect of gemfibrozil is to lower blood levels of VLDL cholesterol and triglyceride. As the blood VLDL and triglyceride levels fall, the HDL cholesterol level increases. There is usually a modest fall of about 10 percent in the total and LDL cholesterol levels as well.

The men treated with gemfibrozil had a 34 percent reduction in coronary heart disease compared with those on the placebo. The conclusions regarding the causal association of HDL cholesterol and coronary heart disease from this study are tentative because so many lipid and lipoprotein variables in the blood were being changed at one time. Nevertheless, the results from the Helsinki Heart Study suggest the following relation between the HDL cholesterol level and coronary heart disease:

For each 1 percent increase in your HDL cholesterol level, there is about a 3 percent decrease in your risk of coronary heart disease.

Many cholesterol specialists believe that if your HDL cholesterol level is too low (below 35 mg/dl), or even borderline low (between 35 mg/dl and 45 mg/dl), you and your doctor should make an effort to increase it through proper diet, aerobic exercise, and weight control. In the later chapters of this book, you will find out how to accomplish this goal.

As noted in Chapter 3, the Helsinki Heart Study also found that for each 1 percent reduction in total and LDL cholesterol there was a 2 percent decrease in the risk of coronary heart disease. Clearly, *both* LDL cholesterol and HDL cholesterol are important for you.

The LDL/HDL Ratio

The higher your HDL cholesterol level, the lower your risk of coronary heart disease; the lower your HDL cholesterol level, the higher your risk. Conversely, the higher your LDL cholesterol level, the higher your risk of coronary heart disease; and the lower your LDL cholesterol level, the lower your risk. This suggests, as Dr. William Castelli of the Framingham Heart Study, among others, has noted, that the ratio of LDL cholesterol to HDL cholesterol can be used to assess the risk of coronary heart disease. If your LDL cholesterol level has not been measured, you can use the ratio of total cholesterol to HDL cholesterol.

In Table 4-2, I have summarized the Framingham Study's rankings (by percentiles of degree of risk of coronary heart disease) for the ratios of LDL cholesterol to HDL cholesterol and of total cholesterol to HDL cholesterol in men and women. You and your doctor can determine your ratio and discuss what it means. In general, the lower your ratio, the lower your risk of coronary heart disease; the higher your ratio, the greater your risk. For example, if your ratio of total cholesterol to HDL cholesterol exceeds 6.0, or your ratio of LDL cholesterol to HDL cholesterol exceeds 4.0, you are at high risk. And as the next chapter makes clear, if you also have other risk factors for coronary heart disease, your risk will be even higher.

What Factors Can Raise or Lower Your HDL Cholesterol Level?

Since it is likely that increasing your HDL cholesterol level will help you prevent coronary heart disease, it is important that you understand what factors can affect that level.

Gender. In general, men have lower HDL cholesterol levels than women. The average is about 45 mg/dl for men and about 55 mg/dl

Table 4-2. Rankings of the Ratios of Blood Total Cholesterol
to HDL Cholesterol and of LDL to HDL Cholesterol

Rankings by selected percentiles		Total/HDL ratio	LDL/HDL ratio
		MEN	
Lowest	5%	2.94	1.53
	10%	3.30	1.90
	25%	3.95	2.49
	50%	4.88	3.19
	75%	6.09	4.10
	90%	7.30	4.92
Highest	95%	8.02	5.48
		WOMEN	
Lowest	5%	2.57	1.33
	10%	2.90	1.65
	25%	3.48	2.13
	50%	4.23	2.74
	75%	5.17	3.54
	90%	6.39	4.38
Highest	95%	7.25	5.05

Source: Data for adults from the Framingham Heart Study, as reported by
W. P. Castelli et al. in *Circulation* 67 (1983): 730–734.

for women. Men and women have similar levels of the HDL subfamily called HDL_3, but women have higher levels of another HDL subfamily, HDL_2, which is believed to be the critical factor making for a lower risk of coronary heart disease. (Women also have higher levels of the major protein of HDL, called apolipoprotein A1 or apoA1.) Information on how your level of HDL cholesterol compares with that of other men or women can be found in the Cholesterol and Triglyceride Tables at the back of the book.

Weight. There is a strong and consistent relation between your HDL cholesterol level and how much you weigh relative to your height. In both men and women, and both young adults (20–39 years) and middle-aged adults (40–59 years), those who are too heavy have lower HDL cholesterol levels than those who are of average weight or lean (Figure 4-3). In Chapter 5 you will find how to determine whether your weight is appropriate for your height.

Cigarette smoking. If you smoke cigarettes, you will have a lower HDL cholesterol level than someone who does not smoke. Since cigarette smoking itself is an important risk factor for coronary heart disease, the additional burden of a low HDL cholesterol level will add considerably to your risk of developing coronary heart disease.

Sugar. Too much table sugar or sucrose can lower your HDL cholesterol level. In the diet recommended for you in Chapter 11, the simple sugars and sucrose are decreased and the complex carbohydrates are increased.

Alcohol. In contrast to sucrose, alcohol consumption is associated with higher HDL cholesterol levels in both men and women, and for all adult age groups. A number of other studies have found that drinkers had higher HDL cholesterol levels than abstainers. Some studies have suggested that the increase in HDL cholesterol produced by alcohol is primarily found in HDL_3 rather than HDL_2. Since HDL_2 rather than HDL_3 is thought to be the "good" or protective component of HDL cholesterol, it is not clear that alcohol-produced increases in the HDL cholesterol level are as effective as other increases in reducing the risk of coronary heart disease.

Dr. Richard Moore, Dr. Thomas Pearson, and I have recently completed a study in which 56 men with low HDL cholesterol levels were assigned to one of two groups, one whose members abstained completely from alcohol for eight weeks and one whose members

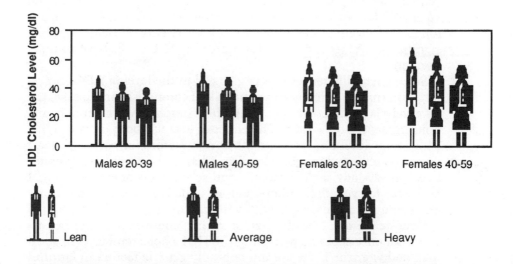

Fig. 4-3. Relation between HDL cholesterol level and body mass. (The women were not on hormones.) Quetelet Body Mass (QBM) index numbers: Lean, 19.0; Average, 25.0; Heavy, 31.0.
From the Lipid Research Clinics Prevalence Study, as reported by G. Heiss et al. in *Circulation* 62 (1980): Supplement IV, pp. IV116–IV128.

drank one beer a day. At the end of the study, we found no difference between the two groups either in HDL cholesterol level or in the blood levels of HDL_2 and HDL_3. However, the beer drinkers showed a significant increase of 10 percent in the level of the major apolipoprotein of HDL, called apoA1. Since apoA1 can help to remove cholesterol from your cells and transport it back to your liver for disposal, such an increase in the level of apoA1 *may be* beneficial, although we do not have direct evidence to that effect.

Doctors have been reluctant to recommend that their patients have a drink a day, since some people may decide that if one is good, two or even more will be better. And this may even be true within the limited context of HDL cholesterol levels; we cannot now say it is or it isn't. What we *can* say with absolute certainty is that whatever the effect of alcohol on cholesterol levels, its other effects, both physical and social, argue very powerfully for moderation in its use.

Exercise. The Lipid Research Clinics studies found a positive and significant association between amount of exercise reported and HDL cholesterol level in men aged 20–39 and 40–59 years. No such association was found in women. Dr. Peter Wood and co-workers found that the average HDL cholesterol levels of men and women runners were 64 and 75 mg/dl, respectively, compared with 43 and 56 mg/dl for male and female nonrunners. Ratliff and colleagues found that jogging three times a week for twenty weeks produced a significant average increase of 8 mg/dl in HDL cholesterol in male firemen.

Since small differences of 3 to 4 mg/dl in the level of HDL cholesterol can make a difference in your risk of coronary heart disease, the relatively large differences in HDL cholesterol between runners and nonrunners is noteworthy. The effect of exercise both on your HDL cholesterol level and on your other risk factors for coronary heart disease is reviewed in more detail in Chapter 15. Strenuous exercise is not always advisable, however, and some kinds of exercise might be better for you than others. Before undertaking an exercise program, you should discuss it with your doctor.

Genetic factors. Obesity, diet, smoking, and exercise together account for only about 20 percent of the HDL cholesterol level of adult men and women. There are undoubtedly genetic factors in families that control HDL cholesterol levels. Dr. Terri Beaty and I, together with our associates at Johns Hopkins, determined the HDL cholesterol levels of 402 persons from 62 normal families in Columbia, Maryland, and found those levels strongly influenced by genetic factors. For example, the similarity between parents and their children was greater on average than the similarity between the mothers and fathers, who were not genetically related. In the Framingham Off-spring Study, children of parents with coronary heart disease had lower HDL cholesterol levels on average than children of parents without coronary heart disease. This means that in all likelihood your HDL cholesterol level will be similar to your parents', and that your child's HDL cholesterol level will be similar to yours.

HDL Cholesterol Level: An Interaction of Factors

To what degree might important factors such as body weight, smoking, and exercise actually influence your HDL cholesterol values? This question was addressed by Dr. Gerardo Heiss and associates, using data from the Lipid Research Clinics Population Surveys. The HDL cholesterol levels of men aged 40 to 59 were measured. Information on their age, alcohol consumption, dietary intake of sucrose, starch, and cholesterol, and educational level was taken into consideration so that the HDL cholesterol levels were comparable within the group.

The men were divided into four different groups: active nonsmokers, inactive nonsmokers, active smokers, and inactive smokers (Figure 4-4). The relation of the average HDL cholesterol levels of the four groups to their body mass was then determined. For example, an inactive man with an average body mass who smokes will generally have an HDL cholesterol level of about 45 mg/dl. If that same man did not smoke, his HDL cholesterol level would be closer to 48 mg/dl. If he became active, his HDL cholesterol level would be around 52 mg/dl. As the figure shows, similar relationships for the four different groups hold at the extremes of the body mass index (i.e., 35.0 and heavy, 17.5 and lean). In summary, these data indicate that you can achieve a better HDL cholesterol level if you are a lean, active nonsmoker. (The body mass index is discussed in detail in Chapter 5).

Hulley and co-workers in the Multiple Risk Factor Intervention Trial (MRFIT) found that a weight loss of about eight pounds produced an increase of 3 mg/dl in HDL cholesterol level; conversely, a gain of eight pounds produced a decrease of 2 mg/dl. The MRFIT study also found that those who stopped smoking cigarettes had about a 4 mg/dl increase in their HDL cholesterol levels.

Doctors at the Hadassah University Hospital in Jerusalem found

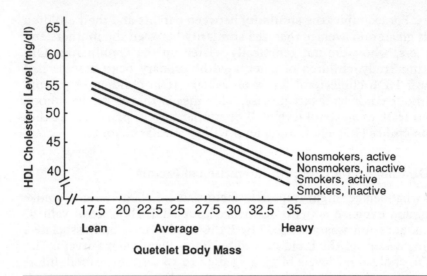

Fig. 4-4. HDL cholesterol levels in men aged 40–59 by cigarette smoking, re-ported physical activity, and body mass.
From the Lipid Research Clinics Prevalence Study, G. Heiss et al. in *Circulation* 62 (1980): Sup-plement IV, pp. IV116–IV128, by permission of the American Heart Association, Inc.

that a weight loss of about 10 percent in moderately obese but oth-erwise healthy subjects resulted in a higher HDL cholesterol level, and that the level remained higher if the lost weight was not re-gained. Once you lose those excess pounds, you must keep them off to maintain your healthier HDL cholesterol level.

Shepherd, Gotto, and co-workers showed that a diet *very high* in polyunsaturated fat and low in saturated fat (a ratio of polyunsatu-rated fat to saturated fat, or P/S ratio, of 4) lowered the HDL choles-terol and apoA1 levels too much. In other words, the decrease in LDL cholesterol was offset by a decrease in HDL cholesterol. Ernst and co-workers found that a less extreme P/S ratio (of 2.0) produced about equal percentage decreases in LDL and HDL cholesterol in patients with high blood cholesterol levels.

The Action Plan that you will find in Chapter 11 emphasizes a decrease in the saturated fat and cholesterol in your diet. A marked increase in your intake of polyunsaturated fat is *not* recommended; rather, the idea is to replace some of the saturated fat in the average diet with unsaturated fat, a category that includes both monoun-saturated and polyunsaturated fat. *If you follow this diet, you will have the right P/S ratio* (not above 1.0).

HDL and Blood Clotting

In 1988 Japanese investigators found that the major apolipoprotein of HDL, apoA1, was identical to another factor in the blood referred to as the prostacyclin stabilizing factor (PSF). PSF binds with prostacyclin (PGI$_2$) to facilitate prostacyclin's protective effect against blood clot formation and blood vessel narrowing. Thus patients with low levels of HDL and apoA1 may tend to form blood clots more easily and constrict their blood vessels more readily. These exciting new data offer a possible explanation of why a low level of HDL is an independent risk factor for the development of coronary heart disease and why a high level of HDL may help to protect against coronary heart disease.

Summary and Recommendations

1. A strong relationship between the blood level of HDL cholesterol and coronary heart disease has been established. A low level of HDL cholesterol is associated with a higher risk of coronary heart disease; a high HDL cholesterol level is associated with a lower risk.

2. A low HDL cholesterol level increases the risk of coronary heart disease even after the effect of other risk factors such as high blood levels of total and LDL cholesterol, high blood pressure, obesity, and cigarette smoking have been considered.

3. A low HDL cholesterol level is a risk factor for coronary heart disease in both men and women and appears to be a powerful predictor, if not the most powerful predictor, of coronary heart disease in people older than 50.

4. The combination of a low HDL cholesterol level with a high total or LDL cholesterol level increases the risk of coronary heart disease substantially. A high ratio of total cholesterol to HDL cholesterol or of LDL cholesterol to HDL cholesterol indicates a high risk of coronary heart disease.

5. Very low levels or very high levels of HDL cholesterol can run in families. Families with low HDL cholesterol levels have a high rate of early coronary heart disease; those with high HDL cholesterol levels tend to be long-lived and have a reduced incidence of coronary heart disease.

6. A number of factors influence HDL cholesterol levels. On average, women have HDL cholesterol levels about 10 mg/dl higher than men. Persons who are overweight, who smoke, who eat a lot of sugar,

and who are inactive will have lower average HDL cholesterol levels than those who do not have these problems or habits.

7. You can increase your HDL cholesterol level by regular aerobic exercise, drinking alcohol in moderation, giving up cigarettes, and losing weight.

8. In trials designed to test the cholesterol (or LDL cholesterol) hypothesis, increasing the HDL cholesterol level had a beneficial effect over and above that of decreasing the total and LDL cholesterol levels. Since this effect, until recent decades altogether unknown, is now beyond dispute, it is clear that efforts directed at increasing the HDL cholesterol level are very much a part of the battle against coronary heart disease.

CHAPTER 5

Your Risk Profile

What are your chances of being stricken by coronary heart disease? To help you arrive at the best possible answer to this question, various yardsticks are provided in this chapter. They are listed for your quick review in Table 5-1.

1. Your Diet

High amounts of total fat, saturated fat, and cholesterol in your diet elevate your blood levels of cholesterol and LDL cholesterol, increasing your risk of coronary heart disease. To help you assess the status of your current diet, consider the following questions. Do you think about what you eat? Do you know which foods are high in cholesterol? Do you know which foods are high in saturated fat? Do you know the difference between saturated fat and unsaturated fat, including monounsaturated fat and polyunsaturated fat? Do you know how to read labels to determine how much fat and what kind of fat a product contains? Do you know the differences between foods from animals and those from plants?

Here a brief quiz is presented to help you to determine the status of your current diet. These questions were prepared by Ginny Hartmuller, R.D., M.S., the chief nutritionist in our Lipid Clinic at Johns Hopkins. This questionnaire is an abbreviated and modified form of a more detailed test provided in the book *The New American Diet*, by Sandra Connor and William Connor.

For each question below, select the answer that best describes your eating habits in the last month. The number at the left of each possible answer is the point score. Put your score in the blank after each

Table 5-1. Your Risk Profile

YOUR	
1. Diet	7. Blood pressure
2. Family history	8. Cigarette smoking status
3. Blood total cholesterol level	9. Weight
4. Blood LDL cholesterol level	10. Blood sugar
5. Blood HDL cholesterol level	11. Stress level
6. Blood triglyceride level	12. Physical activity

question. If you checked more than one answer for each question, put the lowest score checked in the blank.

1. What kind of milk do you usually use for drinking or cooking?
    1. Whole milk _____
    2. Two percent milk _____
    4. One percent milk or buttermilk _____
    5. Skim milk or no milk _____
    SCORE: _____

2. Check the type and number of "visible" eggs you eat each week.
    1. Six or more whole eggs per week _____
    2. Three to five whole eggs per week _____
    3. One to two whole eggs per week _____
    4. One whole egg per month _____
    5. Egg white, egg substitute, or none _____
    SCORE: _____

3. Which frozen desserts are you most likely to eat at least once a month, if any?
    1. Ice cream _____
    2. Frozen whole milk desserts such as milk sherbet _____
    3. Ice milk or Tofutti _____
    4. Sorbet or sherbet without milk, or low-fat frozen yogurt, or ices _____
    5. None _____
    SCORE: _____

4. What kind of cheese do you use for snacks or sandwiches?
    1. Cheddar, Swiss, Brie, American, cream cheese, or regular cheese slices or spreads _____

2. Part-skim-milk mozzarella, neufchatel, creamed cottage cheese, or cheese that has half the fat content of regular cheese _____
4. Low-cholesterol filled cheese such as Cheezola _____
5. Very-low-fat process cheese or no cheese _____
SCORE: _____

5. *Estimate the number of ounces of meat, regular cheese, fish, and poultry you eat in an average day. Include all meals and snacks.*
   1. Eleven or more ounces per day _____
   2. Nine to ten ounces per day _____
   3. Six to eight ounces per day _____
   4. Four to five ounces per day _____
   5. Three ounces or less per day _____
   SCORE: _____

6. *What kind of fats are used most often to cook your food?*
   1. Butter, shortening, lard, meat fat; or eat in restaurants at least four times per week _____
   2. Shortening _____
   3. Inexpensive stick margarine _____
   4. Tub or soft margarine; vegetable oil _____
   5. None (use nonstick pans or spray) _____
   SCORE: _____

7. *What is your daily use of fat—for example, margarine, butter, mayonnaise, or salad dressing)—added at the table? (Take all meals and snacks into account. One teaspoon of fat equals one serving.)*
   1. Use ten servings or more _____
   2. Use eight to nine servings _____
   3. Use six to seven servings _____
   4. Use four to five servings _____
   5. Use three servings or less _____
   SCORE: _____

8. *Do you add salt to your food at the table?*
   1. Always _____
   2. Frequently _____
   4. Occasionally _____
   5. Never _____
   SCORE: _____

9. How often do you eat dessert or baked goods such as sweet rolls, doughnuts, cookies, and cakes?

1. Three or more times per day _____
2. Two times per day _____
3. One time per day _____
4. Four to six times per week _____
5. Three times per week or less _____

SCORE: _____

10. Which snack items are you most likely to eat in an average week?

1. Potato chips, corn chips, chocolate, nuts, snack crackers, doughnuts, peanut butter _____
3. Combination of high-fat and low-fat snacks _____
4. Air-popped popcorn, low-fat crackers _____
5. Fruit or no snacks _____

SCORE: _____

TOTAL SCORE: _____

Here is how to interpret your score:

0–20: *Need diet modification.* You should particularly consider diet modifications in areas with lowest scores.

20–30: *Good diet.* Close to the diet reviewed for you in Chapter 11. Similar to the Step One Diet of the Adult Treatment Panel of the National Institutes of Health and the American Heart Association.

30–40: *Very good diet.* Similar to the stricter version of the diet found in Chapter 11. Close to the Step Two Diet of the Adult Treatment Panel.

40–50: *Excellent diet.* Even stricter than the Step Two Diet.

If your score is 40–50, you have already substantially modified your intake of cholesterol, total fat, and saturated fat. If your score is less than 20, you will need to make a significant number of changes. To help you make these changes, a comprehensive Action Plan is presented in Chapter 11, a two-week menu plan is offered in Chapter 14 to help you get started, and nearly 100 quick and easy recipes for delicious low-cholesterol, low-saturated-fat food will be found at the back of the book.

2. Your Family History

What you have inherited plays a key role in determining your risk of coronary heart disease. Studies of families in which coronary heart disease is common before age 55 make it clear that if one of your relatives has premature coronary heart disease, you are at risk of an early heart attack yourself. This strong tendency for coronary heart disease to run in families manifests itself even after blood total cholesterol levels, blood pressure, cigarette smoking, and other risk factors are taken into consideration.

What do you know about the presence of coronary heart disease in your family? Many of my patients are initially unaware that their family has a history of early coronary heart disease. They may know that blood relatives have died at relatively young ages, but have never asked why or related the death or deaths to their own prospects.

To help you determine your family history, a sample diagram, called a pedigree, has been drawn for you (Figure 5-1). Males are depicted as squares, females as circles. Substitute your own parents, your brothers and sisters, your children, your four grandparents, and the brothers and sisters of both your mother and your father (that is, your uncles and aunts). You have now drawn the pedigree of your own more or less immediate family. Follow these quick and easy steps to complete the family history:

1. Which of your relatives are alive and which have died? Indicate those who are deceased by drawing an X inside the square or circle.

2. Determine the age at which these relatives died.

3. Determine the causes of death if you can. Did any of your relatives die from a heart attack, sudden unexplained death, a stroke, diabetes, or complications of high blood pressure?

4. If so, find out *how old* your deceased relatives were when they *first developed* these conditions. For example, your grandfather may have had a heart attack at 49 but lived another fifteen years.

5. Now determine whether any of your living relatives has coronary heart disease or vascular problems. Has any of them undergone coronary artery bypass surgery or balloon angioplasty? Has any of them had a heart attack, angina pectoris, a stroke, or poor circulation?

6. Is any family member known to have a high blood cholesterol (or triglyceride) level? Do any of your relatives have flat or wart-like yellow deposits around or under their eyes? These are signs of an underlying lipid problem.

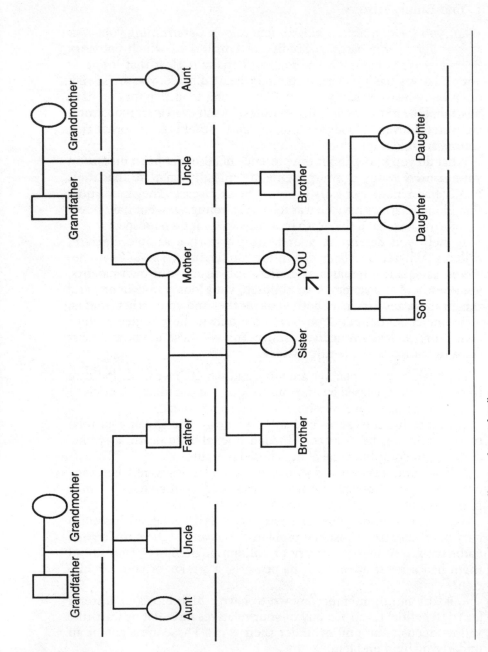

Fig. 5-1. How to draw a pedigree of your family.

7. Do any of your relatives have high blood pressure or diabetes? Are any seriously overweight?

8. A helpful clue is whether any of your relatives are taking medicine for elevated cholesterol or triglyceride, for high blood pressure, or for coronary heart disease (for example, nitroglycerine for chest pain or angina pectoris).

Completing your family's pedigree is an important step in assessing your risk profile for coronary heart disease. You may need to do some additional homework to find the facts to complete this part of your risk profile. If one or more of your relatives had coronary heart disease before the age of 55, you will want to pay particular attention to Chapters 7–9, which discuss the various blood fat problems that run in families who are predisposed to coronary heart disease.

3. Your Blood Total Cholesterol Level

It is a good idea for all adult Americans to have their blood cholesterol levels checked from time to time, even if they are feeling great. Take the case of Patricia Everett, an 18-year-old who was consuming a diet very high in cholesterol and saturated fat, eating meat at least twice a day, frequently indulging in fast foods, and eating lots of candy bars. She was also getting no regular exercise and smoked cigarettes—all this in spite of the fact that her father had a history of high cholesterol.

While at a Johns Hopkins Health Fair, she had her blood cholesterol checked and it was very high. She was sent to the Johns Hopkins Lipid Clinic, where I found that her cholesterol level was 374 mg/dl, with a very high LDL cholesterol level of 291 mg/dl. Not only did she have a cholesterol problem, but her triglyceride level was elevated at 357 mg/dl. In addition, her "good" HDL cholesterol level was very low at 25 mg/dl. In short, this young adult had a very high risk profile. Had it not been for cholesterol screening, she would have gone on for an undetermined amount of time without receiving the proper dietary treatment and, in this case, drug treatment as well.

Most doctors and specialists in the cholesterol field now recommend that all adult Americans have their blood cholesterol level checked. How often it should be rechecked after that depends on the result (see below). It is not necessary for you to be fasting to have this blood test. Your doctor may routinely measure your blood cholesterol level at your annual physical examination. Often the level of

Table 5-2. Guidelines to Help You Interpret Your Blood Cholesterol Level

	Level of blood cholesterol (mg/dl)					
	Males			Females		
Age (years)	Lowest quartile	Average	Highest quartile	Lowest quartile	Average	Highest quartile
	Below		Above	Below		Above
20–29	153	172	194	152	172	192
30–39	172	194	218	161	180	201
40–49	185	207	231	175	197	221
50–59	188	211	235	196	219	244
Over 60	189	210	234	204	226	252

Source: *Lipid Research Clinics Population Studies Data Book,* Vol. I, *The Prevalence Study* (NIH Publication No. 80-1527, July 1980).

blood cholesterol is determined when your doctor obtains a general battery of blood tests to assess your general health status. Although the blood cholesterol level is highest in winter and lowest in summer, the average seasonal difference is relatively small (about 7 mg/dl).

Is it easy to get a reliable blood cholesterol measurement? Not always. Ask your doctor whether the laboratory he uses is standardized by the CDC (Communicable Disease Center) in Atlanta; results from such laboratories tend to be more reliable. If you have your blood cholesterol level checked by screening programs at fairs, at your workplace, or in a special program to promote heart health, the result may be useful in a general way, as it was for Pat Everett. But for a truly accurate reading, you should be prepared to have a second measurement performed by your doctor using a standardized laboratory.

Have you had your level of blood total cholesterol tested? If so, do you know what the result was, and what it means in regard to your risk of coronary heart disease? Your life could depend on the answer, as Pat Everett's did.

How does your blood cholesterol level compare with that of other Americans? You will find in Table 5-2 blood total cholesterol levels for the top quartile, the average, and the lowest quartile of American males and females of various age groups (as the table shows, such levels increase with age). More detailed information is provided in the Cholesterol and Triglyceride Tables at the back of the book; and guidelines for people under twenty are presented in Chapter 6.

Three broad categories of blood cholesterol levels have been defined by the NIH's Adult Treatment Panel:

High blood cholesterol: 240 mg/dl or higher.

Borderline high blood cholesterol: between 200 and 239 mg/dl.

Desirable blood cholesterol: below 200 mg/dl.

If you are between 20 and 29 years old, subtract 20 mg/dl from these values. If you are over 65, discuss your result with your doctor, since more than one in four women but less than one in four men in your age group will have a blood cholesterol level above 240 mg/dl.

If you are in the high blood cholesterol group, you are one of 40 million adult Americans in this situation. Don't be surprised if you are in the high or borderline high group, since *only one out of every two Americans has a blood cholesterol level below 200 mg/dl.* Four out of every five heart attacks occur to people with blood cholesterol levels above 200 mg/dl.

These three broad categories were recommended by the Adult Treatment Panel in 1988 to provide a simple but still meaningful scheme for you and your doctor to follow. As recently as 1984, most laboratories used by doctors reported results for total cholesterol using even broader ranges: for example, 150 to 300 mg/dl was often given as the normal range for all adults. These standards did not give adequate weight to the risk of coronary heart disease at blood total cholesterol levels much lower than 300 mg/dl. They have now been superseded by the categories of the Adult Treatment Panel.

If you are a woman, you are at a lower risk for coronary heart disease than a man; but this does not mean that your blood cholesterol level is unimportant. The blood cholesterol levels are similar in men and women; it simply takes, on average, ten years longer for a woman to develop coronary heart disease than a man. As indicated below, this may be due in part to women's generally higher HDL cholesterol levels.

4. Your Blood LDL Cholesterol Level

LDL carries most of the cholesterol in your blood and is responsible for the cholesterol deposits on the inside of your arteries. If your total blood cholesterol is in the borderline high or high category, it will be important for you and your doctor to determine your LDL cholesterol level.

Your LDL cholesterol level is determined by a blood test that is sometimes referred to as a "lipid profile" or a "lipoprotein profile." You must be fasting for twelve hours for this test. The cholesterol in your blood is carried on the three major lipoprotein families:

Blood cholesterol = [Cholesterol on LDL] +
                    [Cholesterol on HDL] + [Cholesterol on VLDL]

LDL is not usually measured directly, but by ordering a test for blood cholesterol, HDL cholesterol, and triglyceride, you and your doctor can estimate your LDL cholesterol level fairly accurately. How? Let us take an example.

Suppose that the following results are obtained from your blood test: cholesterol 240 mg/dl, HDL cholesterol 45 mg/dl, and triglyceride 150 mg/dl. The steps to be taken to estimate your LDL cholesterol level are as follows:

1. Divide the triglyceride level by 5 to get the VLDL cholesterol level: 150/5 = 30 mg/dl.
2. Add the VLDL and HDL levels: 30 + 45 = 75 mg/dl.
3. Subtract this figure from the total cholesterol level: 240 − 75 = 165 mg/dl. This is your LDL cholesterol level.

This formula, developed by Drs. Friedewald, Levy, and Fredrickson at the National Institutes of Health, works pretty well for about 95 percent of people. It does not work if you have not fasted for at least twelve hours; if your blood triglyceride level is above 400 mg/dl; or if you have a rare condition (one in 2,000 people) called type 3 disease. The chances are small that your blood triglyceride is above 400 mg/dl, or that you have type 3 disease. But if your doctor has told you that you have one or the other of these conditions, you will find them discussed at length in Chapter 8.

A more recent report suggests that dividing the triglyceride level by 6, rather than 5, to get VLDL may provide a more accurate estimate of the LDL cholesterol level. Further studies may validate the use of triglyceride ÷ 6 as the preferred way of estimating LDL. It

Table 5-3. Guidelines to Help You Interpret Your LDL Cholesterol Level

	Level of blood LDL cholesterol (mg/dl)					
	Males			Females		
Age (years)	Lowest quartile	Average	Highest quartile	Lowest quartile	Average	Highest quartile
	Below		Above	Below		Above
20–29	91	109	128	86	105	122
30–39	109	128	149	94	113	134
40–49	118	138	160	105	125	148
50–59	121	144	165	116	140	164
Over 60	123	145	168	126	150	176

Source: see Table 5-2.

should be understood in either event that the LDL level arrived at this way is only an estimate; when the actual LDL level in the blood is measured by a laboratory, it is likely to be a slightly different figure.

How does your blood LDL cholesterol level compare with that of other Americans? You will find in Table 5-3 values for the top quartile, the average, and the lowest quartile of American males and females of various age groups. Once again, more detailed information is provided in the Cholesterol and Triglyceride Tables.

How can you determine if your LDL cholesterol level is too high? The Adult Treatment Panel has defined three categories for LDL cholesterol:

High LDL cholesterol: 160 mg/dl or higher.

Borderline high LDL cholesterol: between 130 and 159 mg/dl.

Desirable LDL cholesterol: below 130 mg/dl.

If you are between 20 and 29 years old, subtract 20 mg/dl from these values. Again, if you are over 65 and female, there is more than a one in four chance that your LDL cholesterol level will be above 160 mg/dl.

What is the advantage of having your level of LDL cholesterol measured? For one thing, if your blood total cholesterol is borderline high, you and your doctor will want to know whether this result is due primarily to a high LDL level or a high HDL level. Most often it will be due primarily to a high LDL level. But if you are in the 10 to 15 percent of cases in which a borderline high total cholesterol level reflects an unusually high HDL level, your LDL cholesterol may actually be in the desirable range; and since a high HDL level is in itself desirable, the news in this event is doubly good.

Conversely, despite a total blood cholesterol level in the desirable range (less than 200 mg/dl), you may have a family history of premature coronary heart disease or you may yourself already have coronary heart disease. In this event, despite a desirable total blood cholesterol level your LDL cholesterol may be borderline high or even high. Under these circumstances, your HDL cholesterol level will be low.

Clearly, then, your total blood cholesterol level can be misleading, particularly if you carry more of your cholesterol on LDL, and less on HDL, than the average person. As noted earlier, about one in five persons who develop coronary heart disease has a blood cholesterol level less than 200 mg/dl. This matter is discussed further in Chapter 9, "Are You at Risk if Your Cholesterol Level Is Normal?"

Table 5-4. Guidelines to Help You Interpret Your HDL Cholesterol Level

	Level of blood HDL cholesterol (mg/dl)					
	Males			Females		
Age (years)	Lowest quartile	Average	Highest quartile	Lowest quartile	Average	Highest quartile
	Below		Above	Below		Above
20–29	38	45	51	46	53	63
30–39	37	44	51	45	54	64
40–49	37	44	52	48	57	67
50–59	37	45	53	50	61	72
Over 60	40	49	62	50	61	74

Source: see Table 5-2.

5. Your Blood HDL Cholesterol Level

In Chapter 4 the point was made that your HDL cholesterol level is an independent predictor of your risk of coronary heart disease: the higher the HDL level, the lower the risk. HDL cholesterol is thus important in its own right. In Table 5-4 you will find figures for HDL cholesterol levels that will show how you compare with other Americans.

What level of HDL cholesterol will place you at particularly high risk of coronary heart disease? The Adult Treatment Panel defined this level as below 35 mg/dl, and that is the definition I use in this book. As you can see from Table 5-4, about one in four American men has an undesirably low HDL cholesterol level; only one in ten American women has this problem. Because less scientific information is available about HDL cholesterol than about LDL cholesterol, I use the following guidelines for my patients:

Low HDL cholesterol: less than 35 mg/dl.

Borderline low HDL cholesterol: between 35 and 45 mg/dl.

Desirable HDL cholesterol: Above 45 mg/dl.

6. Your Blood Triglyceride Level

Triglyceride is the fat in your blood that your body uses to carry the fatty acids from your diet or those made in your liver through your bloodstream. Triglyceride from your diet is carried from your intestines on lipoproteins called chylomicrons. After you eat a meal containing fat, the triglyceride level in your blood will increase to about double that obtained when you are fasting; that's why it is necessary for you to fast twelve hours before taking a blood test for triglyceride. When you are fasting, most of the triglyceride in your blood is carried on VLDL (very low-density lipoprotein), the lipoprotein made in your liver and released into your bloodstream.

A number of factors can influence your level of blood triglyceride. These factors include obesity, diets high in simple sugar, fat, or alcohol, and weight loss. Your weight should be stable for at least one month before the triglyceride test. The level of blood triglyceride can fluctuate considerably, and it will be important for you to have at least two measurements made by your doctor after an overnight fast.

Some researchers have found that a high blood level of triglyceride in fasting people is associated with an increased number of cases of coronary heart disease; others have not found such an association. But the most recent results from the Framingham Heart Study reaffirm the importance of a high blood triglyceride level as a factor in the development of coronary heart disease.

Unlike cholesterol, triglyceride does not accumulate in the build-up of atherosclerosis inside the coronary artery. Rather the importance of your blood triglyceride level is that it often provides a signpost, or indicator, of an underlying problem. The measurement of your blood level of triglyceride is important for three reasons:

1. Your blood triglyceride level is a factor in estimating your LDL cholesterol level (see above).

2. Even if your LDL cholesterol level is in the desirable range (below 130 mg/dl), a high triglyceride level may be an indicator that you are at increased risk of coronary heart disease. This is particularly true if your HDL cholesterol level is low, if you have a positive family history of premature coronary heart disease, or if you already have coronary heart disease.

3. There are also several genetic conditions of blood lipids in which a high blood triglyceride level signals the kind of problem with processing blood fats and lipoproteins that often leads to premature coronary artery disease. These matters are reviewed further for you in Chapter 8.

Table 5-5 presents average triglyceride values and those for the lowest and highest quartiles of Americans by gender and age group. You can see that males generally have higher triglyceride levels than females, and that the levels increase with age in both sexes, with some exceptions for men over 50. More details will be found in the Triglyceride Tables at the back of the book.

Table 5-5. Guidelines to Help You Interpret Your Triglyceride Level

	Level of blood triglyceride (mg/dl)					
	Males			Females		
Age (years)	Lowest quartile	Average	Highest quartile	Lowest quartile	Average	Highest quartile
	Below		Above	Below		Above
20–29	67	91	128	59	80	108
30–39	78	109	160	59	79	110
40–49	88	123	174	67	91	127
50–59	87	122	175	79	105	145
Over 60	85	116	159	82	110	153

Source: see Table 5-2.

How can you and your doctor decide whether your blood triglyceride level is too high? I use the following guidelines for my patients:

Very high triglyceride: above 500 mg/dl.

High triglyceride: between 250 and 500 mg/dl.

Borderline high triglyceride: between 150 and 249 mg/dl.

Desirable triglyceride: below 150 mg/dl.

With more knowledge and research in the future, more precise definitions will be possible.

A Consensus Development Conference on Hypertriglyceridemia at the National Institutes of Health considered definitions of high blood triglyceride and made recommendations for its treatment in 1984. Diet and weight reduction are the first forms of treatment for a high blood triglyceride level, and these two measures often do the job. Medication is recommended only if your level remains above 500 mg/dl after diet and weight reduction. The Action Plan diet reviewed for you in Chapter 11 can also be used if you have a blood triglyceride problem. Chapter 16 is devoted to medications for blood lipid problems of all sorts, including a high blood triglyceride.

7. Your Blood Pressure

High blood pressure, or hypertension, is a strong risk factor for coronary heart disease and stroke. Your risk increases gradually as your blood pressure rises. However, after your blood pressure increases to above 140/90 mm Hg (millimeters of mercury) your risk increases more dramatically. High blood pressure is important for you in your risk profile. Consequently, certain basic information is reviewed for you here as a starting guide to help you and your doctor assess your risk of cardiovascular disease from high blood pressure.

Do you know what your blood pressure is? Actually, many more Americans know their blood pressure than know their blood cholesterol level. Has your blood pressure been measured by a competent health professional on at least three different occasions? Do you know the meaning of the two numbers that constitute your blood pressure reading? If you know what your blood pressure is, do you know if it is too high, i.e., do you know if you have hypertension? If you have high blood pressure, have you and your doctor considered appropriate dietary treatment, and if necessary drug treatment?

Your blood is pumped from your heart into a large artery called the aorta with sufficient force to make your blood travel through the various arteries to deliver oxygen and nutrients to your cells. This force is called the systolic blood pressure. It is measured as the top number of a blood pressure determination (e.g., 120 of a 120/80 reading). The very small blood vessels in your body, called capillaries, are an extensive network covering hundreds of miles. The opening inside your capillaries is quite narrow, about the size of a pin, and consequently capillaries provide resistance to the flow of blood from your heart. Such resistance is recorded as the diastolic blood pressure. It is the lower number (e.g., 80 of 120/80).

You can have an elevation in your systolic blood pressure, in diastolic blood pressure, or in both. What constitutes high blood pressure, or hypertension? The 1988 report of the Joint National Committee on Detection, Evaluation, and Treatment of High Blood Pressure recommends certain categories to classify blood pressure (Table 5-6).

If you are eighteen or older, a diastolic blood pressure less than 85 and a systolic blood pressure less than 140 are considered normal. Just as with blood cholesterol, the diagnosis of hypertension in adults needs to be confirmed by your doctor by determining the average of two, or preferably three, blood pressure levels; two or more measurements are desirable because blood pressure can vary widely according to circumstances, so that a single measurement is more subject to error than an average of two or more. If your blood pressure is 140/90 or higher, and thus in one of the risk categories summarized in Table 5-6, you have a lot of company: approximately 60 million persons in the United States.

Even if your blood pressure has previously been found to be normal, you should have it measured at least once every two years in the future. If it is in the high normal range, it should be rechecked every

Table 5-6. Guidelines to Help You Interpret Your Blood
Pressure Levels

Range (mm Hg)	Category
Diastolic blood pressure	
Below 85	Normal blood pressure
85 to 89	High normal blood pressure
90 to 104	Mild hypertension
105 to 114	Moderate hypertension
Above 114	Severe hypertension
Systolic blood pressure	
(when diastolic below 90)	
Below 140	Normal blood pressure
140 to 159	Borderline isolated systolic hypertension
Above 159	Isolated systolic hypertension

Note: Categories are those recommended by the 1988 Report of the Joint
National Committee on Detection, Evaluation and Treatment of High Blood
Pressure in *Archives of Internal Medicine* 148 (1988): 1023–1038.

year. Severe hypertension (that is, a diastolic blood pressure above
115) requires immediate attention by your doctor; moderate hypertension (diastolic between 105 and 114) should be evaluated within
several weeks, and a mild hypertension (diastolic between 90 and
104) confirmed within a month or so.

If you do have hypertension, your doctor will want to make sure
that it is not caused by certain diseases (for example, of the kidney)
or other medical conditions. In addition, some medications may
raise blood pressure, among them oral contraceptives, steroids, nasal
decongestants, appetite suppressants, and certain antidepressive
medications.

A plan for the treatment of hypertension can be developed by your
doctor. Some of the major aspects of treatment will include the following:

Obesity. A strong correlation exists between body weight and
blood pressure. As the body weight increases, so does the blood pressure, on average, particularly in young to middle-aged adults. Weight
reduction often results in a decrease in the blood pressure.

Sodium restriction. It has been previously shown that moderate
restriction in the sodium content of your diet (to approximately two
grams of sodium or five grams of salt per day) may reduce your high
blood pressure. It appears that certain patients are more responsive
than others to the dietary restriction of sodium.

Alcohol. Heavy consumption of alcohol (for example, more than 4 ounces of 100-proof whiskey, 16 ounces of wine, or 48 ounces of beer a day) may elevate your blood pressure. Therefore you should drink only in moderation if you have hypertension—or even if you don't.

Dietary fats. In some recent studies, a reduction of dietary saturated fat and an increase of polyunsaturated fat have been found to lower blood pressure levels. Restricting your dietary fat may help lower your blood pressure as well as your blood cholesterol level. Thus the Action Plan diet presented in Chapter 11 may help on both counts.

Cigarette smoking. Your risk factors for coronary heart disease are additive. Thus, if you are hypertensive, you should particularly avoid cigarette smoking.

Exercise. A regular exercise program involving walking, jogging, and swimming, in addition to weight control, may be useful in reducing your blood pressure. Exercise is reviewed for you further in Chapter 15. As noted above, an exercise program should be undertaken only after discussion with your doctor.

Behavioral modification. You may also benefit from behavioral modification, such as learning to relax and other methods of "biofeedback." With the assistance of your doctor, these approaches may produce a modest but significant reduction in your blood pressure, particularly if you have mild hypertension.

The medications used for the treatment of hypertension, and their benefits, side effects, and effectiveness, will not be reviewed here. Should you not respond to diet, salt restriction, and weight control, your doctor can decide if medication is necessary. Reducing your blood pressure with drugs, if necessary, will decrease your risk of death and complications from cardiovascular disease.

Even if you have mild hypertension, treatment with anti-hypertensive drugs will provide protection for you against stroke and enlargement of the heart. In one study (the Hypertension Detection and Follow-Up Program), there was a 20 percent reduction in the total number of deaths in patients with mild hypertension (diastolic blood pressure 90–104 mm hg); this included a significant reduction in both fatal and nonfatal coronary heart disease events.

If you do have a blood cholesterol or blood triglyceride problem, certain medications that are used to treat high blood pressure or hypertension can adversely affect your blood lipid and lipoprotein levels. The effects of these anti-hypertensive medications on blood lipid and lipoprotein levels are reviewed for you in Chapter 16, where the drug treatment of blood cholesterol and triglyceride problems is also considered.

If you are over 65, you may experience an increase in systolic blood pressure to 160 or higher while your diastolic blood pressure remains below 90, a condition often referred to as "isolated systolic hypertension." It is not clear what effect this condition has on your risk of coronary heart disease; this question is currently being evaluated by a study called the Systolic Hypertension in the Elderly Program. Therefore, if you are over 65, your doctor will need to decide on a treatment tailored to your particular risk profile.

If you have a positive family history of premature coronary heart disease or of stroke due to hypertension, and you also have hypertension, this combination puts you in a high-risk category. Other high-risk groups include blacks and obese people. If you have a high blood cholesterol level, or smoke cigarettes, or have both these risk factors, an elevated blood pressure is even more serious. With such a combination of risk factors, your risk of coronary heart disease would be ten times that of someone with none of these risk factors.

If you know your blood pressure level and its relationship to health and disease, you are one step further ahead in preventing not only coronary heart disease but also other common complications of hypertension such as stroke and kidney disease.

8. Your Cigarette Smoking Status

In 1979 the Surgeon General's Report on Smoking and Health summarized over 30,000 studies that implicated cigarette smoking as a significant cause of early death and disability in the United States. Indeed, about 10 percent of all hospital admissions in our country can be attributed to cigarette smoking. In addition to the relation between cigarette smoking and coronary heart disease, other health problems related to cigarette smoking include various cancers (especially of the lung, mouth, throat and larynx, and bladder) and several lung diseases (such as emphysema and chronic or long-standing bronchitis). In addition, smoking can also complicate pregnancy and produce infants whose weight at birth is lower than normal.

Smoking cigarettes is associated with excessive coronary heart disease risk even when other risk factors such as high blood cholesterol and hypertension are absent. When combined with other cardiovascular risk factors, cigarette smoking multiplies your risk. If you smoke cigarettes, your HDL cholesterol will be lower than that of a nonsmoker. It is imperative that you stop smoking if your program to decrease your risk of coronary heart disease is to be successful.

The more cigarettes you smoke, the greater your risk of coronary heart disease. This "dose-response" relationship is determined by the number of years you have smoked, the number of cigarettes you smoke per day, and the amount of tar, nicotine, and carbon monoxide contained in the cigarettes. If you have switched from cigarettes to a pipe or cigars but still inhale, you are also at increased risk.

In addition to the strong association between cigarette smoking and fatal and nonfatal heart attacks, workers from the Framingham Heart Study showed that *those who continue to smoke after their first heart attack had an increased rate of death when they suffered their second heart attack.* If you have had a coronary artery bypass operation and you continue to smoke more than a pack a day, you have three times as great a risk of developing atherosclerosis in your bypass graft as a person who doesn't smoke.

The final report of the Pooling Project Research Group, published in 1978, showed that middle-aged men who had stopped smoking had an incidence of coronary heart disease only slightly greater than those who had never smoked. Those who smoked over one pack a day had over three times as many heart attacks as those who had never smoked. Thus, *if you stop smoking, your risk of coronary heart disease decreases with time and eventually approaches that of those who never smoked.*

In addition, if you smoke cigarettes, you increase your chance of developing hardening of the arteries or atherosclerosis in the blood vessels of your legs. You may have heard this condition referred to as "poor circulation." Doctors call it "peripheral vascular disease."

In the Oslo Heart Study, men with high blood cholesterol levels had a significant decrease in their rate of coronary heart disease when they changed to a diet low in total fat, saturated fat, and cholesterol and stopped smoking cigarettes. There is absolutely no question that these two lifestyle changes complement each other, and that making them will be of significant benefit for you. If you follow the diet found in Chapter 11 but do not stop smoking cigarettes, or alternatively if you stop smoking cigarettes without changing an excessive dietary intake of total fat, saturated fat, and cholesterol, you will not achieve an optimal decrease in your risk of coronary heart disease. You can't do anything about your family history, but smoking and diet are both in your power to change.

9. Your Weight

What is a "normal" weight? The answer is not simple. For example, what one society considers normal another society may consider too fat. The concept of "ideal" weight is easier to handle, the ideal weight being the weight most conducive to good health and long life. The well-known body weight tables of the Metropolitan Life Insurance Company were developed with this idea in mind. These tables, however, have several drawbacks. One is that they predominantly reflect statistics from an upper-middle-class white group. Another is that they do not take age into account, thus implying the doubtful proposition that a weight deemed ideal at age 21 is also ideal at 45 and 65.

To help you determine whether your weight is in the desirable range for a person of your height, I have used here the classification of J. S. Garrow as put forward by Dr. F. Xavier Pi-Sunyer in the book *Modern Nutrition in Health and Disease.*

First weigh yourself without clothing and measure your height without shoes. Now go to Figure 5-2. Using your height in inches and your weight in pounds, you can place yourself in one of four categories: desirable weight (0), mild obesity (I), moderate obesity (II), marked obesity (III). There is also a fifth category, less than desirable weight for height, but not many of us fall into that group.

Figure 5-2 also has scales for weight in kilograms (kg) and height in meters (m) because Garrow's classification is based on the Body Mass Index (BMI) originally proposed by a French doctor named Quetelet in 1871; the French then as now used the metric system. The Quetelet BMI, which you encountered earlier in Figures 4-3 and 4-4, is simply the weight (in kilograms) divided by the height (in meters) squared (kg/m^2). Using the Quetelet BMI, Garrow proposed the following classification for both males and females:

Grade	Quetelet BMI
III (marked obesity)	Over 40
II (moderate obesity)	30–40
I (mild obesity)	25–29.9
0 (desirable weight)	20–24.9

Garrow's desirable range corresponds nicely with the lowest mortality range in life insurance tables. Mortality begins to increase at a BMI above 25. The greatest risks occur in those with Grade II or III obesity.

The ranges of this classification are broad enough to work pretty

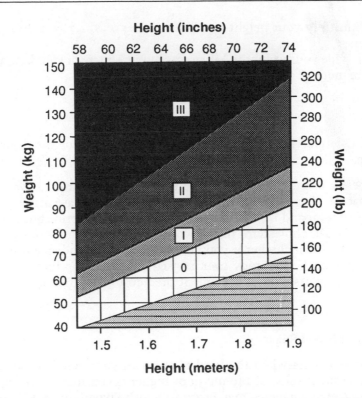

Fig. 5-2. Use of height and weight to determine whether you are in the desirable range (0), mildly obese (I), moderately obese (II), or markedly obese (III). From J. S. Garrow, *Treat Obesity Seriously* (Edinburgh: Churchill-Livingstone, 1981), p. 3; modified from the version in M. E. Shils and V. R. Young, eds., *Modern Nutrition in Health and Disease* (Philadelphia: Lea and Febiger, 1988) with permission from Churchill-Livingstone.

well for both sexes and all ages. The major weakness of the Quetelet BMI is that very muscular people such as professional football players and weight lifters may be classified as obese when they are not.

If you wish to calculate your own Quetelet BMI, the calculation is simple enough:

1. Determine your weight in pounds and divide by 2.2 to convert to kilograms. For example, if you weigh 160 pounds, divide 160 by 2.2, giving 72.7 kilograms.

2. Measure your height in inches, multiply by 2.5 to convert to centimeters, and divide by 100 to get your height in meters. Thus if you are five feet eight inches tall, multiply 68 inches by 2.5, giving 170 centimeters; then divide 170 by 100, giving 1.7 meters.

3. Multiply your height by itself. Thus 1.7 × 1.7 = 2.89 square meters.

4. Divide your weight in kilograms by the square of your height (in square meters):

$$\frac{72.7 \text{ kilograms}}{2.89 \text{ square meters}} = 25.2$$

Your Quetelet BMI is 25.2, a little above the top of the desirable range.

Obesity is a significant adverse promoter of other cardiovascular risk factors. For example, if you are obese, you will have higher blood levels of total and LDL cholesterol and total triglyceride but a lower level of HDL cholesterol than if you are not obese. Your blood pressure will also be higher if you are obese. Finally, evidence from the Framingham Heart Study over 26 years of follow-up indicates that obesity is by itself an independent predictor of the risk of coronary heart disease.

10. Your Blood Sugar

Diabetes occurs when the level of sugar in your blood is too high. A blood sugar value of 140 mg/dl or higher is commonly used to define diabetes. Diabetes may begin in youth (Type I) or in adulthood (Type II).

Juvenile onset or Type I diabetes is ordinarily manifested in the first or second decade of life. It is caused by the production of antibodies against the patient's own tissues, particularly the islet cells in the pancreas, those cells responsible for the body's production of insulin.

Adult onset or Type II diabetes characteristically occurs in the fourth, fifth, and sixth decades of life. Type II diabetes has a genetic component: people from certain families produce insulin less efficiently, particularly as they get older. If a person is obese, the fat cells in the body respond less well to insulin, causing the pancreas to produce a greater amount of insulin to compensate for this inefficiency. Eventually, the pancreas cannot produce enough insulin to overcome the resistance in the fat cells and the blood sugar rises.

Diabetes is associated with atherosclerosis in the coronary arteries, the aorta, and the arteries of the brain and kidney. If you have diabetes, you are at increased risk of coronary heart disease, stroke, kidney disease, and peripheral vascular disease. Even after all the other risk factors are considered, total cardiovascular disease is about twice as common in diabetics as in nondiabetics.

In addition to abnormalities in the processing of blood sugar in diabetes, many diabetic patients also have abnormalities in their blood lipids, notably a high blood triglyceride level. If you have diabetes, you should work with your doctor to control your condition. It will be important for you to maintain normal levels of blood sugar over a 24-hour period of time, reduce to ideal body weight, and control any blood lipid problem you may have. The Action Plan diet in Chapter 11 will also be an important part of controlling your blood lipid levels.

11. Your Stress Level

When people are asked to rank the leading causes of heart disease, stress almost always ranks first, yet there is little research to support this ranking. Since stress cannot be measured directly like blood cholesterol, blood pressure, and the number of cigarettes a person smokes in a day, it is difficult to demonstrate a relationship between heart disease and stress.

Research on stress and heart disease at one time focused on so-called Type A versus Type B behavior patterns. Type A people are competitive, impatient, always pressed for time, doing many things at the same time, and motivated by achievement. Type B people are more relaxed and tend to take things in stride. Some early studies indicated that the Type A pattern was associated with coronary heart disease, but more recent studies have failed to confirm this relationship. Experts now generally consider the whole notion of Type A behavior unhelpful.

More recently this type of research has changed focus, and some newer ideas about stress are being examined. A tendency to react to various situations with anger or frustration has proved to be easier to measure than Type A behavior, and has shown a relationship to coronary heart disease in initial studies. Similarly, people whose heart rates and blood pressure increase a great deal when they are exposed to a frustrating situation may also be more likely to develop heart disease. Both of these approaches to stress now appear more fruitful than the Type A behavior approach.

In summary, current studies now suggest that people who anger easily or have a low tolerance for frustration may be more likely to develop coronary heart disease. Those who are more "reactive"— that is, have a greater change in their heart rate and blood pressure—

may also be more likely to develop coronary heart disease, especially if they are exposed to situations where this occurs frequently. What we do not know is how to alter these reactions to stress, or even whether altering them would in fact lower a person's chance of getting coronary heart disease.

Much more research is needed before we have answers to many of our questions about stress and heart disease. However, it seems a matter of common sense to keep your stress levels low by making time for pleasurable leisure-time activities and trying to minimize frustrations and angry situations. As part of this approach, a good exercise program can help a lot.

12. Your Physical Activity

Recently, there has been a trend in this country toward increased physical activity, particularly of the aerobic variety, for example, running, jogging, walking briskly, swimming, and cycling. Regular aerobic activity produces better cardiovascular conditioning, can increase your level of HDL cholesterol, and decreases body weight. It improves your sense of well-being and your energy level. Regular exercise is also a great reliever of stress. In Chapter 15 the relation between exercise and decreased risk of coronary heart disease is reviewed for you, and you will learn about the beneficial effects of exercise on your blood cholesterol and lipoprotein levels.

Yet physical activity and exercise are not the only answer, or even the main answer, if you wish to reduce your risk of coronary heart disease. Before the writer Jim Fixx took up marathon running, he had smoked two packs of cigarettes a day for twenty years and was as much as 60 pounds overweight. Putting these factors together, Fixx was particularly at risk of coronary heart disease for a number of years. At about the age of 35, he stopped smoking, followed a good low-fat diet, took off weight, and exercised. Why then did he die suddenly? Is vigorous aerobic exercise detrimental, or even dangerous, in middle-aged adults? *It can be.*

If you modify a number of your risk factors for cardiovascular disease, such as diet, blood pressure, and smoking, are you "safe" from coronary heart disease? Not entirely. Jim Fixx made all these changes, but apparently ignored a warning sign of coronary heart disease, namely angina pectoris.

Perhaps the greatest lesson that Jim Fixx can teach you is the importance of evaluating your family history of coronary heart disease and making sure that you do not have a genetic problem involving your blood cholesterol and lipoproteins. His father had his first heart attack at 36, and died of his second at 43. Yes, a person with a family history of coronary heart disease should have all his or her risk factors evaluated, but in particular he or she should be thoroughly evaluated for the presence of any underlying inherited disorders of cholesterol and lipoprotein processing. Those who have inherited abnormalities in their blood lipid or lipoprotein profiles should be rigorously treated, often with medication, and followed. "Genes and cholesterol" is the subject of Part II of this book (Chapters 7, 8, and 9).

Summary

If you were already knowledgeable about each of the twelve risk factors discussed in this chapter, you get an "A" for awareness. If you are generally unaware of your levels of blood lipids and lipoproteins, of your family history, of your blood pressure, and of dietary factors associated with the development of cardiovascular disease, you need to act now. If you do, you will be well on your way toward decreasing your risk of coronary heart disease, and toward a longer and healthier life.

CHAPTER 6

Are Your Children at Risk?

$\mathbf{T}$here may be coronary heart disease or blood cholesterol problems in your family. Does this mean that your children are likely to develop premature coronary heart disease in their thirties, forties, or fifties? How can you tell whether your child is likely to have a blood cholesterol problem or some other lipid problem? When and how often should the blood cholesterol level be checked? What can be done about these problems if they exist? Should all children modify the cholesterol and saturated fat content of their diet? At what age should such a diet be started?

This chapter will help you to answer these questions. You will learn that blood cholesterol measurements obtained in childhood predict adult levels. In fact, many of the harbingers of risk factors for coronary heart disease are present in childhood.

Is this so surprising? Obesity acquired in childhood is highly predictive of obesity in adult life. Smoking habits are often established by the beginning of high school. The preference of Americans for foods rich in cholesterol and saturated fats and high in calories is determined early in life, when children are strongly influenced by the family's eating habits. These acquired lifestyle selections adversely influence the blood lipid and lipoprotein levels, producing higher concentrations of cholesterol, LDL cholesterol, and triglyceride but lower levels of HDL cholesterol.

When such a poor lifestyle is combined with a genetic predisposition to a blood cholesterol problem or to premature coronary heart disease, the process of atherosclerosis is likely to accelerate, further increasing the risk that such a child will develop premature coronary heart disease as an adult.

By understanding what precursors of adult disease can be detected in children, what can be done to modify or prevent them, and what kind of nutritious, modified-fat diet works best for children, you will be in a position to start your child on the way to a healthier life. This chapter will help you achieve this goal.

Does Coronary Atherosclerosis Begin in Childhood?

When autopsies were performed on young soldiers killed in action, a surprising degree of coronary atherosclerosis was found. For example, in soldiers killed in the Vietnam and Korean conflicts, 45 percent and 77 percent, respectively, of the coronary arteries had atherosclerosis, which varied in extent from deposits blocking over 50 percent of an artery, to smaller raised deposits called fibrous plaques, to flat deposits called fatty streaks.

How early did coronary atherosclerosis in these young soldiers begin? In the International Atherosclerosis Project, Drs. Strong and McGill studied the relation between fatty streaks and fibrous plaques in the coronary arteries from 4,737 autopsies of people of both sexes, aged 10–39 years, from six different geographic and racial groups. There were several major findings:

1. Fatty streaks in the coronary arteries were rare before ten years of age, quite frequent between ten and twenty years, and nearly always present after twenty.

2. Some fatty streaks became fibrous plaques, a transition that began in some cases before the age of twenty and increased quite rapidly in the following two decades.

3. Countries such as the United States, where fatty streaking was more extensive in childhood, had more advanced lesions of coronary atherosclerosis in middle age.

These observations suggest that atherosclerosis begins in childhood and slowly progresses through the adult years, leading to significant blockages in the arteries that result in heart attack, sudden death, angina pectoris, stroke, or poor circulation.

Are the blood cholesterol levels of American children generally too high? Dr. Knuiman and associates studied the cholesterol levels of 560 seven- and eight-year-old boys in sixteen countries from various regions of the world with different rates of coronary heart disease. The highest cholesterol levels were found in boys from the European countries and the United States, where coronary heart disease is most common (Figure 6-1). The average blood cholesterol lev-

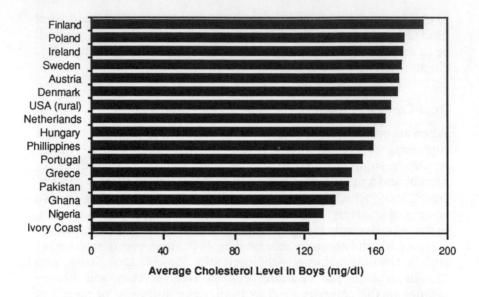

Fig. 6-1. Blood cholesterol values of boys aged seven and eight from sixteen countries.
Data from J. T. Knuiman et al. in *Atherosclerosis* 36 (1980): 529–537.

els were the lowest in three West African countries and in Pakistan, where coronary heart disease is rare. In countries such as Greece, Portugal, and Hungary, modern-day societies where coronary heart disease is less of a problem, the children had levels of total cholesterol in between the United States and the African countries.

The proportion of the total cholesterol carried on HDL was about one-third and was similar in the various groups of boys except for the Asians, whose HDL proportion was lower. About two-thirds of the blood cholesterol was therefore carried on LDL, meaning that LDL accounted for most of the difference in cholesterol levels in the boys from the various countries. VLDL and triglyceride levels were not measured.

Great differences were found among the sixteen countries in their children's fat intake. A very high association ($r = 0.91$) was found between the average blood cholesterol levels and the per capita availability of animal products. Those countries that consumed a greater percentage of calories as fat had children whose average cholesterol levels were higher.

Blood Cholesterol Levels in Children

In 1985, Drs. Newman, Berenson, and colleagues published an important paper in the *New England Journal of Medicine* from the Bogalusa Heart Study. Total blood cholesterol, LDL cholesterol, HDL cholesterol, and VLDL cholesterol levels, blood pressure, and weight were measured in a large population of children in Bogalusa, Louisiana, over fifteen years. During this time about three dozen children and young adults died accidentally, and the amount of atherosclerosis in their aortas and coronary arteries was assessed at autopsy.

Those who had had higher levels of blood cholesterol and LDL cholesterol years before had more extensive fatty streaks in their aortas. For the coronary arteries, the level of VLDL cholesterol at entry into the study was the strongest predictor of cholesterol deposits. An opposite relationship was found for HDL cholesterol. Children who had lower amounts of HDL cholesterol relative to their blood cholesterol had greater amounts of cholesterol deposited in their arteries as fatty streaks.

This study provided the first evidence that the levels of blood cholesterol, LDL cholesterol, HDL cholesterol, and VLDL cholesterol in children can *predict the degree of early atherosclerosis in the blood vessels of young persons.*

In Chapter 5 you learned about the importance of a positive family history of premature coronary heart disease. Does such a positive family history have implications for your child? *Definitely.* If any of a child's parents or grandparents developed coronary heart disease before the age of 55, there is about a one in three chance that the child has a blood cholesterol problem. If either you or your spouse has a high level of blood cholesterol or LDL cholesterol, your children are two to five times more likely to have a high blood cholesterol level than children whose parents have normal cholesterol levels. The genetic nature of some of these blood lipid problems in children is reviewed for you in more detail in Chapters 7, 8, and 9.

If your child has a cholesterol problem, should you be checked? By all means, as the case of John Covington (pp. 17–18) makes clear. His sons David and Michael had been referred to me by their pediatrician, and were found to have high (266 mg/dl) and borderline high (177 mg/dl) cholesterol levels, respectively. In such cases I make it a practice to screen the parents, and I almost always find that one or both also have some blood lipid abnormality. Usually the parents have not had their blood lipids measured before, nor do they know whether anyone in their family developed coronary heart disease. Sometimes they are generally aware of a problem but have not been adequately treated.

John, as we have seen, proved to have a total blood cholesterol of 313 mg/dl, an LDL cholesterol of 252 mg/dl, and an HDL cholesterol of only 30 mg/dl; he had an LDL/HDL ratio of over 8 and a triglyceride of 203 mg/dl. As also noted, he had a family history of coronary heart disease, and an angiogram showed a total blockage in the right coronary artery and less severe atherosclerosis in many of the other coronary arteries. The family had already made some diet changes, but other diet changes and drug treatment were necessary. John is better now: his LDL/HDL ratio is down to 3.0. But if it were not for his sons' doctor, he would be in imminent danger of a heart attack.

Can your child have too little of the good HDL cholesterol? Apparently so. Dr. Charles Glueck and colleagues, and other researchers, have found low levels of HDL cholesterol in children from families with a pronounced history of coronary heart disease. If your child is found to have a low level of HDL cholesterol and early coronary heart disease runs in your family, your child may well have inherited a genetic trait that will place him or her at increased risk for coronary heart disease as an adult. Examples of such families are discussed in Chapter 9.

Should Your Child's Blood Cholesterol Be Checked?

When is it a good idea to check a child for high blood cholesterol? Two general approaches have been taken: (1) check only those children with a positive family history of premature coronary heart disease; (2) check all children.

The advantage of the first approach is that the yield is high: about one in three such children will have a high blood cholesterol level. The disadvantage is that many parents are too young to have developed premature coronary heart disease, and many more are unaware of heart problems in their own parents or other relatives. For these reasons, this approach will miss many children with blood cholesterol problems.

The advantage of the second approach, general screening, is that potentially all children with problems can be detected. The disadvantage is that general screening would single out a very large number of children for repeat testing, dietary counseling, and follow-ups. Not only might this large number exceed the capacity of doctors to handle, but it would almost certainly include some inaccurate measurements leading to incorrect diagnoses, putting a further burden on all concerned.

Finally, if a nutritious, balanced, modified-fat diet is recommended for all healthy children over two years of age, why check children's blood cholesterol at all? The answer is: so that those children who need closer attention to their diet and closer follow-up as they grow older can be identified. I propose the following approach for you and your children, one that goes beyond the positive family history approach but stops short of general screening:

1. First, the blood cholesterol level of both parents should be tested. If either one's level is above 200 mg/dl, it should be rechecked by your doctor and further testing for LDL cholesterol, HDL cholesterol, and triglyceride levels should be performed.

2. Second, if either parent has any one of the following findings, your child should have his or her blood cholesterol level checked.

(a) Parent's LDL cholesterol is borderline high (130 to 159 mg/dl) or high (above 160 mg/dl).

(b) Parent's HDL cholesterol is low (less than 35 mg/dl).

(c) Parent's triglyceride level is high (above 250 mg/dl).

3. Third, if either parent or another blood relative has developed coronary heart disease before age 55, your child should have *more than a blood cholesterol test;* blood cholesterol, LDL cholesterol, HDL cholesterol, and triglyceride should all be measured.

At what age should your child's blood cholesterol be checked? Any time after the age of two years. At birth a child's blood cholesterol level is only about 70 mg/dl, and over 50 percent of the total cholesterol is carried on HDL. In the first few weeks of life, LDL increases significantly, to the point where about two-thirds of a child's total blood cholesterol is carried on LDL and only about one-third on HDL. When your child reaches the age of two, his or her blood cholesterol and LDL cholesterol reach levels that will be essentially maintained until the late teens.

Your child's physician can either do a blood cholesterol test in the office or send the blood out to a hospital laboratory; it is not necessary for your child to fast for this test. Many doctors simply prick the child's finger, take a few drops of blood, and use a desk-top analyzer to get a reading. This method is not as accurate as a laboratory analysis. It may be sufficient when the resulting cholesterol level is reassuringly low, but if it is borderline or high the results must be followed up with more detailed testing.

Table 6-1. How to Interpret Total, LDL, and HDL
Cholesterol Levels in Children and Adolescents
Aged 2–19

Category	Level (mg/dl)
Blood cholesterol	
High	200 or higher
Borderline high	170–199
Desirable	Below 170
LDL cholesterol	
High	130 or higher
Borderline high	110–129
Desirable	Below 110
HDL cholesterol	
Low	Below 35
Borderline low	35–45
Desirable	Above 45

How Can You Know if Your Child's Blood Cholesterol Level Is Too High?

Table 6-1 shows desirable, borderline, and high levels of total, LDL, and HDL cholesterol for children and adolescents. Assuming that the results of an initial fingerstick or other test for total blood cholesterol are known, your child should have further blood tests if the following circumstances apply:

1. The total cholesterol is 170 mg/dl or higher. There is a one in four chance that your child will have a value of 170 mg/dl or higher on the initial test. (This is not surprising, since American children in general have blood cholesterol levels that are too high.)

2. The total cholesterol is less than 170 mg/dl, but there is a family history of premature coronary heart disease.

The second test can be ordered by your child's doctor. For this test it will be necessary for your child to fast (nothing to eat or drink except water or clear juice for twelve hours). This time the blood will be drawn from a vein in your child's arm by the doctor or an assistant, and will be used to measure the following: (1) total cholesterol; (2) triglyceride; (3) HDL cholesterol. From these three measures, you and your child's doctor can estimate the LDL cholesterol level by using the formula from Chapter 5:

$$LDL = \text{Total cholesterol} - [HDL + \tfrac{1}{5}\,\text{Triglyceride}]$$

This test is important because it will enable you and your doctor to make the following assessments:

1. If the blood cholesterol is above 170 mg/dl, is it that high because of a high LDL cholesterol (which is bad) or because of a high HDL cholesterol (which is good)?

2. If the blood cholesterol is above 170 mg/dl, is the triglyceride level also too high? If so, your child may have a blood lipid problem called "familial combined hyperlipidemia" (FCH), which is reviewed for you in Chapter 8.

3. If the blood cholesterol is below 170 mg/dl, a high triglyceride may still be present. A high triglyceride level is often accompanied by a low HDL cholesterol level. Such children may have a triglyceride problem (Chapter 8) or an HDL problem (Chapter 9).

4. If the blood cholesterol is below 170 mg/dl and the triglyceride level is also normal, is the HDL cholesterol level too low? This situation can occur in children from families with premature coronary heart disease (Chapter 9).

5. Finally, if both the blood cholesterol and LDL cholesterol levels are very high (above 230 mg/dl and 160 mg/dl, respectively)—only one child in a hundred has such elevated levels—your child's doctor will need to consider the possibility that your child has inherited the genetic cholesterol problem called familial hypercholesterolemia (see Chapter 7).

Occasionally, high levels of blood cholesterol and LDL cholesterol are due to other health problems, such as low thyroid activity, diabetes, and disease of the liver or kidney. Your child's doctor will know how to check out these possible explanations for high blood cholesterol levels.

About one in twenty children has a high LDL cholesterol (130 mg/dl or higher), and about one in four is borderline high (between 110 and 129 mg/dl). Sometimes the LDL cholesterol level is high despite a borderline high or even desirable blood cholesterol level. This situation particularly occurs when a high LDL cholesterol is accompanied by a low HDL cholesterol.

The figures for children with undesirable or borderline HDL cholesterol levels are the same as for LDL levels: about one in twenty is low (under 35 mg/dl) and one in four is borderline low (between 35 and 45 mg/dl). After adolescence, HDL cholesterol levels are generally higher in females than in males (see also the Cholesterol and Triglyceride Tables at the back of the book).

Table 6-2. How to Interpret Blood Triglyceride Level
in Children and Adolescents (mg/dl)

Category	Age	
	Under 10	10–19
High	100 or higher	130 or higher
Borderline high	75–99	90–129
Desirable	Below 75	Below 90

From 10 to 15 percent of children with high blood cholesterol levels have them for the best possible reason: a high HDL cholesterol level. Thus when a two-year-old girl was sent to me because of a history of a high cholesterol, I found that her cholesterol level, 199 mg/dl, was primarily due to an excellent HDL cholesterol level of 94 mg/dl (the average for her age is 55). In fact, her HDL cholesterol was even higher than her LDL cholesterol, which was entirely normal at 87 mg/dl.

The triglyceride level of a child under ten has to be only about 100 mg/dl to fit into the high category (Table 6-2). Once again, about one in twenty children has a value this high, and about one in four is borderline high. As the table shows, the cutpoints for blood triglyceride levels are higher for children over nine years old. After fifteen years of age, males generally have a significantly higher triglyceride level than females, and this difference persists throughout adult life.

If your child has a high triglyceride level, this may be a tipoff that your family has a genetic condition associated with premature coronary heart disease. Such a finding should not be ignored; it should lead you and your doctor to review your family history and decide whether you and your spouse and your other children should be tested. Alternatively, a high triglyceride may also be due to your child's being too heavy, to your daughter's use of oral contraceptives, or to the use of such drugs as Accutane (used for acne) and prednisone. Your doctor can help you to assess these factors.

What if your child's blood cholesterol level is desirable (less than 170 mg/dl) and there is no family history of premature coronary heart disease? In this case, you need only do your best to see that he or she acquires good habits: eating properly, exercising, not smoking. Eating properly means that your child, along with the rest of the family, follows the prudent Action Plan diet found in Chapter 11. I'd also recommend that the blood cholesterol level be checked again in five years.

A further check in adolescence is a good idea. Adolescence is a trying time for both parent and child. Three factors that warrant special attention in the cardiovascular area are:

1. *Smoking.* Adolescents who smoke already have lower levels of HDL cholesterol than those who do not smoke.

2. *Oral contraceptives.* Adolescents on birth control pills have higher levels of blood cholesterol, LDL cholesterol, and triglyceride but lower levels of HDL cholesterol than those who are not. Young women with a positive family history of premature coronary heart disease should obtain a lipid profile prior to starting oral contraceptives. If your daughter's profile is abnormal, it will usually be worsened by the use of oral contraceptives; and this is clearly something to be discussed with her doctor.

3. *Exercise.* Adolescents who are physically fit generally have lower levels of blood cholesterol, LDL cholesterol, and triglyceride but higher levels of HDL cholesterol than those who are less fit. Their blood pressure will be lower as well. This is a time of life when exercise habits can be formed for a lifetime.

Relationship Between Cholesterol Levels in Childhood and Adulthood

If your child's level of blood cholesterol is too high, will he or she become an adult with a high level of blood cholesterol and thus at increased risk of coronary heart disease? Twenty-five percent of adult Americans fall into this category.

In an impressive study in Muscatine, Iowa, Dr. Ronald Lauer and associates examined the relationship between childhood and adult cholesterol levels. They initially tested 2,446 subjects at ages eight to eighteen and later retested them as young adults at ages 20–25 or 26–30. The following results were obtained:

1. The initial childhood blood cholesterol level was the major predictor of the adulthood cholesterol level.

2. Of children with blood cholesterol levels initially found to be "high" (greater than the 90th percentile) on a single measurement, 43 percent were found to be "high" (greater than the 90th percentile) at ages 20 to 30 years; 62 percent had levels greater than the 75th percentile, and 81 percent had levels greater than the 50th percentile.

3. There was little risk of finding high adult levels (above the 90th percentile) when childhood levels were less than the 50th percentile.

4. Blood cholesterol levels in childhood were also a predictor of

Table 6-3. Changes in Blood Cholesterol
Level in Childhood and Adulthood (mg/dl)

Age group	Lower level	Average level	Higher level
	Below		Above
5–14	143	158	171
25–29	154	176	199
40–44	179	204	229
50–54	189	211	237

Source: Lipid Research Clinics Population Studies.
  Note: A lower level is defined as a value in the lowest quartile (below the 25th percentile); a higher level as a value in the highest quartile (above the 75th percentile).

adult LDL cholesterol levels and the ratio of LDL cholesterol to HDL cholesterol, but not of adult HDL cholesterol levels.

5. LDL cholesterol and HDL cholesterol levels and the ratio of LDL cholesterol to HDL cholesterol were adversely affected by a number of acquired lifestyles or conditions, including obesity, smoking, and the use of oral contraceptives.

6. A family history of coronary heart disease was an important correlate of elevated blood cholesterol levels in both children and young adults, *indicating further that inherited factors play an important role in the control of blood cholesterol levels, even in children.*

In summary, the evidence for tracking of the blood cholesterol level is strong. A child's blood cholesterol level may not perfectly predict his or her blood cholesterol level as an adult, but a child with a blood cholesterol level above 170 mg/dl is much more likely as an adult to have a level above 240 mg/dl (Table 6-3), which is well outside the desirable range and indicative of a higher risk of coronary heart disease.

A child in the high range who adopts a diet lower in cholesterol and saturated fat will have lower blood cholesterol and LDL cholesterol levels throughout childhood, and very probably a lower blood cholesterol level as an adult as well. Children in the low range, as the table shows, are less likely to develop borderline high or high blood cholesterol levels as adults. However, a "heart-healthy" lifestyle makes sense for both groups, including a nutritious modified-low-fat diet, the avoidance of obesity and cigarette smoking, and good habits of exercise.

Will your child's HDL cholesterol level persist into adult life?

Probably, though more research on this point is needed. As we have seen, average HDL levels are about 55 mg/dl for both boys and girls. In the second decade of life, this average falls to about 45 mg/dl for boys but remains unchanged for girls; and these second-decade averages persist into adulthood, where they probably explain, at least in part, the much higher incidence of coronary heart disease in men.

Averages are one thing, individuals another. In a large study in the Princeton, Ohio, School District, about two-thirds of the children with low HDL cholesterol levels had low or borderline low HDL levels when they were retested five years later. The available evidence suggests that a low HDL level as a child does predict a lower HDL cholesterol level later in life, and that children with low HDL levels seem destined to become adults at higher risk of coronary heart disease.

What about your child's triglyceride level? Does it predict his predisposition as an adult to coronary heart disease? Here again we need more information than we have. Based on our current understanding, the importance of triglyceride levels in children is primarily confined to children born in families where there is a history of premature coronary heart disease. In these children, a high blood triglyceride level is presumptive evidence of a faulty gene predisposing them to coronary heart disease as adults.

Obesity in Children

At least 10 percent of American children aged five to fourteen weigh far too much for their height. These obese children are generally less physically fit than leaner children; they also have higher blood levels of cholesterol, LDL cholesterol, and triglyceride but lower levels of HDL cholesterol than leaner children, and higher blood pressure levels. Moreover, studies show that obese children are likely to become obese adults. You can help your child avoid becoming a high-risk candidate for coronary heart disease by seeing that he or she stays fit and lean.

How can you tell if your child is obese? Usually you can tell just by looking. If you are not sure, measure the child's height and weight; have your child's doctor check the measurements and assess whether he or she is too heavy. Often such an assessment is made in terms of percentiles. Thus children whose height is in the 50th percentile (average) but whose weight is in the 90th percentile are clearly far too heavy.

Weight reduction in children can be tricky because unlike adults children are still growing taller. Too much restriction in calories can temporarily decrease the velocity of growth. My advice is to have an obese child engage in aerobic exercise for at least 30 minutes four times a week. A reasonable goal is to maintain current weight; as the child grows taller, he or she will "thin out." If moderate exercise and restrictions on especially fattening foods like candy bars, pizzas, and desserts don't do the job, a program of weight control for your child should be undertaken under a doctor's supervision.

Can Diet Affect Your Child's Cholesterol Levels?

If your child is less than two years old, no change should be made in the fat content of his or her diet unless such a change is recommended by the child's physician.

In a 1972 study of 484 adolescent males with an average age of fifteen years (range twelve to eighteen years) at St. Paul's School in Concord, New Hampshire, Ford and co-workers substituted low-cholesterol, low-saturated-fat foods for the high-cholesterol, high-saturated-fat foods ordinarily eaten by American children. The nutritionists found out what the boys had been eating by recording their food intake over five or seven days. The differences between the two diets are summarized for you in Figure 6-2.

Their total fat intake decreased from 39 to 33 percent of total calories, and saturated fat from 15 to 10 percent of calories. Polyunsaturated fat increased from 3 to 10 percent of total calories, giving an equal proportion of saturated and polyunsaturated fat (P/S ratio of 1.0). Their cholesterol intake decreased by 44 percent, down to 300 mg/day.

Did this low-fat diet contain enough protein? Definitely. The total daily protein intake in the low-fat diet was estimated at 111 grams, nearly double what the National Academy of Sciences recommends as a minimum for boys this age and actually a little more than the boys' previous diet contained.

The percent of calories from carbohydrates increased from 48 to 53 percent. Since carbohydrates replaced some of the calories lost from saturated fat, the decreased fat intake did not compromise the number of calories needed for growth; as Figure 6-2 shows, the boys continued to eat over 3,000 calories per day.

All these changes in the diet are similar to those you can make by putting your child on the Step One Action Plan diet in Chapter 11. This diet is similar to that recommended for all healthy American children over two years old both by the American Heart Association

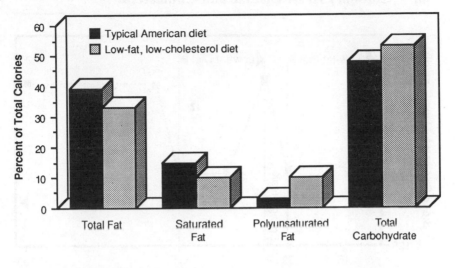

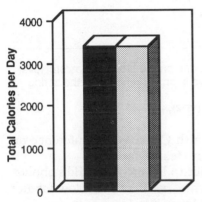

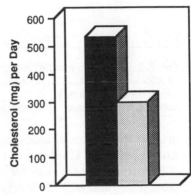

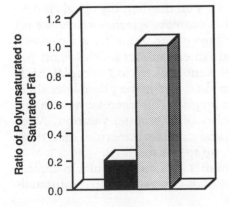

Fig. 6-2. Some nutrient differences between a typical American diet and a low-fat, low-cholesterol diet. Data from C. H. Ford et al. in *Preventive Medicine* 1 (1972): 426–445.

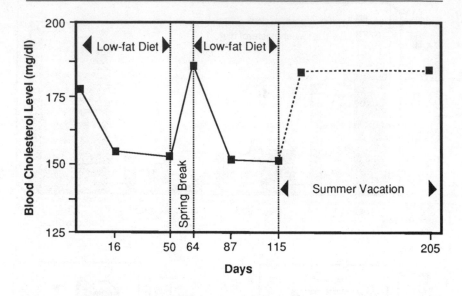

Fig. 6-3. Effect of a low-fat, low-cholesterol diet on the blood cholesterol level of adolescent boys. (The figure for 129 days is an inference from the spring break measurements.)
Data from C. H. Ford et al. in *Preventive Medicine* 1 (1972): 426–445.

and by the National Institutes of Health Consensus Conference on Lowering Blood Cholesterol to Prevent Heart Disease.

How long does it take for such a diet to lower your child's cholesterol level, and will the level stay down? The effect of the low-fat diet reviewed in Figure 6-2 is summarized for you in Figure 6-3.

Before the boys began the diet, their average blood cholesterol level was 178 mg/dl. After only sixteen days on the diet, the blood cholesterol level fell about 15 percent. This decrease was maintained for up to 50 days, after which time the boys went home for a two-week spring break. After eating a typical American diet for this short period, their average cholesterol level went back up to 186 mg/dl. Back at school they resumed the low-fat diet; and just 23 days later their cholesterol level was down to 152 mg/dl. This decrease was maintained up to the time they left school for summer vacation. After three months of summer vacation and a regular American diet, their average blood cholesterol was back up to 183 mg/dl.

Clearly a low-fat, low-cholesterol diet gets quick results in adolescents. So does a return to a typical high-cholesterol, high-saturated-fat diet!

Let's take an example of an all too common American child. Holly Collins, a twelve-year-old girl, was found by her pediatrician to have a blood cholesterol level of 241 mg/dl and proved to have a dismaying family history. Her mother's father had had a stroke and a heart attack. Her father's mother had had an elevated blood cholesterol level and had died from coronary heart disease in her early sixties. To top it off, her father's father had had early coronary heart disease. Although she looked healthy and had a perfectly normal physical exam, she was somewhat overweight (119 pounds) for her height (about 5'2").

I found that her diet was very high in fat with plenty of cheese, potato chips, pizza, and ice cream; she also ate a lot of candy and used many spoonfuls of sugar in her iced tea. I put her on an Action Plan diet that included some reduction in total calories. Here are her lipid profiles before the diet, after two months on the diet, and after six months on the diet:

Lipid profile	Average before diet	After two months	After six months
Cholesterol	228	168	158
LDL cholesterol	158	113	97
HDL cholesterol	43	40	49
LDL/HDL ratio	3.8	2.8	2.0
Triglyceride	134	75	61

After two months on the diet and a weight reduction of about nine pounds, her blood cholesterol, LDL cholesterol, and triglyceride levels fell significantly. Her HDL cholesterol was still borderline low, but her ratio of LDL cholesterol to HDL cholesterol had improved. Six months later, she had lost another ten pounds and her blood lipid profile was excellent.

As a result of losing about twenty pounds, her weight dropped from the 90th percentile to the 50th. She gained an inch of height as well, putting her between the 50th and 75th percentiles in that respect. As so often happens, a sensible diet improved her appearance as well as her health.

Suppose your doctor has found that your child has a high LDL cholesterol, but the good HDL cholesterol is also high. What should you do? It depends. Here is one example where the child required closer attention. Lori Alleva was sent to our clinic by her pediatrician at the age of eleven because a high blood cholesterol level was found during routine screening in the office. I found her blood cholesterol high, the LDL cholesterol borderline high, but the HDL cholesterol also high. Because of the borderline high LDL cholesterol and a very positive family history of premature coronary heart disease (her father had died at 44 of a heart attack), she was put on the Action Plan diet (Chapter 11). When she returned two months later, all her worrisome values had improved and her excellent level of HDL cholesterol persisted. Here are her lipid profiles before and after the diet:

Lipid profile	Before diet	After diet
Cholesterol	204	177
LDL cholesterol	116	94
HDL cholesterol	73	72
LDL/HDL ratio	1.6	1.3
Triglyceride	77	57

Is a Diet Low in Cholesterol and Saturated Fat Safe for Your Child?

An important question, and one often heard, is whether changing a child's current diet might adversely affect his or her growth and development. To answer this question, let's start from the beginning.

During its first nine months in the womb, your child's blood cholesterol level is quite low, reaching its lowest point of about 30 mg/dl in the second trimester. This low cholesterol level occurs, in part, because the fetus is not eating any cholesterol or saturated fat and the blood lipoproteins in the mother are too large to cross over the placenta from the mother's blood into the baby's. During this period of very active growth and development, the fetus utilizes sugar (i.e., glucose) and fatty acids from the mother's blood for its energy needs. The fetus relies almost entirely on the synthesis of its own cholesterol; it has been estimated that only 20 percent of the cholesterol in the fetus comes from the mother. It also appears that the fetus preferentially utilizes glucose to make cholesterol in its brain. The sugar and fatty acids from the mother can also be used by the fetus to make other lipids such as triglyceride and phospholipid. The brain and other organs develop normally.

The commercial formulas fed to babies, such as SMA® and Enfamil®, contain little cholesterol; an infant drinking one quart of formula per day would ingest only about 20 mg of cholesterol per day. (For comparison, a similar amount of human milk would provide 100–200 mg of dietary cholesterol per day.) Commercial formulas have been fed to infants in this country for 30 to 40 years without ill effects. An entire generation of Americans given commercial formulas has grown into healthy adults.

Dr. Samuel Foman and co-workers in a hospital research unit in Iowa intensively studied 469 infants aged from eight to 112 days, then examined them again when they were eight years old. Those who had been breast-fed were compared with those who had been bottle-fed, and no differences in height, weight, or blood cholesterol levels were found between the two groups.

Drs. Friedman and Goldberg, two pediatricians in Scottsdale, Arizona, found that a group of 51 children who from birth were prescribed a diet low in cholesterol and saturated fat, with a ratio of polyunsaturated to saturated fat of 1.0, had the same average height, weight, and head size at three years of age as a control group of 420 children fed a "regular American diet" from birth. But those on the low-fat, low-cholesterol diet had a lower average blood cholesterol level (145 mg/dl) than those eating a regular diet (154 mg/dl).

"Experiments of nature" are often informative in helping you to assess whether a certain treatment or diet is effective and safe. Seventeen-year-olds in Mediterranean countries such as Greece, Turkey, and Israel get only about 30 to 35 percent of their calories from total fat, as compared to an American percentage of about 40; and their diet has a ratio of polyunsaturated to saturated fat of about 0.85, as compared to an American P/S ratio of 0.43. The consumption of such a relatively low-total-fat, low-saturated-fat diet by Mediterranean youngsters is not associated with changes in growth in the preceding adolescent period. For example, for the ages 15–19 the average heights of Israeli males (69.1 inches) and females (64.9 inches) are very similar to those of American males (69.4 inches) and females (65.1 inches). Plainly, then, eating less total fat and less saturated fat does not stunt one's growth.

The National Heart, Lung, and Blood Institute is currently sponsoring a major study called the Dietary Intervention Study in Children (DISC), whose purpose is to determine the safety, effectiveness, and feasibility of a diet for children that is relatively low in total fat, saturated fat, and cholesterol and moderately enriched in polyunsaturated fats and complex carbohydrates. The subjects are nine- and ten-year-old boys and eight- and nine-year-old girls, identified through cholesterol screening programs, who have borderline high to high blood cholesterol levels (170 to 230 mg/dl). Children with markedly high levels (above 230 mg/dl) are not eligible for the study.

Half the children are assigned to a special dietary intervention group, and half are assigned to a "usual care group" and referred back to their doctors. The diet for the special intervention group is designed to reduce their total and saturated fat intake to 28 percent and 8 percent of calories, respectively, and their dietary cholesterol intake to less than 150 mg/day.

Medical centers in six areas of the country are participating in the study: Baltimore; Newark, New Jersey; Chicago; New Orleans; Portland, Oregon; and Iowa City, Iowa. The children will be monitored very carefully as they progress through adolescence, a period of very rapid growth and development. This study is looking carefully at their growth and their school performance as well as their general health. The intent is to determine once and for all whether this low-fat, low-cholesterol diet contains enough minerals, vitamins, and protein for optimum results on all three counts.

Do you need to wait until the results of the DISC study are in before you change your child's eating habits? No. The Step One diet reviewed for you in Chapter 11 is a nutritious, well-balanced diet containing adequate calories, protein, minerals, and vitamins to promote growth. This low-fat, low-cholesterol diet is not as restricted as the one being used in the DISC study, but it is similar to the diet recommended by the American Heart Association and the NIH Consensus Conference on Lowering Blood Cholesterol to Prevent Heart Disease.

Is there any rational basis for thinking that a low-cholesterol, low-fat diet may adversely affect the growth and development of your child? I have found none. Some argue that the "brain needs cholesterol to grow." But by the age of two years about 90 percent of the growth of the brain is completed. Further, the brain and other organs and tissues in your child can manufacture as much cholesterol as is needed. The cells in your child's body are not dependent on the cholesterol in the diet to meet their need for cholesterol. *Cholesterol is not an essential dietary nutrient.*

The cells of the body can also manufacture their own saturated fats. One fatty acid that the body cannot make is linolenic acid, a polyunsaturated fat found in vegetable oils. The body can use linolenic acid to make other unsaturated fats.

What about protein? The Action Plan diet proposed in Chapter 11 *contains as much protein* as a high-fat, high-cholesterol diet. Lean meat, fish, and poultry provide sufficient protein from animal sources, with the remainder of the protein derived from vegetable sources. All the essential amino acids are present.

Of more concern is whether your child will get enough calories. Fat contains nine calories per gram and is an important source of calories for growing children. Your child needs calories, may even need fat, to grow, but not the kind of fat that will raise his or her cholesterol level. What kind, then? As we have seen, the thing to do is replace saturated fat, so far as possible, with unsaturated fat. For example, snacks are an important source of calories for your child. Snacks need not be doughnuts or ice cream or pizza; they can be fresh fruits, yogurt, or popcorn made with a vegetable oil margarine. Low-fat milk, low-fat cheeses, and low-fat desserts are preferable to high-fat alternatives and still provide needed calories. (The meal plans in Chapter 14 list a variety of acceptable snacks; see also the Recipes at the back of the book, especially the breads and the desserts.)

But can't a child eat too much polyunsaturated fat? Yes, that is possible. But if your child follows the Step One Action Plan diet in Chapter 11, he or she will get the proper balance between saturated fats, monounsaturated fats, and polyunsaturated fats, as well as a sufficient number of calories to grow and thrive.

Remember that if your child is a very active adolescent male, he will require as many as 3,000 calories a day to meet his energy needs. In the study of Ford and associates summarized in Figure 6-2, adolescent boys on a diet low in total fat and saturated fat put away over 3,000 calories a day.

Will your child get enough minerals such as iron, calcium, and zinc from a low-fat, low-cholesterol diet? Almost certainly yes, says Dr. Joanne Dwyer, a nutritionist at Tufts University, although care must be taken with children between two and five years old to see that their mineral intake is sufficient. For older children the increase in fresh fruits and vegetables in the low-fat diet usually provides *more* minerals and vitamins than a diet full of fast food, potato chips, candy bars, pies, cakes, and ice cream. Lean red meats provide ample zinc and iron, and low-fat or skim milk and low-fat cheeses provide calcium.

Does a low-fat diet increase a child's risk of cancer? Quite the reverse. It has been found that a high total fat intake (*not* a low total fat intake) is associated with increased risk of cancers, for example, those of the breast and colon. In fact, the Committee on Diet, Nutrition, and Cancer of the National Academy of Sciences has recommended that Americans reduce their total fat intake to about 30 percent of calories, and increase their consumption of fiber and complex carbohydrates.

Table 6-4. Dietary Guidelines for Healthy Children Older Than Two Years

Recommendations	Practical implications
1. Nutritionally adequate diet consisting of a variety of foods.	1. Satisfies Recommended Dietary Allowances of the Food and Nutrition Board of the National Research Council for protein, vitamins, and minerals.
2. Calorie intake based on growth rate and activity level.	2. Have your child's doctor measure his or her height and weight at regular intervals.
3. Decrease total fat intake to approximately 30% of calories, and saturated fat to about 10% of calories.	3. Emphasize consumption of lean meat, fish, and poultry and decreased use of fatty meats: substitute vitamin D–fortified skim milk or low-fat milk for whole milk; broil or bake rather than fry foods.
4. Increase use of polyunsaturated fats (to no more than 10% of calories).	4. Use vegetable oil margarine rather than butter; use vegetable oils such as safflower, olive, canola, or corn oil rather than lard for cooking or salads.
5. Lower cholesterol intake to less than 300 milligrams a day.	5. Limit eggs to 2 or 3 a week; also items 3 and 4 above.
6. Maintain protein at about 15% of calories.	6. Protein of both animal and vegetable sources will provide all essential amino acids.
7. Increase percentage of calories from carbohydrates to 50–55%, derived primarily from complex carbohydrates, and emphasize an increase in fiber.	7. Increase consumption of whole grain or enriched breads and whole grain, enriched, and fortified cereals; increase consumption of fruits and vegetables; decrease consumption of desserts, snack foods, candy bars, sweets.

General Guidelines for Your Child's Diet

Some general dietary guidelines for healthy children over two years of age are provided for you in Table 6-4. These guidelines are consistent with those of the American Heart Association, the Senate Select Committee on Nutrition and Human Needs, and the recent National Institutes of Health Consensus Development Conference on Lowering Cholesterol to Prevent Heart Disease.

The 1982–83 Committee on Nutrition of the American Academy of Pediatrics stopped short of these recommendations, stating only that "current dietary trends in the United States toward a decreased consumption of saturated fats, cholesterol, and salt, and an increased intake of polyunsaturated fats, should be followed with moderation. Diets that avoid extremes are safe for children." More recent statements by this committee in 1986 and 1989 did not differ substantially from this earlier statement.

When Should Medication Be Used for a Child with a Cholesterol Problem?

In general, if a child's levels of blood cholesterol and LDL cholesterol after three to six months on a low-saturated-fat, low-cholesterol diet remain above 230 mg/dl and 160 mg/dl, respectively, consideration should be given to using a bile acid resin drug—particularly if the child has a positive family history of coronary heart disease or a low HDL cholesterol level. Medications to lower the blood triglyceride level are not used for children.

For example, Kevin Fura, a 15-year-old boy, had a blood cholesterol level of 236 mg/dl even after three months on a diet low in cholesterol and saturated fat. His LDL cholesterol was very high at 190 mg/dl, and his HDL cholesterol was very low at 21 mg/dl; his LDL/HDL ratio was above 9. His mother's father had died at the age of 35 from a heart attack. Putting all these things together, I did not hesitate to add treatment with cholestyramine, starting with one scoop twice a day.

Upon follow-up, his values had improved noticeably: blood cholesterol 210 mg/dl; LDL cholesterol 157 mg/dl; HDL cholesterol 42 mg/dl; LDL/HDL ratio 3.7; and triglyceride 42 mg/dl. The next step will be to increase his cholestyramine to one scoop three times a day to lower his LDL cholesterol to below 130 mg/dl.

Is the Cholesterol Hypothesis "Proven" in Children?

Not definitely. A definitive proof of the cholesterol hypothesis in childhood would require two major long-term studies. One would take the blood cholesterol levels of a large number of children and see how well those levels predict which children develop coronary heart disease as adults. The other would be a diet intervention study in which children were divided into two groups, one on a low-cholesterol, low-saturated-fat diet, the other on a regular American diet high in cholesterol and saturated fat. The rate of heart attacks in the two groups would be compared when they became middle-aged adults.

Since such studies would require tens of thousands of children and a follow-up of 40–50 years, it is unlikely that they will be carried out. In the circumstances, the best advice I have is that you and your child's doctor consider the available evidence reviewed here and decide whether a diet lower in total fat, saturated fat, and cholesterol makes sense for your child. I need scarcely add that to me the evidence points overwhelmingly in that direction.

Summary

1. A child with a high blood cholesterol level is likely to become an adult with a high blood cholesterol level.

2. Your child should have a blood cholesterol test if either parent has a blood cholesterol level above 200 mg/dl, an HDL cholesterol level less than 35 mg/dl, or a triglyceride level above 250 mg/dl, or if there is a positive family history of premature coronary heart disease.

3. This blood test can be obtained any time after the age of two. Your child does not have to be fasting for a blood cholesterol test.

4. If your child has a blood cholesterol level above 170 mg/dl, *or a* positive family history of premature coronary heart disease, a follow-up blood test for cholesterol, HDL cholesterol, LDL cholesterol, and triglyceride should be obtained. Your child will need to fast twelve hours for this test.

5. A diet low in total fat, saturated fat, and cholesterol will lower your child's levels of blood cholesterol and LDL cholesterol.

6. Since nutritional habits are formed in childhood, it makes sense to start dietary changes early in life (after the age of two) even if your child's cholesterol level is normal.

7. There is no evidence to indicate that a low-fat, low-cholesterol diet is harmful or inconsistent with the principles of good nutrition. Such a diet is already consumed by children in a number of modern-day societies, for example, in Mediterranean countries, where the incidence of coronary heart disease is one-half that in the United States.

8. The avoidance of obesity and cigarette smoking, attention to weight control, and good habits of exercise acquired in childhood are important to the prevention of coronary heart disease later in life.

Genes and Cholesterol

PART TWO

Genes and Cholesterol

CHAPTER 7

Do You Have Familial Hypercholesterolemia?

I saw him from across the hospital room at the clinical center at the National Institutes of Health. He was sitting on the edge of the bed. Large orange bumps the size of baseballs protruded underneath the skin of both his elbows. His face was thin, and orange wartlike growths were present under his eyes and over both eyelids. This was my first exposure to a patient with the most severe kind of cholesterol problem.

At that time, in 1967, it was not understood why such patients had blood cholesterol levels of almost 1,000 mg/dl and LDL cholesterol levels above 900 mg/dl. It was clear, however, that such profound increases led to severe atherosclerosis and coronary heart disease, often before the age of twenty. Both parents of such children have less extreme but significantly elevated levels of total and LDL cholesterol in their blood. Now, two decades later, the reason why this happens is well understood. Indeed, this kind of cholesterol problem—called familial hypercholesterolemia, or simply FH—is the best understood of the inherited lipid disorders.

FH is one of the most common inherited diseases in humans, affecting about one in every 500 people. (In comparison, such well-known inherited diseases as phenylketonuria [PKU] and cystic fibrosis occur in about one in 10,000 and one in 2,000 humans, respectively.) About half the men and half the women who have the less extreme form of FH develop coronary heart disease by the average ages of 40 and 50 years, respectively. By 65 years of age, almost 90 percent of such patients will develop coronary heart disease.

By understanding the basic problem that causes FH, you will gain insight into how and why a low-cholesterol, low-saturated-fat diet lowers your blood total and LDL cholesterol. Thus, even if you and your family do *not* have FH, you can improve your understanding of

Table 7-1. Average Blood Cholesterol, LDL, HDL, and Triglyceride Levels in FH Heterozygous Children and Adults and in FH Homozygotes (mg/dl)

Category	Total cholesterol	LDL cholesterol	HDL cholesterol	Triglyceride
Children				
Normal children	158	94	53	60
FH heterozygotes	299	242	43	82
FH homozygotes	678	625	34	101
Adults				
Normal adults	194	123	53	83
FH heterozygotes	367	298	44	148

Source: Data from P. O. Kwiterovich et al. in *Journal of Clinical Investigation* 53 (1974): 1237–1249. Data for normal children from *Lipid Research Clinics Population Studies Data Book*, Volume I, *The Prevalence Study* (NIH Publication No. 80-1527, July 1980).

how your diet and even certain drugs work for you. You will learn that the diet in Chapter 11, and certain drugs reviewed in Chapter 16, are effective for very specific reasons.

How Is FH Inherited?

Genes for a specific trait are inherited in pairs: that is, we receive one gene for the trait from our mother and another gene for the trait from our father. If you have the less extreme form of FH, you have inherited a normal gene from one parent and an abnormal gene for FH from the other. The abnormal FH gene will be expressed by rather high blood total and LDL cholesterol levels (Table 7-1). Such elevations often lead to accelerated depositing of cholesterol in the coronary arteries, and in tendons of the hands, elbows, knees, and heel cords. FH is an example of a *dominant genetic trait:* that is, you need only one abnormal gene to have the condition.

It is unlike most dominant genetic traits, however, in that those unfortunate children who inherit two abnormal genes for FH (one from each parent) survive. Such children have blood total and LDL cholesterol levels that are astronomically high (Table 7-1). They usually develop coronary heart disease before the age of twenty and cholesterol deposits under the skin.

Those with the less extreme form of FH, i.e., those who carry one abnormal gene for FH and one normal gene, are called FH heterozygotes (het'-aro-ZYE-goats), from the Greek *heteros*, meaning the other (of two), and *zygosis*, meaning joining. There is a 50:50 chance that an FH heterozygote will pass the abnormal FH gene to his or her child. When the spouse of an FH heterozygote is normal, half of their children, on average, will also be FH heterozygotes. Those with the most extreme form of FH carry two abnormal genes for FH and are known as FH homozygotes (ho'-ma-ZYE-goats), from the Greek *homos*, the same, and *zygosis*, joining.

When both parents are FH heterozygotes, their children have one chance in four of inheriting both FH genes, one chance in two of inheriting one FH gene and one normal gene, and one chance in four of inheriting two normal genes.

In Figure 7-1 you see the pedigree of Tracey's family, which was assembled when it was found that Tracey (T.B.) was an FH homozygote. Her blood cholesterol and LDL cholesterol levels were both sky-high. The levels of her parents, Steven and Kathy Bechard (S.B. and K.B.), were both high also, but not as high as Tracey's. Both passed on their abnormal FH gene to Tracey; neither passed it on to Tracey's brother Steven.

Looking back a generation, you can see that Tracey's father received one abnormal FH gene from his mother, Jessie (J.B.), and one normal gene from his father, Ernest (E.B.), and that Tracey's mother received an abnormal gene from her father, John Slater (J.S.), and a normal gene from her mother.

Why are the total and LDL cholesterol levels so high in FH? Thanks to the pioneering work of Drs. Michael Brown and Joseph Goldstein at the Southwestern University School of Medicine in Dallas, we know the answer to this question. This outstanding work, for which these two medical scientists received the Nobel Prize for Medicine and Physiology in 1985, led to the discovery of a protein called the LDL receptor.

The LDL receptor is responsible for removing LDL from your blood at a normal rate. FH heterozygotes have only half the normal number of LDL receptors and thus remove LDL at only half the normal rate, leading to about a twofold increase in their blood total and LDL cholesterol levels. FH homozygotes have few if any functioning LDL receptors and remove LDL at only about one-fourth the normal rate, leading to at least a fourfold increase in their total and LDL cholesterol levels (Table 7-1).

How Do You Know Whether You Have FH?

How can you determine whether your high blood cholesterol indicates that you have inherited FH? There are several important clues and one test that can help you and your doctor answer this question.

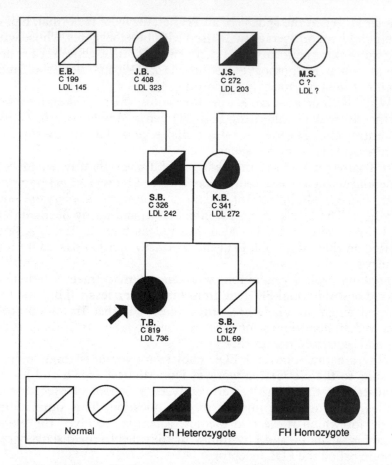

Fig. 7-1. Pedigree of a family with familial hypercholesterolemia: squares are males, circles females. Blood levels of cholesterol (C) and LDL cholesterol are provided where known. The arrow points to Tracey, whose plight brought the family to medical attention.

Cholesterol deposits under the skin. One important clue is the presence of cholesterol deposits under the skin. These deposits, called "xanthomas," usually start in the patient's twenties or thirties. They often occur as round, hard bumps under the skin and within the tendons in areas of increased friction, notably the tendons in the hand (particularly over the knuckles), the tendons over the elbow, and the Achilles tendon in the heels. The finding of both xanthomas and elevated blood total and LDL cholesterol levels argues that FH is present until proven otherwise.

Cholesterol deposits can also occur in the clear outer layer of the eye, called the cornea; such deposits have the shape of a half moon and are called "corneal arcus." Or there can be flat or slightly raised orange-colored deposits under the eyes or on the eyelids, called "xanthelasmas."

Very high blood total and LDL cholesterol levels. The higher your blood cholesterol level, the less likely it is due to diet alone and the more likely it is due to FH. The average total and LDL cholesterol levels for FH heterozygotes and FH homozygotes are summarized for you in Table 7-1. These values are in the top 1 percent of the general population. If you have similar total and LDL cholesterol elevations, there is about a one in five chance that you have FH. Another clue, though not always a very helpful one, is that the triglyceride level is usually normal in patients with FH.

Relatives with FH. Half of the relatives of patients with FH are also affected. If one of your parents, about half your brothers and sisters, and half your children have elevated blood total and LDL cholesterol levels but normal triglyceride levels, it is very likely that FH is present in your family. On average, the other half of your first-degree relatives will have normal lipid levels. On the other hand, if both cholesterol and triglyceride problems are present in your family, another inherited lipid problem, called "familial combined hyperlipidemia," may be present. This disorder is reviewed for you in the next chapter.

Coronary heart disease. If very premature coronary heart disease is present in your family, afflicting men in their thirties and women in their forties, there is a strong possibility that the FH gene is present in the family.

Test for activity of LDL receptors. A definite diagnosis of FH requires a clear demonstration that the number of LDL receptors working in your cells is decreased. To perform this test, cells must be grown from a small piece of skin taken from your arm using a procedure called a biopsy. From the piece of skin, cells, called fibroblasts, are grown in cell culture in a research laboratory. Alternatively, cells from the blood, called lymphocytes, may be obtained and grown in cell culture.

The cells are grown under special conditions that stimulate the number of LDL receptors on their surface. LDL cholesterol is removed from blood of a donor and made radioactive, and the actual binding of LDL to the LDL receptors on the cells is measured. Unfortunately, this test to determine whether a normal number of LDL receptors is working is expensive, time-consuming, and laborious, and is not routinely available to practicing physicians or their patients.

If your doctor suspects that you carry the FH gene but cannot be certain, this does not alter the principles underlying your treatment. Treatment starts with a good low-cholesterol, low-saturated-fat diet as outlined in Chapters 11 and 14. If necessary, drugs can be used to increase the number of LDL receptors that are working on the surface of your cells.

If you have other risk factors such as cigarette smoking, obesity, and hypertension, they will need to be modified because they will increase even further your already higher risk of premature coronary heart disease. Like all other patients with a significant blood cholesterol problem, those with FH need to be treated and followed for a lifetime.

What Happens if Your Child Has FH?

In normal infants the average blood cholesterol and LDL cholesterol levels are quite low at birth (Table 7-2). In FH heterozygotes, by contrast, the LDL cholesterol level is about twice as high at birth in blood taken from the umbilical cord. For example, Andrea was sampled at birth because her mother, Donna, has tendon xanthomas and a high blood cholesterol level. Andrea's grandfather had died at 49 of coronary heart disease. At birth, her total cholesterol was high at 97 mg/dl, her LDL cholesterol elevated at 47 mg/dl, and her HDL cholesterol low at 28 mg/dl. She was an obvious candidate for a diagnosis of FH.

If it is known that either you or your spouse has FH, the finding of a high LDL cholesterol in the cord blood indicates that your baby has inherited the abnormal gene for FH. If you suspect as prospective parents that either of you has FH, a cord blood sample can be obtained by your doctor.

As we have seen, blood cholesterol and LDL cholesterol levels increase rapidly in the first few weeks of life, reaching a plateau by the age of one to two years. It is important that a follow-up blood sample be obtained at this time; indeed, if you and your doctor suspect that your child is at risk of FH, a blood test can be obtained any time after the child's first birthday. At the age of two, Andrea's blood cholesterol was 276 mg/dl and her LDL cholesterol was 222 mg/dl. Despite a good low-cholesterol, low-saturated-fat diet, by the time she was

Table 7-2. Average Blood Cholesterol, LDL, HDL, and Triglyceride Levels at Birth in FH Heterozygotes and Normal Infants (mg/dl)

Category	Total cholesterol	LDL cholesterol	HDL cholesterol	Triglyceride
Normal infants	74	31	37	37
FH heterozygotes	100	62	30	47

Source: Data from P. O. Kwiterovich et al. in *Lancet* 1 (1973): 118–122.

nine her blood cholesterol had increased to over 300 mg/dl, and I started treatment with a bile acid resin. On just one packet per day, her blood cholesterol fell to 253 mg/dl. Recently I increased her dose to two packets per day, and I now expect that we will be able to lower her cholesterol to below 200 mg/dl.

A child with only one abnormal FH gene does not develop coronary heart disease before the age of twenty. Because the early stages of atherosclerosis in such FH heterozygous children are more accelerated than in normal children, the early diagnosis and treatment of FH is important. The goal of treatment is to lower the total and LDL cholesterol levels early in life so as to retard the development of more advanced atherosclerosis and decrease the risk of heart attacks and death in middle age.

In contrast to the child with one abnormal FH gene, the unfortunate FH homozygous child, who has two, will almost surely develop significant atherosclerosis before the age of twenty; and about one in four of these children will die before that age from cholesterol deposits in the coronary arteries or the aortic heart valve. Treatment of such children is more difficult; indeed, heroic measures are necessary, as discussed below.

How common are children who are FH homozygotes? Since the frequency of FH heterozygotes is one in 500, the chance that two persons with one abnormal FH gene will marry is only one in 250,000. Further, when two FH heterozygotes have a child, there is only one chance in four that the child will receive an abnormal FH gene from both the father and the mother. By multiplying 1/250,000 × 1/4, you can see that *FH homozygous children are very rare, indeed, one in a million.* In the United States, where there are approximately 240 million people, only about 240 children are FH homozygotes.

Children who are FH homozygotes often develop cholesterol deposits under their skin by the time they are five years old, and occasionally these deposits are present even at birth. These very early cholesterol deposits are often flat, orange, raised, "coin-like" deposits that differ from those that begin later in the tendons.

Kathy Baker had an "orange bump" removed from her right index finger at the age of six, but her blood cholesterol level was not measured by her doctor. When I first saw her, at the age of nine, she had many cholesterol deposits, some between her fingers, others as fairly large bumps over her elbows and in the tendons of her toes and both Achilles tendons. Her total cholesterol was 849 mg/dl, LDL cholesterol 818 mg/dl, HDL cholesterol 25 mg/dl, and triglyceride 110 mg/dl.

This condition can be detected as a result of chest pain or heart attack. Jerome Jennison, or "J.J.," a nine-year-old boy from India with a cholesterol of about 1,000 mg/dl, complained to me that he woke out of a deep sleep and felt like "two walls were closing in on me, one against my chest, the other against my back." Coronary angiography showed that all three of his major coronary arteries were blocked, and he underwent triple-vessel coronary artery bypass surgery several days later. Today he is doing better, but I am concerned about blockages developing in his bypasses and whether he will be able to lead a full and productive life.

Tracey and Barbara, on the other hand, developed severe cholesterol deposits in their aortic valves. The deposits appeared to be getting smaller after a special operation called a portacaval shunt; but under stress these deposits limited the flow of blood to the coronary arteries, and the girls' hearts could not pump normally. They died from heart failure and shock.

Because of the severity of the FH homozygous condition, such patients are usually treated at a major medical center accustomed to dealing with this condition. Treatment with a low-cholesterol, low-saturated-fat diet and LDL-lowering drugs normally increases the number of a patient's LDL receptors, but FH homozygous children have few if any LDL receptors to begin with and often do not respond to such treatment.

More heroic measures are often necessary. In one procedure, called plasmapheresis, the cholesterol-enriched blood is removed from the FH homozygote and replaced with a plasma substitute that contains no cholesterol. Plasmapheresis often lowers the total cholesterol to less than 200 mg/dl on the day the procedure is performed. However, it rises very rapidly over the next week or so, and the procedure must therefore be repeated approximately every two weeks.

Certain major operations have also been performed in an attempt to lower the blood cholesterol in these children. Two of these operations, called partial ileal bypass and portacaval shunt, have not proved successful and I will not discuss them further. Another, which *has* been successful, is liver transplantation. The liver is a key organ involved in both the production of cholesterol by the body and the removal of cholesterol (on LDL) from the blood. Since the FH homozygote has no LDL receptors on the surface of the liver cells, LDL cannot be taken up from the blood into the liver for disposal. When the liver from an FH homozygous child is replaced by a normal liver from a donor, the patient obtains LDL receptors, and these can then remove LDL from the blood and dispose of it properly.

In one case, that of a six-year-old FH homozygous child studied by a group of medical scientists in Dallas and Pittsburgh, liver transplantation lowered the total cholesterol in the blood from 1,000 to 300 mg/dl. The cholesterol did not return entirely to the normal range because some LDL is processed by cells other than the liver, and these other cells still do not function normally in this child.

The LDL Receptor and Its Role in Controlling Cholesterol

Even if neither you nor anyone in your family has or seems likely to have FH, the elegant work in this area of Drs. Brown and Goldstein and other researchers is worth a few minutes of your time. Their findings offer new and precious insights into the normal processing of cholesterol by your body, and into the way treatment with diet and certain medications works.

What causes a particular human disease? One way this question can be answered is to grow cells from patients affected with the disease and study them in cell culture. By altering the nutrients in the liquid (medium) that bathes the cells, the cells can be grown under different conditions. The processing of cholesterol and lipoproteins such as LDL can also be studied in cultured cells. One cell type that has been grown in culture for this purpose is the fibroblast, a large spindle-shaped cell grown from a piece of human skin removed by biopsy.

Brown, Goldstein, and their co-workers first used cultured fibroblasts from FH homozygotes, FH heterozygotes, and unrelated normal persons. They found that the cells from normal persons manufactured their own cholesterol, the amount varying with the amount of cholesterol in the culture medium outside the cells. When enough cholesterol was present outside the cells, the cells used this cholesterol and manufactured very little of their own. Conversely, when no cholesterol was present outside the cells, the amount made by the cells increased at least 50-fold. In contrast, cultured fibroblasts from FH homozygotes manufactured the maximum amount of cholesterol even when there was ample cholesterol in the medium outside the FH cells.

It was next shown that LDL cholesterol (and not HDL cholesterol) was responsible for regulating the synthesis of cholesterol by the cells. The inability of the FH homozygous cells to use LDL cholesterol in the media indicated that the cells were not capable of taking up the LDL particles normally. Subsequent studies demonstrated clearly that the FH homozygous cells were incapable of moving LDL from outside the cell into the cell. Whereas in normal cells the LDL particles were bound to the cell by a specific protein on the cell's surface, little if any of this protein was present in FH homozygous cells and only half the normal amount in FH heterozygous cells. This protein is now called the LDL receptor.

What is the role of the LDL receptor in processing your LDL cholesterol? In normal cells, the binding of LDL to the LDL receptor permits the removal of LDL from the blood (Figure 7-2). Following the uptake of LDL by the cell, the LDL particles are then transported to special cell components (called lysosomes), which break them up into smaller pieces. Some of these smaller pieces are then released from the lysosomes and transported within the cell to various places where this cholesterol is used to decrease the production of cholesterol by the cell itself.

The number of LDL receptors that the cell makes is also decreased, thus preventing further entry of LDL from the medium after a sufficient amount has been received. Most excess cholesterol is prepared for storage in the cell, although some may be used for the assembly of the outer coating or membrane around the cell.

When a medium containing LDL cholesterol is replaced by a medium containing no cholesterol, the production of LDL receptors is no longer suppressed and the number of LDL receptors on the surface of the normal cell increases. In states of cholesterol "starvation," LDL receptor production increases in an effort to get more cholesterol from outside the cell; in states of cholesterol "excess" in the medium, LDL receptor production decreases to prevent too much cholesterol from entering the cell.

To determine the maximum number of functioning LDL receptors, normal cells are grown for 24 or 48 hours in a cholesterol-free medium. A normal cell has about 10,000 functioning LDL receptors on its surface, an FH heterozygous cell about half this number. Thus

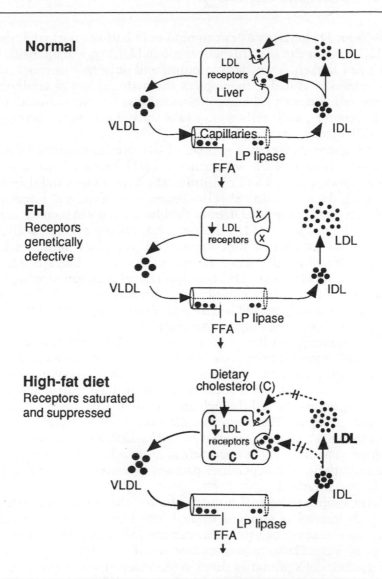

Fig. 7-2. Scheme for the production of cholesterol-rich LDL from triglyceride-rich VLDL and IDL, and the removal of LDL by the LDL receptors in the liver (*top*). In patients with FH, the LDL receptors are genetically defective (*middle*), leading to high LDL levels in the blood. A high-fat diet can saturate and suppress the LDL receptors (*bottom*), and the LDL level will increase as a result.

cells from FH heterozygotes can bind only half the normal amount of LDL to their surface, only half as much LDL is taken up inside the cells and broken down by lysosomes, and only half as much LDL cholesterol is available to suppress the manufacture of cholesterol by the cell. Since an FH homozygous cell has few if any functioning LDL receptors, such cells do not take up and process LDL through the LDL receptor pathway.

Subsequent studies by a number of laboratories examined the actual processing of LDL within normal, FH heterozygous, and FH homozygous patients and confirmed the hypothesis established by the work done on cultured cells. People with a normal number of LDL receptors removed LDL from the blood at a normal rate, and had a normal blood level of LDL cholesterol. FH heterozygotes, with half the normal number of functioning LDL receptors, removed LDL from the blood at half the normal rate and had LDL cholesterol levels twice as high as normal. FH homozygotes, with no functioning LDL receptors (Figure 7-2), removed LDL from their blood at about one-fourth the normal rate and had total cholesterol and LDL cholesterol levels four to six times higher than normal.

If FH homozygotes have no functioning LDL receptors, how is any LDL at all removed from their blood? The answer is important, and the clue to it first came from studies of cultured cells. When LDL is present in very high concentrations in the media of cultured cells, it primarily enters the cell through another route that does *not* involve the LDL receptor. This route is called the "LDL receptor *independent* pathway" to distinguish it from the LDL receptor *dependent* pathway. The independent pathway is more active at very high LDL concentrations; the dependent pathway operates primarily at low LDL concentrations.

Later studies in normal humans showed that about two-thirds of LDL cholesterol is removed through the LDL receptor dependent pathway and about one-third through the LDL receptor independent pathway. Since FH homozygotes have few if any LDL receptors, LDL enters their cells primarily through the independent pathway. In FH heterozygotes, the proportion of LDL removed through the independent pathway is in between that in normal persons and FH homozygotes.

The Importance of the LDL Receptor

As noted, the entry of cholesterol into the cell on LDL through the LDL receptor dependent pathway is "regulated," providing a balance between the amount of cholesterol manufactured by the cell and the amount of cholesterol taken in from outside the cell. The LDL receptor helps the body to keep up with the constant demand to remove LDL cholesterol from the blood. In its twenty-hour lifespan, the LDL receptor makes one round trip into and out of the cell every ten minutes, for a total of several hundred trips.

In contrast, LDL that enters the cell through the LDL receptor *independent* pathway does not do so through the LDL receptor. It is not regulated by the LDL receptor or any other balancing mechanism, and will continue to enter unimpeded, facilitating the buildup of cholesterol in the cell. The higher the level of LDL cholesterol in your blood, the greater the amount of LDL that will enter your cells through the LDL receptor independent pathway. By lowering the LDL cholesterol in your blood, you decrease the amount of LDL entering your cells through the LDL receptor independent pathway. Where large amounts of LDL enter by this pathway, as in the FH homozygote and heterozygote, we find the accumulation of cholesterol in xanthomas, and more importantly in the arteries, leading to atherosclerosis and coronary heart disease.

Even if you do not have FH, your LDL receptors are very important. The number of functioning LDL receptors in a normal person can vary up to threefold depending on diet and other factors. *Factors that decrease the number of your LDL receptors will produce an increase in your LDL cholesterol level and increase your risk of atherosclerosis and coronary heart disease.* Factors that increase the number of your LDL receptors will decrease your LDL cholesterol level and decrease your risk of atherosclerosis and coronary heart disease.

Studies by Dr. Daniel Steinberg and colleagues at San Diego, and by others, indicated that about 70 percent of the removal of LDL by LDL receptors occurs in the liver. Other organs also take up LDL; for example, your adrenal gland uses cholesterol from LDL to make cortisone and other adrenal steroids. In summary, most of the cells in the body have LDL receptors; but the majority of LDL that is cleared by LDL receptors occurs in your liver.

Cholesterol in your diet enters your bloodstream from the intestine on lipoprotein particles called chylomicrons. As the triglyceride in the chylomicrons is broken down in your blood, a particle is produced, called a chylomicron remnant, that is enriched in cholesterol. The chylomicron remnant is cleared rapidly by the liver. When this happens, as Drs. Brown and Goldstein showed, the amount of cholesterol in the liver is increased; the action of the LDL receptors in the liver is decreased, and less LDL is then removed from the blood (Figure 7-2); and the production of cholesterol by the liver is decreased.

It follows that the degree to which the LDL cholesterol level increases on a high-cholesterol diet is determined, in part, by how efficiently the production of cholesterol by the liver is suppressed. One person in five does not suppress the production of cholesterol very well, and such people experience a significantly greater increase in LDL cholesterol levels than those with more efficient livers.

Too much saturated fat in your diet will also interact with dietary cholesterol to further decrease the number of LDL receptors in your liver. If you decrease the saturated fat and cholesterol in your diet, the number of LDL receptors in your liver will increase and your blood LDL cholesterol level will fall.

Drugs and the LDL Receptor

Certain cholesterol-lowering drugs, including the bile acid resins and the inhibitors of cholesterol production, have their effect by increasing the number of LDL receptors in the liver (Figure 7-3). These and other drugs are reviewed for you in Chapter 16.

The bile acid resins lower your blood total and LDL cholesterol in the following manner:

1. After bile acids are released from the gall bladder into the intestine, they are normally taken back up by the intestine and delivered to the liver for re-use. But the bile acid resins bind bile acids in the intestine, preventing their reabsorption into the blood and causing their excretion into the stool.

2. The liver normally changes some of its cholesterol into bile acids. When fewer bile acids are returned to the liver, the liver compensates by changing more of its cholesterol into bile acids.

3. The amount of cholesterol in the liver thus decreases, leading to an increased production of LDL receptors. The amount of LDL removed from the blood through the LDL receptors is accordingly increased and the blood level of LDL cholesterol decreases.

Other drugs act on a key enzyme that controls the manufacture of cholesterol. This enzyme, called HMG CoA reductase, facilitates the conversion of a precursor, HMG CoA, to a product called mevalonic acid, which is used by the body to make cholesterol. A drug called lovastatin (Mevacor®) "looks like" HMG CoA. The enzyme is fooled by the resemblance and binds the drug by mistake. As a re-

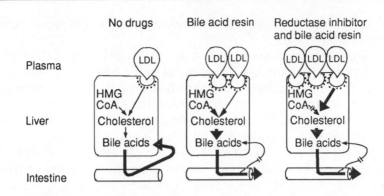

Fig. 7-3. Effect of two LDL-cholesterol-lowering drugs on LDL receptors on the surface of liver cells. One class of drugs, called bile acid resins, binds bile acids in the intestine and prevents their normal return to the liver (*middle*); more cholesterol is used to make bile acids, and LDL receptors are increased in number. Another class of drugs, called HMG CoA reductase inhibitors, blocks the ability of the liver to make cholesterol, further increasing the production of LDL receptors.
Reproduced with permission from M. S. Brown and J. L. Goldstein in *Science* 234 (1986): 44.

sult, less HMG CoA is converted into mevalonic acid and the body's production of cholesterol is decreased. The amount of cholesterol in the liver decreases, leading to an increase in LDL receptors; thanks to the ensuing significant uptake of LDL from the blood into the liver, the level of LDL cholesterol in the blood falls (Figure 7-3).

The effective drug treatment of elevated LDL levels is aimed at increasing the number of LDL receptors and speeding the removal of LDL cholesterol from the blood. A low-cholesterol, low-saturated-fat diet will also increase the number of LDL receptors in your liver and is an important first step in the treatment of a cholesterol problem. Finally, some patients will also require that the synthesis of cholesterol, triglyceride, and lipoproteins in their liver be decreased by drugs to prevent an overproduction of VLDL and the subsequent release of excessive amounts of VLDL into the blood. Since VLDL is changed into LDL in your blood, a decrease in VLDL is often accompanied by a decrease in LDL.

HDL Cholesterol and FH

As Table 7-1 shows, children and adults with FH also have lower than normal HDL levels. The lower HDL cholesterol level is found in both FH heterozygotes and FH homozygotes, and is present even at birth (Table 7-2).

HDL removes cholesterol from cells, and ultimately such cholesterol is delivered to the liver for disposal in the bile or for re-use. Drs. George Steiner, Dan Streja, and I studied several hundred members of a large, fascinating family in Newfoundland with FH. Considering only those members with FH, we found significantly more coronary heart disease in those with an LDL/HDL ratio of 4.0 or higher than in those with an LDL/HDL ratio below 4.0. Clearly patients with FH who also have low HDL levels require even more aggressive treatment.

Summary

1. Familial hypercholesterolemia (FH) is one of the most common inherited diseases in humans, affecting about one in every 500 people.

2. FH is inherited as a dominant genetic trait. Genes for a specific trait are inherited in pairs. If you have inherited a normal gene from one parent and an abnormal gene for FH from the other, you will have high levels of blood total cholesterol and LDL cholesterol; 350 mg/dl and 280 mg/dl, respectively, are average levels in adults with FH. A person with one abnormal FH gene is called an FH heterozygote.

3. FH heterozygotes can be detected at birth and early in childhood by screening the offspring of parents known to have the disorder.

4. A child who has inherited an abnormal gene for FH from both his parents will have blood total and LDL cholesterol levels close to 1,000 mg/dl and 900 mg/dl, respectively. A person with two abnormal FH genes is called an FH homozygote. Only one American in a million has this disorder.

5. One out of two FH heterozygotes will develop coronary heart disease by the age of 40 years in males and 50 years in females. FH homozygotes usually develop coronary heart disease before the age of twenty, and many die before that age.

6. FH heterozygotes often develop cholesterol deposits (xanthomas) in their tendons in adulthood. FH homozygotes usually have visible cholesterol deposits in their skin by the age of five.

7. The basic problem in FH resides in a defect in a protein called the LDL receptor. Normal cells have about 10,000 LDL receptors, FH heterozygotes 5,000 LDL receptors, and FH homozygotes few if any functioning LDL receptors.

8. The LDL receptor is responsible for removing LDL cholesterol from the blood, and for the proper processing of cholesterol after it is inside the cell. A diet high in cholesterol and saturated fat decreases the number of LDL receptors and increases the LDL cholesterol level; a diet low in cholesterol and saturated fat increases the number of LDL receptors, leading to a decrease in the blood LDL cholesterol level.

9. Certain medications, notably the bile acid resins and the inhibitors of cholesterol production (HMG CoA reductase inhibitors), increase the number of LDL receptors, decreasing the level of LDL cholesterol in blood.

10. In persons with FH, a low HDL cholesterol level, or such other risk factors as cigarette smoking and high blood pressure, can increase the risk of coronary heart disease even further.

CHAPTER 8

Do You Have a Triglyceride Problem?

You are probably less familiar with the blood fat triglyceride than you are with cholesterol. Unlike cholesterol, triglyceride has received little attention in the press, or on radio and television. In this chapter you will learn more about triglyceride, where it comes from, how it is processed by your body, and how important it is as a risk factor for coronary heart disease.

What Is Triglyceride?

Triglyceride is a fat that contains three fatty acids, each attached to a backbone provided by glycerol. It is a completely different fat from cholesterol, but like cholesterol it is a normal component of blood and can either come from your diet or be manufactured by your body.

Most of the fat you eat is in the form of triglyceride. After you eat a meal, the triglyceride and cholesterol in your diet are taken up by your intestine and "packaged" into round particles called chylomicrons. The chylomicrons are released into your bloodstream, where their triglyceride is broken down by removing the fatty acids from the glycerol backbone (Figure 8-1). This occurs along the lining of the blood vessels through the action of a protein, an enzyme called lipoprotein lipase, and a helper protein, apoC2. A smaller particle, the chylomicron remnant, is produced, which contains proportionately more cholesterol and less triglyceride than the original chylomicron, and this smaller particle is taken up immediately by the liver.

When you get up in the morning, all the triglyceride from your diet is gone. You are fasting, and the only triglyceride in your blood has been made by your liver. While you slept, your liver packaged its

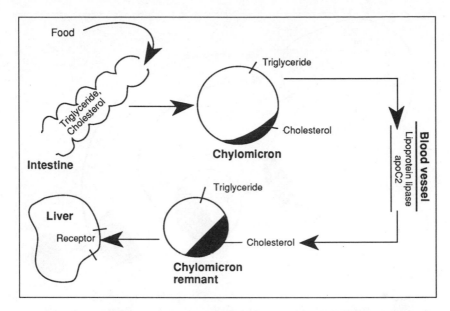

Fig. 8-1. The processing of dietary triglyceride and cholesterol in the blood. After the triglyceride in the chylomicron is broken down by lipoprotein lipase with the help of apoC2, a chylomicron remnant is produced and is then removed by the chylomicron receptor in the liver.

triglyceride into particles called VLDL (very-low-density lipoproteins) and released them into your bloodstream.

As with chylomicrons, the triglyceride inside VLDL is then broken down in the blood, producing a smaller VLDL remnant particle (Figure 8-2). The VLDL remnant may be either taken up by the liver or modified further into IDL (intermediate-density lipoproteins). IDL particles are then at a crossroad; they may be taken up by the liver, or the remaining triglyceride may be further broken down, producing the final product in the process, the cholesterol-rich LDL. The remodeling of lipoproteins at the surface of the liver occurs through the action of an enzyme called hepatic triglyceride lipase.

The fatty acids released from the triglyceride in chylomicrons or VLDL are taken up by either your muscles, where they are used for energy, or your fatty tissue, where they are reincorporated into triglyceride and stored for future use. In between meals, the fatty acids are again released from triglyceride and then transported as "free" fatty acids on albumin from the fatty tissue back to the liver. In the

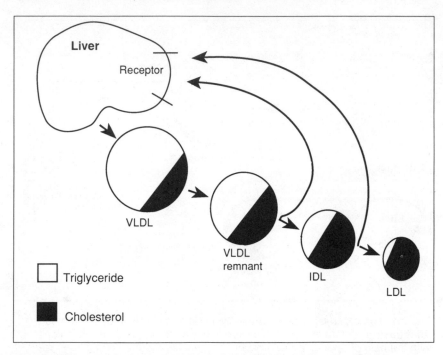

Fig. 8-2. The processing in the blood of triglyceride-rich lipoproteins from the liver and their change into cholesterol-rich LDL. The triglyceride-rich VLDL is produced in the liver and released into the bloodstream, where the triglyceride is broken down, producing a smaller VLDL remnant. The VLDL remnant may be taken up into the liver through the LDL (B,E) receptor, or may be broken down further into IDL. IDL may also be taken up by the same receptor, or may be converted into cholesterol-rich LDL, the final product of this pathway.

liver these fatty acids may be reattached to glycerol, forming triglyceride for VLDL, or they may be broken down into smaller fragments producing energy. One of these fragments can also be used by the liver to make cholesterol.

Will a high triglyceride level increase your risk of coronary heart disease? There is no simple answer to this question. The blood level of triglyceride in humans varies over a wide range. As we have seen, triglyceride levels are generally higher in males than in females, and increase with age. Patients with coronary heart disease often have high, or borderline high, levels of blood triglyceride. However, patients with an elevated blood triglyceride level often have, in addition, higher levels of total cholesterol and lower levels of HDL cholesterol and suffer from obesity, diabetes, and high blood pressure.

Because of the frequent presence of these other risk factors for coronary heart disease, it has been difficult to determine whether a high blood triglyceride level *causes* coronary heart disease, or whether it is simply *associated with* coronary heart disease.

As you will learn in this chapter, it is *the company that triglyceride keeps in the blood* that is important in determining whether an increased triglyceride level places you at increased risk of coronary heart disease.

Measuring and Interpreting Your Triglyceride Level

Your triglyceride level is determined by a blood test that can be ordered by your doctor. The blood must be taken after an overnight fast (nothing to eat or drink but water) for twelve hours. Unlike your cholesterol levels, your blood triglyceride level can be influenced dramatically if you are not fasting because of the presence of chylomicrons. After you eat a meal containing fat, the triglyceride level in your blood gradually increases, reaching its highest level four hours after eating. It then begins to fall. Although most of the triglyceride on chylomicrons from a meal is cleared from the blood after six or seven hours, it takes at least ten hours for it to be cleared completely.

Your blood triglyceride level should be measured after your weight is stable for at least one month. While you are losing weight, your blood triglyceride level will be much lower than it is when your weight is stable. Conversely, if you are gaining weight, your triglyceride level may be higher.

Your blood triglyceride should be determined in any of the following circumstances.

1. Your blood cholesterol level is above 200 mg/dl.

2. You have coronary heart disease.

3. You have a positive family history of premature (before 55 years of age) coronary heart disease.

4. One of your blood relatives is known to have an elevated blood triglyceride.

5. You have diabetes.

6. You have suffered from a condition called pancreatitis, discussed below.

How do you know whether you have a blood triglyceride problem? You can interpret your triglyceride value by referring to Table 8-1, or to the more detailed Table 5-5 in Chapter 5, which takes into ac-

Table 8-1. Simplified Guidelines for
Interpreting Your Blood Triglyceride
Level

Blood triglyceride level (mg/dl)	Interpretation
Above 500	Very high
250–500	High
150–249	Borderline high
Below 150	Desirable

count your age and sex. If your blood triglyceride level is normal, the plasma from your blood will have a clear appearance; no VLDL will be seen. Above 250 mg/dl the plasma will have a cloudy appearance due to the elevated VLDL levels; and above 500 mg/dl the appearance will be milky. When the triglyceride level reaches the thousands, both chylomicrons and VLDL are visible and the blood plasma is "creamy."

If your blood triglyceride is above the desirable level, how can you determine your risk of coronary heart disease? If you are free of coronary heart disease, you can use your levels of HDL cholesterol and LDL cholesterol to assess your risk:

1. The HDL cholesterol level is often low in patients with a high or borderline high level of blood triglyceride. If your HDL cholesterol level is too low (under 35 mg/dl), you should consider this finding as a separate risk factor for coronary heart disease.

2. If your LDL cholesterol is borderline high (130–160 mg/dl) or high (over 160 mg/dl), you are at increased risk of coronary heart disease.

3. If your LDL/HDL ratio is between 4.0 and 5.0 (above average risk) or above 5.0 (high risk), you may be at increased risk even if your LDL cholesterol level is less than 130 mg/dl.

If you already have coronary heart disease and your blood triglyceride level is borderline high or high, you have a blood lipid problem *until proven otherwise.* You should work with your doctor to lower your blood triglyceride level, decrease your blood cholesterol and LDL cholesterol levels, and increase your HDL cholesterol level. You should reduce to ideal body weight, and follow the Action Plan diet reviewed for you in Chapter 11. As you will learn below, you may also require a drug to treat your problem.

Why is a high blood triglyceride level important? A high triglyceride level is important chiefly as a *marker,* an indicator that you may have an underlying problem in the processing of your blood fats and lipoproteins that puts you at increased risk of coronary heart disease.

I first saw John Bistrian when he was 45. He had undergone coronary artery bypass surgery three years earlier, and had recently suffered a stroke. His blood triglyceride level was high at 292 mg/dl, and so was his VLDL cholesterol at 52 mg/dl. His blood cholesterol was only 178 mg/dl, and his LDL cholesterol was normal at 108 mg/dl. However, his "good" HDL was very low at 18 mg/dl, and his LDL/HDL ratio (108/18) was well above 5.0.

He had a history of hypertension, which was successfully treated. He was not a smoker. On a combination of a Step Two diet (Chapter 11) and nicotinic acid (500 mg three times per day), his triglyceride level fell to 166 mg/dl and his HDL cholesterol level rose to 41 mg/dl. His blood cholesterol and LDL cholesterol levels remained much the same at 185 and 111 mg/dl, respectively, but his LDL/HDL ratio, at less than 3.0, was now in the desirable range.

Many times these problems are genetic. Several kinds of genetic triglyceride disorders are discussed below.

Familial Combined Hyperlipidemia (FCH)

Familial combined hyperlipidemia, or FCH, was first described by Drs. Joseph Goldstein, Helmut Schrott, William Hazzard, Edward Bierman, and Arno Motulsky at the University of Washington over fifteen years ago. These researchers studied people who had survived a heart attack and their available first-degree relatives, i.e., parents, brothers, sisters, and children. In about 12 percent of these families, elevated lipids in the affected family members appeared in various combinations. For example, some people had high blood levels of cholesterol, some high levels of triglyceride, some high levels of both. The phrase "familial *combined* hyperlipidemia" was used by these doctors to described the presence of different combinations of elevated lipids in family members.

The most common finding in patients with FCH is premature coronary heart disease. FCH is the most commonly recognized inherited blood lipid problem associated with premature coronary heart disease. In fact, if you have developed coronary heart disease before the age of 55, FCH is a possibility that you and your doctor should not overlook. Patients with FCH do not have the cholesterol deposits under their skin and in the tendons (xanthomas) that are commonly found in patients with familial hypercholesterolemia (Chapter 7), but they may have deposits of cholesterol in the cornea of their eye, called corneal arcus.

As its name makes clear, FCH runs in families. If you have FCH, it is currently thought, you probably inherited a faulty gene from one of your parents and a normal gene from the other. The gene for FCH causes an elevated blood level of triglyceride and/or cholesterol when it is present in a single dose, and its effect is not canceled out by the presence of the companion normal gene. As noted in Chapter 7, a condition that causes disease when only one faulty gene is present is called a dominant trait.

If you have FCH, then, on average half of your first-degree relatives will also have FCH. In fact, the only way to determine if your blood triglyceride problem is due to FCH is to find out if your relatives have different combinations of elevated lipids (see below).

What causes FCH? You might think of FCH as a condition in which the "thermostat" that regulates the production of VLDL in the liver is not working properly. By malfunctioning, this thermostat is permitting a high output (at least double the normal) of VLDL particles by the liver, resulting in an increased number of VLDL particles in the blood.

In Figure 8-2 you saw the normal processing of triglyceride-rich VLDL and its products in the blood, ending up with cholesterol-rich LDL: VLDL → VLDL remnants → IDL → LDL. In patients with FCH this normal sequence is speeded up, and the lipoproteins are produced at a rate that exceeds the body's capacity to remove them. The increased production of VLDL in the liver has the following results:

Increased VLDL → Increased VLDL remnants →
Increased IDL → Increased LDL

The patient with FCH may have any one of three lipoprotein profiles, depending upon his or her metabolic state. As an example, let's take the family of William Manlove (Table 8-2).

Because William's VLDL particles were broken down more slowly than normal, his triglyceride level was extremely high. His blood LDL cholesterol level was normal. The combination of high triglyceride and normal LDL gave him what is called a type 4 lipoprotein pattern.

Why was William's blood cholesterol also elevated? VLDL carries five times as much triglyceride as cholesterol; if the level of VLDL is very high, as it was in this patient, the blood cholesterol will also be

Table 8-2. Blood Lipid and Lipoprotein Levels (mg/dl) in a Family with FCH

Category	Male index case (W.M.)	Sister (E.M.)	Sister (K.J.)	Son (C.M.)	Daughter (J.M.)
Age when sampled	46	51	57	29	16
Lipid profile					
Cholesterol	600	357	347	154	197
LDL cholesterol	42	230	213	41	138
HDL cholesterol	23	69	100	38	31
LDL/HDL ratio	1.8	3.3	2.1	1.1	4.5
VLDL cholesterol	535	58	34	75	28
Triglyceride	2,480	238	87	422	172
Lipoprotein pattern	Type 4	Type 2B	Type 2A	Type 4	Type 2B

high. Although William's son Clark (C.M.) also had a type 4 lipoprotein pattern, his cholesterol was normal because he had a less extreme elevation in VLDL.

William's sister Katherine Jester (K.J.) broke down her VLDL very efficiently, with speedy conversion into LDL. Her blood cholesterol and LDL cholesterol levels were high, but her triglyceride level was normal. This combination gives her what is called a type 2A lipoprotein pattern. His other sister, Emily Manlove (E.M.), and his daughter Jane (J.M.) appeared to process the increased VLDL particles at a normal rate, leading to higher VLDL *and* LDL levels (type 2B lipoprotein pattern). Their blood levels of both triglyceride and cholesterol were elevated.

The elevations of cholesterol and triglyceride in children in such families are often milder; sometimes the children start with completely normal lipid levels, which become elevated as they become adults. If you have FCH or premature coronary heart disease, your children should have a blood test for cholesterol, triglyceride, HDL cholesterol, and LDL cholesterol. If a child's total cholesterol is above 170 mg/dl, or the triglyceride above 100 mg/dl, the child should be given the Action Plan diet recommended in Chapter 11 and monitored over the years into young adulthood.

Do your levels of blood cholesterol and triglyceride change dramatically? If they do, and in opposite directions, this may be an indication that you have FCH. I call this hallmark of FCH "bouncing lipids." The lipids often bounce without any explanation. For example, Gerald Grabush developed angina pectoris at the age of 48 and was found to have a complete blockage of his right coronary artery. He had FCH and bouncing lipids:

Lipid profile	Sample 1	Sample 2
Cholesterol	247	306
LDL cholesterol	138	220
HDL cholesterol	24	34
LDL/HDL ratio	5.8	6.5
VLDL cholesterol	85	52
Triglyceride	426	259

The two samples were taken only three months apart. The different profiles cannot be explained by any significant changes in diet or weight, and he was taking no medication.

Other patients with FCH may on occasion have normal blood cholesterol and triglyceride levels. For example, Elliott Fiedler was 35 years old when I first studied him as part of a family with FCH. We took two samples two years apart:

Lipid profile	Sample 1	Sample 2
Cholesterol	198	301
LDL cholesterol	142	246
HDL cholesterol	40	39
LDL/HDL ratio	3.6	6.3
VLDL cholesterol	16	16
Triglyceride	75	118

What accounts for this difference? Elliott had gained twenty pounds.

What is the practical message for you from these two examples? First, if your blood lipid profile "bounces," don't assume that the laboratory is at fault; you probably have FCH. Second, even if your blood cholesterol and triglyceride are normal, you should have them rechecked in a year if you have premature coronary heart disease, a family history of premature coronary heart disease or FCH, or a weight gain of twenty pounds or more.

How Is FCH Treated?

Reduction of dietary cholesterol and saturated fats. Dietary cholesterol and saturated fatty acids end up in the liver, where they provide additional "fuel" for the production of VLDL. If you have FCH, you can follow the Action Plan diet of Chapter 11, which is low in cholesterol and saturated fats. Such a reduced-fat diet may also facilitate the removal of LDL from your blood by increasing the number of LDL receptors in your liver.

Reduction to ideal body weight. If you are overweight, it will be important for you to reduce to a more ideal body weight, since obesity abets the overproduction of VLDL and triglyceride in your liver.

Let's take the example of William Manlove, the W.M. of Table 8-2. When I first saw William, he weighed 216 pounds—too much for his height and build—and ate all the wrong foods. Two months later he had changed his bad eating habits and had lost fifteen pounds, producing a dramatic improvement in his lipid profile. Five months later, his weight had stabilized (at 190 pounds) and so had his lipid profile:

Lipid profile	Baseline	Two months on diet	Five months on diet
Cholesterol	600	212	227
LDL cholesterol	42	150	146
HDL cholesterol	23	39	36
LDL/HDL ratio	1.8	3.8	4.1
VLDL cholesterol	535	23	45
Triglyceride	2,480	116	227

His LDL cholesterol level was now too high; but over the next four years, as he remained on his diet and maintained his new weight, it gradually fell into the desirable range (between 107 and 124 mg/dl). During this time, his LDL/HDL ratio also fell to an acceptable range (from 2.0 to 3.4).

Drugs. If diet and weight control alone are not sufficient to control your blood lipid problem in FCH, your doctor may need to prescribe a drug. Since an overproduction of VLDL is the basis for FCH, nicotinic acid is often the drug of first choice because it specifically decreases the production of VLDL particles in the liver. Decreasing VLDL production slows the subsequent formation of VLDL breakdown products, including LDL. Often treatment with nicotinic acid not only decreases blood cholesterol, LDL, VLDL, and triglyceride levels, but increases the HDL cholesterol level.

Patients with FCH have a *combined* lipid pattern, and this often requires a *combined* drug regimen. For example, gemfibrozil (Lopid®) is often used to treat a high blood triglyceride level; but in patients with FCH the LDL cholesterol level may increase when the triglyceride level decreases. Such patients will require the addition of a second drug. The bile acid sequestrants can be effective when combined with either nicotinic acid or gemfibrozil. In patients with FCH who combine a high LDL cholesterol level with a borderline high triglyceride level, lovastatin (Mevacor®) may also be effective.

Let's take an example. James Bell was 39 years old when he was

referred to me by a vascular surgeon because he had high blood cholesterol and triglyceride levels. The right carotid artery in his neck
and the femoral artery in his right leg were blocked with atherosclerosis. Despite some dietary changes, his cholesterol and triglyceride
levels remained too high and his HDL level too low.

I started him on Lopid, two capsules twice a day, with mixed results: after four weeks his triglyceride level was down to normal, but
his LDL cholesterol was even higher and his HDL cholesterol remained low. I then added cholestyramine (Questran®), two scoops a
day, to his treatment, with the following results:

Lipid profile	Before Lopid	After Lopid	After Lopid plus Questran
Cholesterol	261	284	163
LDL cholesterol	119	237	119
HDL cholesterol	22	24	22
LDL/HDL ratio	5.4	9.9	5.4
VLDL cholesterol	120	23	22
Triglyceride	475	116	109

This was a remarkable response, except that his HDL was still too
low. One reason for this, I'm sure, was that he continued to smoke
cigarettes despite his FCH and his poor circulation.

Familial Hypertriglyceridemia (FHT)

Familial hypertriglyceridemia is an inherited disorder in which the
patient has high blood levels of triglyceride and VLDL cholesterol, a
normal LDL cholesterol level (under 130 mg/dl), usually a low or
borderline low HDL cholesterol level, and an LDL/HDL ratio of 3.0
or less.

Let's take an example. Peter Stokes was a 47-year-old man with a
high blood triglyceride level. He had no coronary heart disease, and
his parents were in their seventies. His lipid profile was as follows,
before and after following the Action Plan diet of Chapter 11:

Lipid profile	Before diet	After diet
Cholesterol	201	201
LDL cholesterol	79	92
HDL cholesterol	35	41
LDL/HDL ratio	2.2	2.2
VLDL cholesterol	87	68
Triglyceride	426	341

Peter was 6'2" and weighed 175 pounds; what he needed was not to lose weight, but to decrease his triglyceride level and increase his HDL cholesterol level. This happened, and his LDL/HDL cholesterol ratio remained in the below-average risk category for coronary heart disease.

Peter had a type 4 lipoprotein pattern (high triglyceride, normal LDL), very like that of William Manlove's son Clark (C.M. in Table 8-2). If you have such a pattern, how can you tell whether your problem is FCH or FHT? There are several ways to tell:

1. FHT is inherited as a Mendelian dominant trait, meaning that half of your adult blood relatives will have a similar type 4 lipoprotein pattern; in other words, FHT "breeds true."

2. With repeated blood samples, your blood lipid profile will not fluctuate, that is, the LDL cholesterol will not change back and forth between normal or low normal and distinctly high.

3. Upon treatment with diet, weight reduction, or triglyceride-lowering drugs, your LDL cholesterol level will not rise significantly, but will remain normal (under 130 mg/dl).

In FHT there is no increased production of LDL as a consequence of increased VLDL production. Instead the liver makes VLDL particles that are larger and contain more triglyceride than normal VLDL. The number of VLDL particles secreted by the liver is not increased in FHT, but each particle is swollen with triglyceride. Such VLDL piles up in the blood without increased conversion into LDL. Factors that increase or abet VLDL production, such as obesity, will further exacerbate the problem.

FHT as such does not increase your risk of coronary heart disease, though it does increase your chance of developing diabetes, which is an element of your risk profile. It also increases your risk of developing gout, a painful arthritic condition. The indicated treatment for FHT is the same as for FCH: a diet low in total fat, saturated fat, and cholesterol, lower in simple sugars (e.g., table sugar, candies, desserts), higher in fiber and the complex carbohydrates found in grains, vegetables, and fruits.

In this condition, reduction to ideal body weight is of utmost importance. The results can be dramatic. Bobby Banks, a 58-year-old man with FHT, was 30 pounds overweight at 212. He had very high blood levels of cholesterol and triglyceride, and his HDL cholesterol was too low. He also had diabetes and was taking the drug Glucotrol® (glipizide), which increases the body's production of insulin. We put him on a diet and he lost 28 pounds in seven weeks, with a remarkable improvement in his lipid profile:

Lipid profile	Before weight loss	After weight loss
Cholesterol	329	204
LDL cholesterol	87	127
HDL cholesterol	25	45
LDL/HDL ratio	3.5	2.8
VLDL cholesterol	217	32
Triglyceride	1,140	162

His diabetes also improved; the blood sugar became normal, so that sugar was no longer spilling into his urine.

At his next visit, two months later, his weight had become stable at 181 pounds. His triglyceride was 225 mg/dl, cholesterol 220 mg/dl, HDL cholesterol 46 mg/dl, LDL cholesterol 129 mg/dl. His blood sugar was down to 56 mg/dl, and his Glucotrol was discontinued. Diet and weight reduction had brought both his triglyceride problem and his diabetes under control.

If after diet and weight control your blood triglyceride level remains above 500 mg/dl, drug treatment for your condition should be considered. The available drugs for blood triglyceride problems are reviewed for you in Chapter 16.

Type 3 Disease

If your cholesterol and triglyceride levels are both very high, your doctor will be evaluating you carefully. For example, Alton Albert, a 35-year-old man, was referred to me with a blood cholesterol of 362 mg/dl and a triglyceride of 558 mg/dl. When I examined him, I found orange streaks in the creases of his palms and raised orange bumps on his elbows, in both cases xanthomas caused by deposits of cholesterol and triglyceride under the skin. These deposits provided a clue that he had inherited a blood fat problem called type 3 disease, or type 3 for short.

Type 3 is one of five general patterns or types of lipid and lipoprotein abnormalities in the blood as described in the late 1960s by Dr. Donald Fredrickson and his associates, Dr. Robert Levy and Dr. Robert Lees, at the National Institutes of Health. The types in the last row of Table 8-2 are from this same classification.

Type 3 is strongly associated with premature atherosclerosis in the arteries of the heart, brain, and legs. Alton was healthy when I saw him, but his family history disclosed a number of early heart attacks on his mother's side and strokes on his father's side. Fortunately, he did not have two common complications of type 3, high blood pressure and high blood sugar.

I ordered a special blood test for Alton, one in which plasma from the blood is placed in a special centrifuge overnight and subjected to forces powerful enough to separate the VLDL particles from the LDL and HDL. Two characteristics of the VLDL particles are then determined: their content of cholesterol and triglyceride, and the distance that the negatively charged particles migrate toward a positively charged electrode (electrophoresis).

The first test showed, as I had suspected it would, that Alton's VLDL contained much more cholesterol than normal VLDL. In normal people, as we have seen, the average ratio of VLDL cholesterol to triglyceride is roughly one over five, or 0.20, and a ratio higher than 0.30 is distinctly abnormal. Alton's ratio was 0.56.

In addition, Alton's VLDL particles migrated in an abnormal manner after electrophoresis. In normal people VLDL travels to the same position as "prebeta" proteins, and LDL migrates with the blood proteins called "beta" globulins; normal VLDL are also referred to as prebeta lipoproteins and normal LDL as beta lipoproteins. In contrast, type 3 VLDL migrate to the beta position, as Alton's did.

Alton was put on the Action Plan diet described in Chapter 11. Here are the results after six months:

Lipid profile	Before diet	After diet
Cholesterol	400	193
LDL cholesterol	123	107
HDL cholesterol	37	35
LDL/HDL ratio	3.3	3.1
VLDL cholesterol	240	51
Triglyceride	428	153

His high initial level of total blood cholesterol was due not to a high LDL cholesterol but to a very high VLDL cholesterol. The triglyceride level was also high, and the HDL cholesterol level was borderline low. Diet and weight loss made a significant improvement in his lipid profile, which was accompanied by a marked decrease in his xanthomas.

Although type 3 affects only one person in 2,000, it is of considerable general interest because *it provides an important insight into how diet and genes interact to produce a blood lipid problem.* In type 3 there is a problem with removing triglyceride-rich lipoproteins from the blood; this includes both those carrying triglyceride from the diet and those carrying triglyceride from the liver.

Triglyceride and cholesterol from the diet. Dr. William Hazzard and others have shown that in type 3 the chylomicron remnant particle (Figure 8-1) is removed too slowly, with the result that these particles build up in the blood. The resulting abnormal condition can be improved by decreasing the amount of cholesterol, total fat, and saturated fat in your diet. This decreases the number of chylomicrons, and consequently the burden of chylomicron remnants that must be cleared by your liver.

Triglyceride from the liver. Normally, some of the VLDL remnants and IDL particles derived from VLDL are removed by the liver (Figure 8-2). In type 3 the uptake of VLDL remnants and IDL by the liver is faulty, leading to an excessive amount of VLDL remnants and IDL in the blood. This problem can be corrected by decreasing the production of their precursor, VLDL, in the liver, and/or by increasing the breakdown of VLDL remnants and IDL in the blood.

Both chylomicron remnants and VLDL remnants are ordinarily removed from the blood by the interaction of apoE with receptors on the surface of your liver (Figures 8-1 and 8-2). In type 3 a genetic defect is present that alters the structure of apoE significantly; as a result, the key (apoE) does not fit the lock (the receptors). Because they cannot fit into the receptors normally, the chylomicron remnants and VLDL remnants cannot enter the liver normally and build up in the bloodstream.

Genetics of type 3. If you have type 3, you have inherited a faulty gene from both of your parents such that all the apoE your body makes is defective. This condition, which is usually only produced when both genes are faulty, is called a recessive trait. Type 3 is even more complicated than the usual blood fat problem, since those affected must also have a separate gene that increases the production of VLDL.

As noted, about one out of 2,000 persons has type 3. If you have premature coronary heart disease, there is about one chance in 100 to 200 that you have type 3. Your parents will probably not have type 3, although they may have some elevation in their triglyceride level; but your brothers and sisters may also have type 3 if they have inherited both faulty genes from your parents. Your children will inherit only one faulty gene from you, and usually a normal gene from your spouse.

Treatment of type 3. A diet low in cholesterol and low in saturated fat decreases the burden of dietary fat on your liver, and may also facilitate the liver's uptake of VLDL remnants and IDL by increasing the number of its LDL receptors. Reduction to ideal body weight will decrease the production of VLDL in your liver.

These measures can help a lot in patients with type 3. For example, Alton Albert followed a good low-fat diet and lost fifteen pounds; six months later his lipid profile was greatly improved. But Alton's case is unusual, and treatment with a drug is almost always needed. Both gemfibrozil (Lopid®) and clofibrate (Atromid-S®) increase the breakdown of chylomicron and VLDL remnants; gemfibrozil decreases the production of VLDL as well.

Sondra Hinckley is a good example of the effect of drug treatment on patients with type 3. She had suffered a heart attack at the age of 48, and several months later had had a two-vessel coronary artery bypass operation. She stopped smoking, having previously smoked a pack a day for 33 years. She was told at the time of the bypass that she had a high blood cholesterol level, and it was even higher three years after the surgery, when I first saw her in clinic.

The low-cholesterol, low-saturated-fat diet that I first prescribed lowered Sondra's blood cholesterol and triglyceride levels, but she still had an abnormal profile. I then added clofibrate (Atromid-S®), two capsules twice daily, which led to a profound improvement in her lipid profile:

Lipid profile	Before diet	After diet	After drug
Cholesterol	389	316	163
LDL cholesterol	147	157	75
HDL cholesterol	56	46	57
LDL/HDL ratio	2.6	3.4	1.3
VLDL cholesterol	186	113	31
Triglyceride	301	156	70

Recently, Sondra's thallium stress test changed from positive to negative, which may indicate improvement in her coronary atherosclerosis. The poor circulation of patients with type 3 generally appears to improve after drug treatment.

What lessons does type 3 teach us? At least the following five:

1. Lipoproteins other than LDL can produce atherosclerosis. Both chylomicron remnants and VLDL remnants can lead to deposits of cholesterol in the arteries of the heart, brain, and legs early in adult life.

2. Type 3 is another example of how *an elevated blood triglyceride problem can be a marker for an important underlying problem*, one

that can produce atherosclerosis and place you at high risk for premature coronary heart disease.

3. The importance of a diet low in saturated fat and cholesterol is clear, since this diet decreases the burden of chylomicrons and chylomicron remnants to be processed by the body and removed from the blood.

4. Such a diet may also increase the number of LDL receptors on the surface of the liver; this will assist in removing VLDL remnants and IDL from the blood.

5. The final lesson is that treatment of type 3 is very effective. Diet and weight reduction, as the first steps of treatment, work very well. Usually the addition of a drug such as gemfibrozil (Lopid®) or clofibrate (Atromid-S®) completes the treatment nicely. Proper treatment often causes xanthomas to disappear or get much smaller, commonly improves the circulation in the legs, and in most cases significantly decreases the risk of coronary heart disease.

Sky-High Blood Triglyceride Level: Type 5 Disease

What if your blood triglyceride level is "sky-high"? If it is higher than 3,000 mg/dl, you have a very serious triglyceride problem. About one man in every 500 and one woman in every 1,000 has such a problem.

Consider the case of Larry Allen, 36 years old when I first saw him, who had all the typical problems associated with type 5 disease. He had almost died from the most serious complication of type 5, pancreatitis, which is due to a swelling of the cells of the pancreas, an organ in the abdomen responsible for producing insulin and certain proteins that are important for digesting food. The swelling is caused by sky-high triglyceride levels. Marked pain in the abdomen is the first sign of pancreatitis.

As usually happens in type 5, Larry's case was complicated by the presence of diabetes. Larry did not need insulin, but his diabetes was serious enough to contribute to his triglyceride problem. At times his triglyceride level was above 3,500 mg/dl, high enough to produce deposits of triglyceride under the skin: small, reddish-yellow raised bumps (eruptive xanthomas) occurring in clusters on his arms, legs, and other portions of his body.

In the beginning, I tried to control Larry's problem with a strict low-fat diet and weight control measures. At times the results were encouraging enough, especially during his hospitalization to the research unit, where an excellent diet brought his triglyceride level as low as 342 mg/dl. But outside the controlled environment of the hospital he did not diet as strictly, and his triglyceride levels ranged from 500 to 2,000 mg/dl. When he really went off his diet, his triglyceride soared above 3,000 mg/dl; and he again developed eruptive xanthomas and abdominal pain. On one occasion his triglyceride went as high as 11,850 mg/dl.

It soon became clear to me that diet alone was insufficient for Larry, and I decided to add a triglyceride-lowering agent, Atromid-S, in a dose of two capsules twice a day. The results were as follows:

Lipid profile	Before drugs	After 1 week on Atromid-S	After 2 months on good diet and Atromid-S
Cholesterol	496	332	174
LDL cholesterol	48	78	107
HDL cholesterol	28	34	38
LDL/HDL ratio	1.8	2	2.5
VLDL cholesterol	420	220	29
Triglyceride	3,465	1,330	217

One could wish for a happier ending to Larry's story. He eventually moved away from Baltimore, abandoned the regimen that had been so successful, and unfortunately succumbed to pancreatitis.

Larry's sky-high triglyceride level was due to abnormally large amounts of chylomicrons (from his diet) and VLDL (from his liver). As noted earlier, the large numbers of chylomicrons and VLDL can actually be seen—without a microscope—in the plasma from the blood of such patients; the problem is a failure to remove these elements efficiently from the blood. For the triglyceride in these lipoproteins to be broken down normally, both lipoprotein lipase and apoC2 must be present in normal amounts and functioning properly (Figures 8-1 and 8-2). Patients with this problem may have a deficiency in either of these proteins. If the liver is also producing VLDL at an accelerated rate, this will worsen the situation.

One of Larry's sons, Steven, also had a type 5 problem before he was ten years old, and several other sons had a milder triglyceride problem, the type 4 lipoprotein pattern. Thus it appears that such triglyceride problems are familial.

Are you at increased risk of coronary heart disease if you have type 5? Yes and no. Larry Allen's high blood cholesterol level was due to his high VLDL. His LDL cholesterol level was low because his VLDL were not being converted into LDL in the normal fashion. His HDL cholesterol level was also low, increasing his risk of coronary heart disease but less so than the same HDL level would for someone who had a high LDL level. As also happens in type 3, Larry had some increase in VLDL remnants and IDL, which contributed to his increased risk of atherosclerosis. Finally, like many other type 5 patients, Larry was too heavy and had diabetes. Since all type 5 patients do not have the same risk profile in these terms, their risk of coronary heart disease will vary.

The important thing to know is that type 5 can be treated successfully. A low-fat diet will decrease the burden of dietary triglyceride; and reduction to ideal body weight, by decreasing the production of VLDL and triglyceride in the liver, will lower the amount of blood triglyceride. (Just as clearly, if patients with type 5 do not follow their diet and reduce to ideal body weight, they will still have very high triglyceride levels even after drug treatment. This was true of Larry Allen.) If diabetes is present, it is important that it be controlled by medication, or if necessary with insulin, to keep the triglyceride level as low as possible.

If after these measures your blood triglyceride level is still above 500 mg/dl, your doctor will need to consider the addition of a triglyceride-lowering drug to your treatment regimen. Nicotinic acid is such a drug, but it can increase both the blood uric acid and blood sugar levels, which already tend to be high in patients with type 5 disease; and since high uric acid levels can lead to gout and high blood sugar levels to diabetes, nicotinic acid should be used only with caution. Gemfibrozil (Lopid®) is often effective. These drugs and others are reviewed for you in Chapter 16.

Summary

1. Triglyceride is a fat in the blood that can come from either the diet or the liver.

2. It is a normal component of your blood, and its level can be determined by a blood test after you have fasted for twelve hours. If you have a total cholesterol level above 200 mg/dl, coronary heart disease, or a positive family history of premature coronary heart disease, or if you are overweight or have diabetes, you should have your blood triglyceride level checked by your doctor.

3. A triglyceride level can be very high (above 500 mg/dl), high, borderline high, or desirable. The triglyceride level varies considerably by age and gender, and both of these factors must be considered in interpreting a given person's triglyceride level.

4. A high or borderline high triglyceride value is associated with increased risk of coronary heart disease when it is accompanied by a borderline high (130–160 mg/dl) or high LDL cholesterol level (over 160 mg/dl), or by a low HDL cholesterol level (under 35 mg/dl). Other risk factors such as hypertension, obesity, and diabetes can accompany a high blood triglyceride level.

5. A high triglyceride level often signals the presence of a blood lipid problem associated with increased risk of coronary heart disease.

6. Familial combined hyperlipidemia (FCH) is the most commonly recognized inherited condition in families with premature coronary heart disease. People with FCH produce VLDL at an accelerated rate in the liver, leading to an increased number of VLDL particles in blood. Such people may have only a high blood triglyceride level, or only a high cholesterol level, or both. Their LDL cholesterol levels are usually high or borderline high, and their HDL cholesterol levels can be low. The levels of cholesterol and triglyceride can fluctuate considerably over time in patients with FCH.

7. Familial hypertriglyceridemia (FHT) is an inherited problem of triglyceride metabolism that is accompanied by an elevated blood triglyceride level, a low HDL cholesterol, but a normal or low LDL cholesterol level. The VLDL particles contain more triglyceride than normal VLDL. The risk of coronary heart disease in FHT is less than in FCH. FHT is often accompanied by diabetes, gout, and obesity.

8. Type 3 disease is an uncommon condition (affecting about one person in 2,000) usually accompanied by high levels of both cholesterol and triglyceride. The lipoprotein particles created by the breakdown of triglyceride in the blood, namely chylomicron remnants, VLDL remnants, and IDL, are not removed by the liver at a normal rate. The pile-up of these remnant lipoproteins can be diagnosed by using special tests to look at the cholesterol and triglyceride content of VLDL and the behavior of VLDL after electrophoresis. Patients with type 3 are at high risk of atherosclerosis of the arteries in the heart, brain, and legs.

9. Type 5 disease occurs when the body cannot normally process triglyceride from the diet or triglyceride from the liver, with the result that chylomicrons and VLDL pile up in the blood. The triglyceride level is usually over 3,000 mg/dl, and can reach 10,000 mg/dl. Diabetes is common in type 5. Although the LDL cholesterol level is low, there is some increased risk of coronary heart disease and poor circulation because the HDL cholesterol level is very low.

10. The first form of treatment for these disorders of triglyceride

metabolism is a diet that is low in total fat, saturated fat, and cholesterol, as presented in Chapter 11. Reduction to ideal body weight is
an important part of treatment.

11. If diet and weight loss do not reduce the blood triglyceride level
to less than 500 mg/dl, a triglyceride-lowering medication should be
considered such as gemfibrozil (Lopid®) or nicotinic acid. If you have
the high LDL level associated with FCH, a second drug such as a bile
acid sequestrant may be necessary to lower the LDL cholesterol to
below 130 mg/dl.

CHAPTER 9

Are You at Risk
if Your Cholesterol
Level Is Normal?

You may have had your level of blood cholesterol measured
as less than 200 mg/dl, the top of the range deemed desirable by the
Adult Treatment Panel of the National Institutes of Health. If so,
your risk of coronary heart disease will depend on the presence of
other factors, including certain inherited blood lipid problems, that
will be reviewed for you in this chapter.

Or you may be the one person in five with known coronary heart
disease who has a cholesterol level less than 200 mg/dl. If so, this
chapter will help you understand why you developed coronary heart
disease despite a desirable blood cholesterol level.

What is your family history? If your blood cholesterol level is less
than 200 mg/dl but you have a positive family history of premature
(less than age 55) coronary heart disease, you should obtain a complete lipid profile. That is, following an overnight fast, you should
have a blood test that measures your levels of total cholesterol, triglyceride, and HDL cholesterol.

If your triglyceride level is high (250–500 mg/dl) or very high (over
500 mg/dl), you have probably inherited one of the blood triglyceride
problems reviewed in Chapter 8. It is the *combination* of a positive
family history of premature coronary heart disease *and* a blood triglyceride problem that places you in this category.

If your HDL cholesterol level is less than 35 mg/dl, it is too low. A
low HDL level combined with a positive family history of premature
coronary heart disease may indicate that you carry a gene for
hypoHDL, a condition discussed below.

When the HDL cholesterol is too low, bad things can happen even
when the blood cholesterol is less than 200 mg/dl. For example, take
the case of Ted Levin, who developed coronary heart disease requiring coronary artery bypass surgery at age 33 despite having a desir-

able cholesterol level. He smoked two packs of cigarettes a day right up to his bypass operation; his blood pressure was normal. Nine years later, a repeat heart catherization showed that one of the bypass grafts was completely blocked, and that the blockages in the native coronary arteries had become narrowed further. When I saw him, his blood cholesterol level was 148 mg/dl, his LDL cholesterol 89 mg/dl, and his triglyceride 180 mg/dl; but his HDL cholesterol was low at 31 mg/dl.

After one year of a good low-fat diet, his triglyceride had increased to 234 mg/dl and his HDL cholesterol remained very low at 32 mg/dl. I couldn't use nicotinic acid because he was being treated with a medicine to decrease the high acid content of his stomach. I prescribed Lopid to try to lower his triglyceride level and increase his HDL. Before I could check him again, he developed more heart trouble and had to have a second triple-vessel coronary artery bypass, at the age of 45.

When I saw him again, Lopid had lowered his triglyceride to 109, but his HDL remained at 31 mg/dl, and his LDL/HDL ratio was above 4.0, indicating that he was still in the higher-risk category for coronary heart disease. I knew I had to do something, particularly in view of the second bypass operation. I stopped Lopid and started Mevacor, one pill with dinner, to see if I could lower his LDL cholesterol and improve his LDL/HDL ratio. This is precisely what happened. On Mevacor, his LDL cholesterol decreased from 132 to 70 mg/dl, and his ratio of LDL/HDL fell to 2.0. A repeat coronary angiogram showed that his new bypass grafts were completely open.

Further, as indicated in Chapter 5, even if your blood cholesterol level is less than 200 mg/dl you are at increased risk of coronary heart disease if you have high blood pressure, smoke cigarettes, are considerably overweight, or have diabetes. If you have even one of these other risk factors for coronary heart disease, you should have your levels of cholesterol, triglyceride, and HDL cholesterol determined, and then estimate your LDL cholesterol using the formula described in Chapter 5.

What is your lifestyle? Do you eat whatever you want? Is your diet high in calories, total fat, saturated fat, and cholesterol? Do you exercise rarely or never? Are you ten to twenty pounds overweight? You are certainly not alone, but with such a lifestyle a blood cholesterol level of less than 200 mg/dl is not particularly reassuring. An assessment by your doctor of your levels of triglyceride, HDL cholesterol, and LDL cholesterol will provide further information, and may suggest modifications that will improve your health.

Coronary Disease But Normal Blood Cholesterol

Do you already have coronary heart disease? If so, even a blood cholesterol level less than 200 mg/dl cannot be taken as completely reassuring, since such a level may mask an abnormal lipid profile that places you at increased risk of further problems.

For example, many patients who have had coronary artery bypass surgery develop atherosclerosis in the bypass grafts themselves, sometimes within two years after surgery although usually after five to ten years. In a study performed at the Royal Victoria Hospital in Montreal, it was shown that in patients who had coronary artery bypass surgery, those who eventually developed blockages in their bypass grafts had not only higher blood cholesterol levels but higher triglyceride levels, lower HDL cholesterol levels, and higher LDL/HDL ratios. They also had higher levels of the major protein of LDL, apoB, and lower levels of the major protein of HDL, apoA1. Obviously, even if your blood cholesterol is less than 200 mg/dl, your doctor will also need to consider the other elements of your lipid profile and take action to modify an abnormal profile.

If you have coronary heart disease, you are undoubtedly under the care of a physician; and even if your blood cholesterol is normal, other risk factors such as high blood pressure and cigarette smoking will have been addressed carefully. Many patients stop smoking cigarettes after they have their first heart attack or coronary artery bypass surgery; all should. High blood pressure, and dietary and drug measures to treat it, are generally better understood by the medical community than blood lipid problems, especially when a patient's blood cholesterol is less than 200 mg/dl.

If you have coronary heart disease, it will be important for you to follow a diet low in total fat, saturated fat, and cholesterol even if your blood cholesterol level is less than 200 mg/dl. The importance of a proper diet is better understood these days; whatever your cholesterol level, you were probably not given a breakfast of bacon and eggs in the coronary care unit or encouraged to eat as you chose when you got home. Diets high in total fat, saturated fat, and cholesterol provide a greater burden of fat for your body to remove from the blood following a meal; they also decrease the ability of your liver to remove LDL cholesterol from your blood. The bottom line is that if you have coronary heart disease, you should follow the Action Plan diet of Chapter 11 even if your blood cholesterol is less than 200 mg/dl.

Indeed, you may need to add one or more drugs to a low-cholesterol, low-saturated-fat diet to lower your lipid levels further and thus decrease your chance of having the disease recur. The benefits of drugs were clearly shown by the Cholesterol-Lowering Atherosclerosis Study discussed in Chapter 3, in which patients with coronary atherosclerosis and coronary bypass grafts who were treated with a low-cholesterol, low-saturated-fat diet plus two drugs (colestipol and nicotinic acid) were compared with patients treated with a low-cholesterol, low-saturated-fat diet alone. Those given drugs had significantly less progression of the blockages in their coronary arteries, and fewer new deposits of cholesterol in their bypasses.

HypoHDL

Your total cholesterol is less than 200 mg/dl, your total triglyceride is less than 250 mg/dl, but your HDL cholesterol is less than 35 mg/dl and you have coronary heart disease or a positive family history of coronary heart disease. You are likely to carry a genetic trait that is the link between a low HDL cholesterol level and coronary heart disease. This inherited problem is called "hypoHDL," from the Greek *hypo*, meaning low.

In 1979, Doctors Vergani and Bettale of Milan, Italy, described a family in which two brothers both had heart attacks: one in his late thirties, the other in his early forties. Both brothers had low HDL cholesterol levels but normal blood cholesterol levels. A number of their relatives had died from premature coronary heart disease, and many of their living relatives also had low HDL cholesterol levels. This family had hypoHDL.

As this history suggests, hypoHDL is a dominant trait, expressed when only one abnormal gene is present. On average, one of the parents and half of the siblings and children of persons affected with hypoHDL also have hypoHDL.

Doctors Jane Third and Charles Glueck and co-workers at the University of Cincinnati studied sixteen families who were discovered because a member (called an index case or proband) had a low HDL cholesterol level along with normal levels of blood cholesterol and triglyceride. All but one or two of the sixteen probands had developed coronary heart disease, usually before age 60; fifteen of the sixteen probands were male. Their blood lipid and lipoprotein levels are summarized in Table 9-1. Although their LDL cholesterol levels were in the normal range, the average LDL/HDL ratio was quite high, close to 5.0, because the HDL cholesterol levels were so low. It

Table 9-1. Average Lipid and Lipoprotein
Cholesterol Levels in Adults with HypoHDL
(mg/dl)

Lipid profile	Average	Range
Cholesterol	180	153–241
Triglyceride	157	58–231
HDL cholesterol	28	18–32
LDL cholesterol	127	87–165
LDL/HDL ratio	4.7	3.1–7.9

Source: Data on 16 probands from J. Third et al., in *Metabolism* 33 (1984): 136–146.

is easy to see why these probands had developed coronary heart disease despite their normal blood cholesterol level.

Almost half of the 60 first-degree relatives of these sixteen hypoHDL probands also had low HDL cholesterol levels. This pattern of inheritance indicates that hypoHDL resulted from the action of one faulty gene.

One finds children as well as adults with hypoHDL. One such child, Jason Marshall, age seven, was referred to me when his father died suddenly at the age of 38 without any warning. Jason's physical examination showed that he was a healthy, normal child, but laboratory studies revealed a problem. His HDL cholesterol was only 13 mg/dl; the repeat value was 15 mg/dl. His blood cholesterol was first borderline high at 177 mg/dl and then normal at 131 mg/dl. His triglyceride level was slightly increased at 101 mg/dl and 91 mg/dl. His HDL apoA1 level was very low at 26 mg/dl (the low end of the normal range for him is about 105 mg/dl). His sister Crystal had a very similar lipid profile; the low end of the normal range for her is about 120 mg/dl. For adult males and females, the lower limits for apoA1 are about 90 mg/dl and 105 mg/dl, respectively.

My challenge will be to try to increase Jason's and Crystal's genetically deficient levels of HDL cholesterol and HDL apoA1. A good Action Plan diet and aerobic exercise will be the first steps in their treatment.

What causes hypoHDL and what lessons can you learn from this inherited problem? Medical scientists are working hard to understand what the underlying causes of hypoHDL are. Our current understanding of the processing of HDL in the blood is summarized in Figure 9-1. The liver is the major source of HDL. When HDL is released from liver into blood, it has a coin-like appearance, like a quarter, round and flat. The major protein of HDL, apoA1, is on the

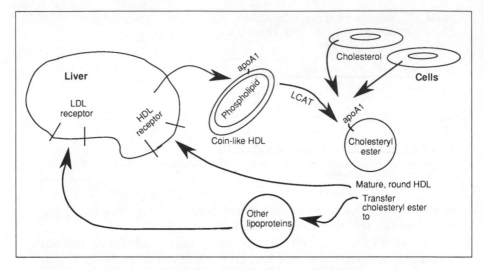

Fig. 9-1. The processing of HDL in the blood. HDL are made in the liver and then released into the blood. The "coin-like" HDL then pick up cholesterol from cells and esterify it through the action of LCAT and its helper protein apoA1, producing a mature, round HDL with cholesteryl ester in the middle. Cholesteryl ester is then transferred to other lipoproteins that are taken up through the LDL receptor, or HDL may deliver the cholesteryl ester directly to the liver through the HDL receptor. This process has been called "reverse cholesterol transport."

surface of HDL; and lipids, such as phospholipid and some cholesterol, are in the inside. Cholesterol is removed from the outer coating or membrane of cells by HDL. Through the action of an enzyme called LCAT (lecithin cholesterol acyl transferase), and its helper protein, apoA1, a fatty acid is removed from the phospholipid lecithin and transferred to cholesterol, changing it into cholesteryl ester. A mature, round-shaped HDL is produced with cholesteryl ester in the middle, surrounded by apoA1. Next, HDL returns cholesteryl ester to the liver for disposal. This occurs either by the interaction of HDL with a receptor on the surface of the liver, or through the transfer of cholesteryl ester from HDL to other lipoproteins, such as VLDL remnants and LDL, which are themselves also taken up by the liver.

Patients with low levels of HDL in their blood do not appear to transport cholesterol from their cells back to the liver as efficiently as patients with normal HDL cholesterol levels. Some of these patients apparently do not make HDL or apoA1 at a normal rate in their liver. Others have difficulty removing the cholesterol from their cells efficiently, including problems with LCAT. Others may not transfer cholesteryl ester efficiently to other lipoproteins, or the HDL may not interact with the liver in a normal fashion. Finally, some patients remove the HDL from their blood too rapidly because of a defect in HDL or in apoA1.

If you or someone in your family has a low HDL cholesterol level for whatever reason, you will want to decrease the burden of LDL cholesterol in the blood by diet and perhaps drugs. You will want to increase the low level of HDL by exercise, weight reduction, and giving up cigarettes. Your doctor may also consider the use of certain drugs such as nicotinic acid and gemfibrozil (Lopid®).

LDL apoB

Sometimes a person develops coronary heart disease and no one can figure out why. With available risk factors, we can account for no more than 50 percent of the variation in the incidence of coronary heart disease. In a number of cases I know of, the blood levels of total and LDL cholesterol were less than 200 mg/dl and 130 mg/dl, respectively, the HDL cholesterol levels were good at 45 mg/dl or higher, the LDL/HDL ratios were not even 3.0, and the triglyceride levels were below 150 mg/dl. The blood pressure was normal, and there was no history of smoking cigarettes. The only possible hint lay in the family history; in one typical case, two relatives had developed coronary heart disease in their fifties. Are there any other tests that can shed light on this kind of mystery?

In the Lipid Clinic at Johns Hopkins, we use a test to measure the amount of LDL apoB in blood. This test is performed at the same time that the LDL cholesterol level is being determined. LDL apoB is the protein component of LDL, the element that enables the lipids (cholesterol, phospholipid, and triglyceride) to mix with the blood (Figure 9-2).

If the relative amounts of the lipids and apoB in LDL were always the same, doctors could estimate the amount of LDL in your blood by measuring any one of its components. However, the amount of cholesterol in LDL varies from person to person; the range of variation in normal people is about 30 percent. In cholesterol problems such as familial hypercholesterolemia (FH), reviewed for you in Chapter 7, LDL is abnormally high in cholesterol. In the condition called "hyperapoB" that will be discussed next, the content of cholesterol in LDL is abnormally low.

Unlike the cholesterol (and cholesteryl ester) in LDL, the apoB

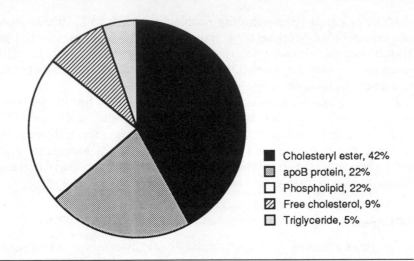

Fig. 9-2. Typical proportions of protein (apoB) and lipids in LDL.

protein in LDL does not vary; that is, on each LDL particle there is always only one molecule of apoB protein. The cholesterol content of LDL may be high, normal, or low, but there is always one particle of apoB protein (Figure 9-3). What does this tell us? That the measurement of LDL apoB provides a better assessment of the number of LDL particles in your blood than the measurement of LDL cholesterol alone.

How can the LDL apoB test help you? If you have coronary heart disease, a blood cholesterol less than 200 mg/dl, and no other risk factors, you may still have an elevated LDL apoB level. This finding would help explain your coronary heart disease because it would indicate that there are too many "bad" LDL particles in your blood. Since these LDL particles contain less cholesterol *per particle* than normal LDL, both the blood cholesterol test and the usual LDL cholesterol test will underestimate their number.

HyperapoB

As Figure 9-3 shows, smaller, cholesterol-depleted LDL particles contain more apoB protein relative to their cholesterol content than normal LDL. This increases their density; hence the phrase "dense LDL." When dense LDL particles are numerous in the blood, the patient is said to have "hyperapoB" (*hyper* meaning increased).

HyperapoB was discovered in 1980 when Dr. Allan Sniderman of the Royal Victoria Hospital in Montreal, our colleagues, and I studied angiograms of men and women admitted to that hospital for evaluation of chest pain to see whether they had any significant blockages in their coronary arteries. Some did, others didn't. The levels of cholesterol, triglyceride, LDL cholesterol, and LDL apoB were measured in the blood of these patients.

As expected, the average levels of cholesterol, triglyceride, and LDL cholesterol were significantly higher in those with coronary blockages than in those without such blockages. What was new was that the level of LDL apoB was also significantly higher in those with blocked arteries, and that the difference between the two groups in average LDL apoB protein level was *more significant* than the difference in LDL cholesterol. In short, the level of LDL apoB predicted the presence of blocked arteries better than the level of LDL cholesterol.

For your review, Figure 9-4 plots the LDL apoB and LDL cholesterol levels of both groups, together with those of an unrelated group of patients with familial hypercholesterolemia, a condition featuring

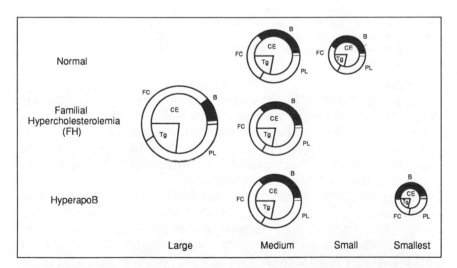

Fig. 9-3. Different sizes of LDL particles in normal persons, patients with familial hypercholesterolemia (FH), and patients with hyperapoB. B = apo B; CE = cholesteryl ester; FC = free cholesterol; PL = phospholipid; Tg = triglyceride.
From A. Sniderman and P. O. Kwiterovich, *Proceedings of the Workshop on Lipoprotein Heterogeneity* (NIH Publication 87–2646, 1987), p. 294.

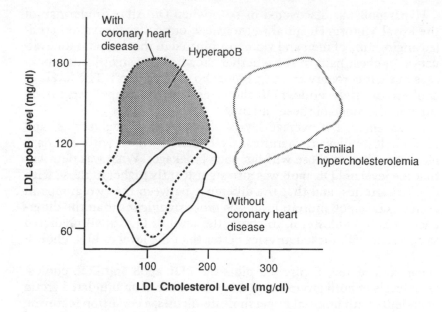

Fig. 9-4. Blood levels of LDL apoB and LDL cholesterol in patients with and without coronary heart disease, and in patients with familial hypercholestero-lemia. Those with hyperapoB are in the shaded area.
Drawn from data from A. Sniderman et al., in *Proceedings of the National Academy of Sciences* 77 (1980): 604–608.

high levels of both LDL cholesterol and LDL apoB. About half the patients with coronary atherosclerosis had high LDL apoB levels (above 120 mg/dl), but their LDL cholesterol levels were mostly normal or borderline high (130–160 mg/dl). It is this combination of high LDL apoB level with a normal or borderline high LDL cholesterol level that we named "hyperapoB."

In hyperapoB, the smaller, cholesterol-depleted LDL particles predominate in the blood, and the ratio of LDL cholesterol to LDL apoB is low (below 1.2). In familial hypercholesterolemia, the larger, cholesterol-rich particles predominate, and the ratio of LDL cholesterol to LDL apoB is often high (above 1.6). Since patients with hyperapoB and those with FH both get premature coronary heart disease, you can see that the number of LDL particles is important, and not just the amount of cholesterol carried by these particles. The goal of treatment must therefore be to decrease the number of LDL particles in the blood.

The elements of hyperapoB. Patients with hyperapoB have two known defects or malfunctions:

1. VLDL and apoB are produced at an accelerated rate in the liver, and an increased number of VLDL particles are released into the blood. This leads to an increased synthesis of the breakdown product of VLDL, namely LDL, and further modeling in the blood produces smaller, denser LDL particles.

2. There is a delayed clearance of dietary fat from the blood. After eating a meal high in fat, the blood triglyceride level increases more dramatically in hyperapoB patients than in normal persons (Figure 9-5). By seven hours after a fatty meal, most of the triglyceride from the diet is cleared in normal persons; but those with hyperapoB still have a significant amount of triglyceride from their diet remaining in their blood.

Can hyperapoB run in families? HyperapoB was present in at least one-third of the offspring of parents with hyperapoB and premature coronary heart disease. In some families, hyperapoB has been passed on from generation to generation as a dominant genetic trait (on average, half of the first-degree relatives are similarly affected).

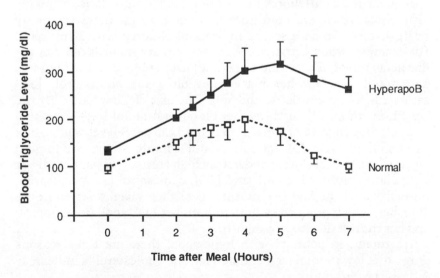

Fig. 9-5. Time of clearance of triglyceride from the diet in patients with hyperapoB and normal persons after eating a meal high in fat.
From J. Genest et al., in *Arteriosclerosis* 6 (1986): 297–304, by permission of the American Heart Association, Inc.

HyperapoB and FCH. Patients with the blood triglyceride problem called familial combined hyperlipidemia (FCH), discussed in Chapter 8, can also have small, dense LDL particles. The following guidelines may help you to distinguish between these two related disorders:

1. If the blood triglyceride level is above 250 mg/dl and the LDL apoB level is above 120 mg/dl, FCH is present.

2. If the blood triglyceride level is below 250 mg/dl and the LDL apoB above 120 mg/dl, hyperapoB is present.

Thomas Ellison, a patient with a high LDL apoB level, had a heart attack at age 44, and a subsequent heart catherization showed blockage in one of his major coronary arteries. He was not a cigarette smoker and his blood pressure was normal, but he had a family history of coronary heart disease. His average cholesterol was 256 mg/dl, LDL cholesterol 135 mg/dl, triglyceride 377 mg/dl, LDL apoB 163 mg/dl, and HDL cholesterol 50 mg/dl. Although his LDL cholesterol was close to the desirable range, his LDL apoB level was almost twice as high as the average in normal adults. His lipid profile indicated that he had FCH.

HyperapoB in childhood. Since the Lipid Clinic at Johns Hopkins also specializes in children from families with premature coronary heart disease, we have seen a number of children with hyperapoB. For example, when Christine Bates was twenty months old, her pediatrician found in a routine screening that her blood cholesterol was 220 mg/dl. Her mother placed her on a low-cholesterol, low-saturated-fat diet similar to the Step One diet of Chapter 11. By the time I saw this child in clinic, her blood cholesterol level was down to borderline high at 175 mg/dl, but her LDL apoB level was high at 129 mg/dl. (A high LDL apoB in a child is a value above 110 mg/dl.) Her triglyceride level was moderately high (140 mg/dl), and both her LDL cholesterol (104 mg/dl) and HDL cholesterol (49 mg/dl) were normal. Christine and her mother were then given a stricter Step Two diet, which produced a drop in both her LDL apoB (to 97 mg/dl) and her triglyceride (to 114 mg/dl).

Treatment. In patients with hyperapoB, there are three reasons why a diet low in total fat, saturated fat, and cholesterol is indicated:

1. Such a diet will decrease the number of lipoprotein particles derived from the diet, since such particles are present for a longer period of time in the blood of these patients.

2. It will decrease the fuel supplied by dietary fat to the liver for the production of VLDL.

3. It will increase the synthesis of LDL receptors to help clear the increased number of dense LDL particles from the blood.

In many cases, diet must be supplemented by drugs. One such case is Gregory McInerny, a 47-year-old dentist who was taking better care of his teeth than his heart. He became concerned when his mother died at 52 of a heart attack and he recalled that two of her brothers had died of heart attacks in their thirties.

He himself had not developed any signs of coronary heart disease. His family physician had found blood cholesterol readings between 200 and 260 mg/dl. He had already been following a low-cholesterol, low-saturated-fat diet, he had stopped smoking ten years earlier, and he exercised by running four to five miles three times a week.

On his first two visits, his average blood cholesterol level was borderline high and his LDL cholesterol was high. His HDL cholesterol was borderline low, and his triglyceride level was normal. However, his LDL apoB level was very high, giving him a very low ratio of LDL cholesterol to LDL apoB (about 1.0). He had hyperapoB, with a significantly large number of smaller, denser LDL particles in his blood.

I recommended that he increase the amount of water-soluble fiber in his diet, especially oat bran, oatmeal, fruits, legumes, and vegetables. This lowered his blood cholesterol and LDL cholesterol levels significantly. However, his LDL apoB remained very elevated and was now actually higher than his LDL cholesterol; his HDL cholesterol and triglyceride levels did not change:

Lipid profile	On low-saturated-fat, low-cholesterol diet	After addition of water-soluble fiber
Cholesterol	230	202
LDL cholesterol	176	145
LDL apoB	173	183
HDL cholesterol	39	39
LDL/HDL ratio	4.5	3.7
Triglyceride	91	90

Because of Gregory's family history of premature coronary heart disease and his persistent very high LDL apoB level, treatment with drugs will be necessary. I considered nicotinic acid, bile acid resins, and lovastatin. Nicotinic acid can lower the LDL apoB level because it decreases the production of VLDL and apoB in the liver. However, because his triglyceride level was ideal, I chose the bile acid resin cholestyramine, which can decrease LDL apoB by increasing the uptake of LDL through the LDL receptors; on four doses per day, his values were: cholesterol 171 mg/dl, LDL cholesterol 111 mg/dl, LDL apoB 117 mg/dl, triglyceride 103 mg/dl. Lovastatin also facilitates the removal of LDL through the LDL receptors, but does so by decreasing cholesterol production in the liver. Lovastatin may therefore be especially effective for those patients who cannot tolerate, or do not respond to, nicotinic acid or the bile acid resins.

HyperapoB and a low HDL cholesterol level. Despite having a desirable or borderline high blood cholesterol, a number of my patients are at high risk for coronary heart disease because they have what I call the "double whammy," a high LDL apoB and a low HDL cholesterol level. One such patient was a pediatrician, Dr. Richard Silberg, who was sent to our clinic by his wife because of "high cholesterol" and a striking family history of premature coronary heart disease. He had made all the appropriate dietary changes outlined in Chapter 11, and this had lowered his cholesterol to a point where he did not believe he needed medication.

When he first came to our clinic, his blood cholesterol was 227 mg/dl and his LDL cholesterol 168 mg/dl. His triglyceride was normal at 135 mg/dl. However, his HDL cholesterol was only 26 mg/dl and his HDL apoA1 level was depressed at 82 mg/dl. His LDL apoB level was very high at 176 mg/dl. Despite a very good diet, he was still at high risk of coronary heart disease.

After confirming his abnormal lipid profile and emphasizing the need for him to continue his good diet, I started treatment with nicotinic acid, 500 mg three times a day, which produced some improvement but not enough. I increased the dose of nicotinic acid to one gram three times a day, and this achieved an excellent result. The patient's cholesterol and LDL cholesterol levels decreased to 164 and 112 mg/dl, respectively; his HDL increased to 35 mg/dl, and his triglyceride level fell to 87 mg/dl. His LDL apoB was considerably improved at 116 mg/dl.

Another interesting case is that of Brian Smith, a 61-year-old man who had been screened for our Coronary Primary Prevention Trial fifteen years ago but did not qualify because his cholesterol was less than 265 mg/dl. He was healthy until two years ago, when he developed chest pain. An angiogram disclosed blocked coronary arteries, and he underwent coronary artery bypass surgery at the Johns Hopkins Hospital. He was also found to have blockages in the arteries in his neck (carotid arteries); these were removed in two further operations six months and one year later.

When I first saw him, after his third operation, he was already on a

modified low-fat diet. His blood cholesterol and LDL cholesterol levels were borderline high. His HDL cholesterol was low and his LDL
apoB very high. His triglyceride level was normal. Because of the
marked hardening of his arteries, his persistent adverse lipid profile
after diet, and a history showing that lovastatin had helped him earlier, I started him on Mevacor, 20 mg with dinner. Only four weeks
later, his abnormal, high-risk lipid profile had improved dramatically:

Lipid profile	After low-saturated-fat, low-cholesterol diet	After addition of lovastatin
Cholesterol	211	170
LDL cholesterol	150	105
LDL apoB	179	119
HDL cholesterol	32	37
LDL/HDL ratio	4.7	2.8
Triglyceride	167	139

Howard Needle, a 53-year-old lawyer who was referred to me because he had a blood lipid problem, had no history of coronary heart
disease. Yet despite his efforts with a low-fat diet, his lipid profile
indicated that he had the "double whammy."

I started him on nicotinic acid, 500 mg three times a day, and his
total and LDL cholesterol levels fell sharply. His HDL cholesterol
increased to 48 mg/dl, his LDL apoB decreased to 144 mg/dl, and his
triglyceride level fell to 156 mg/dl. This was an excellent response.
His new LDL/HDL ratio took him out of the high-risk category and
into a below-average-risk category:

Lipid profile	After low-saturated-fat, low-cholesterol diet	After addition of niacin
Cholesterol	241	188
LDL cholesterol	161	109
LDL apoB	171	144
HDL cholesterol	33	48
LDL/HDL ratio	4.9	2.2
Triglyceride	242	156

Unfortunately, soon afterward he suffered a heart attack. Howard ex-
emplifies well the findings of the major studies reviewed for you in
Chapter 3, namely that *it takes two years for lipid-lowering drugs to
achieve their full benefit in lowering your risk of coronary heart
disease.*

What if the LDL apoB test is unavailable to you? In that case you can use the following guidelines to help you assess your need for drug treatment:

1. If you have coronary heart disease, the Adult Treatment Panel recommends that drugs be used after diet to lower your LDL cholesterol level to less than 130 mg/dl.

2. If your HDL cholesterol is low, your ratio of LDL cholesterol to HDL cholesterol is likely to be 4.0 or higher even if your blood total and LDL cholesterol levels are desirable or borderline high. If you have coronary heart disease, medication can be used to lower your LDL/HDL ratio to 3.0 or less.

3. If you don't have coronary heart disease but have a family history of premature coronary heart disease, drugs should be considered (a) if you are a male and your LDL cholesterol is above 160 mg/dl after diet treatment, or (b) if your LDL cholesterol is borderline (130–160 mg/dl) but your HDL is low (below 35 mg/dl) or your LDL/HDL ratio is above 4.0. If you are a female without coronary heart disease but with a positive family history, the same criteria for considering drug treatment can be used if another risk factor such as hypertension or cigarette smoking is present.

Summary

1. If your blood cholesterol is less than 200 mg/dl but you have a family history of coronary heart disease or you already have coronary heart disease, your HDL, LDL, and triglyceride levels should be measured. You will need to be fasting to have these tests.

2. If your triglyceride level is high (250–500 mg/dl) or very high (over 500 mg/dl), you have probably inherited one of the blood triglyceride problems discussed in Chapter 8.

3. If your blood triglyceride level is less than 250 mg/dl and your HDL cholesterol level is less than 35 mg/dl, you may have inherited a genetic problem called hypoHDL. In this case your parents, siblings, and children also may have inherited hypoHDL.

4. If you have coronary heart disease but all your blood tests (cholesterol, triglyceride, HDL cholesterol, and LDL cholesterol) are normal, your condition may be related to the presence of other risk factors such as hypertension, cigarette smoking, obesity, and diabetes.

5. If you have none of the traditional risk factors for coronary heart disease but have developed coronary atherosclerosis, you and your doctor should try to arrange to have your blood level of LDL apoB

determined. You may have hyperapoB, a condition due to an increased number of LDL particles that are smaller and denser because they contain less cholesterol but relatively more apoB protein than normal LDL. If you have hyperapoB, your children, siblings, and parents may also have hyperapoB.

6. In either hypoHDL or hyperapoB, the first form of treatment is a diet low in cholesterol and saturated fat. Such a diet will decrease the burden of clearing dietary fat and facilitate the removal of LDL from your blood.

7. If you already have coronary heart disease and your blood cholesterol level is less than 200 mg/dl, you and your doctor can review whether medication is indicated. In my view, it probably *is* indicated if your LDL cholesterol level is higher than 130 mg/dl, your LDL/HDL ratio is higher than 4.0, or your LDL apoB level is higher than 120 mg/dl.

PART THREE

Diet and Cholesterol

CHAPTER 10

Blood Cholesterol and Your Diet

Like characters in a play that each influence the outcome of the plot, the various nutrients in your diet affect your blood cholesterol level. Some nutrients have a major part to play; others are in the supporting cast. Major roles are played by these fats in your diet: cholesterol, saturated fat, monounsaturated fat, and polyunsaturated fat. The director of the play is your genetic makeup, which ultimately determines how much influence each of these nutrients has on your blood cholesterol level.

In this chapter you will learn about the individual effects of dietary cholesterol, saturated fats, monounsaturated fats, and polyunsaturated fats. Later chapters will discuss the effects of other dietary nutrients such as fiber and fish oils.

The Nature of Cholesterol and Dietary Fats

Cholesterol. Cholesterol was discovered in 1784 by a French chemist named Poulletier, who first prepared pure cholesterol as a white, waxy powder from a gallstone. It was not called cholesterol until 1816, when another French chemist, Michel Chevreul, coined the word from the Greek *chole,* meaning bile, and *steros,* meaning solid. In this century cholesterol has been the subject of intense study; some thirteen Nobel Prizes have been awarded to scientists working in this area. Thanks to their efforts, the chemical makeup of cholesterol and the way your body makes cholesterol are now well understood.

Cholesterol is composed of 27 carbon atoms in the form of four "rings" with a tail (Figure 10-1, left). A fatty acid can be attached to the third carbon atom (Figure 10-1, right); this form of cholesterol is

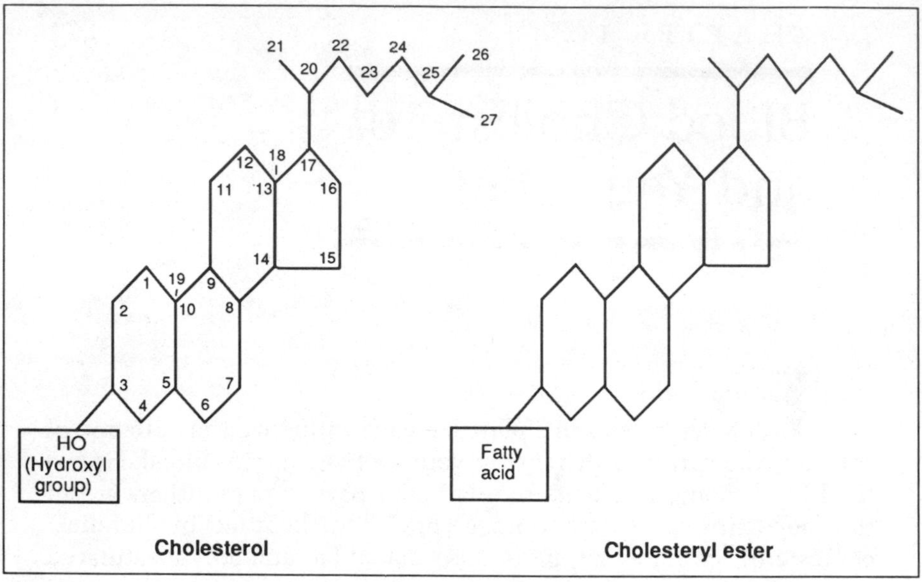

Fig. 10-1. Chemical makeup of cholesterol.

called cholesteryl ester. When there is an excess of cholesterol inside cells, it is stored as cholesteryl ester.

Cholesterol is a natural component of such foods as beef, pork, lamb, chicken, fish, dairy products (milk, butter, cheese, ice cream), and eggs, because it is a normal part of the cells of the animals from which these foods come. Cholesterol is found only in animal cells, not in plant cells. Plants make phytosterol, a compound similar to cholesterol, but humans do not take up phytosterol from their diet into their blood.

Saturated fat. You can actually see saturated fat as the white marbling in red meats, the visible fat around meat or in bacon, and the white layer of fat on the top of gravy after it has stood in the refrigerator overnight. If butter did not have some yellow coloring added, it would appear as a white, solid stick of saturated fat. *All such foods are very high in saturated fat.* They are solid at room temperature.

Animal fats are obvious sources of saturated fat, but there are others hidden in your diet. In whole milk, cheese, ice cream, and vegetable oils such as coconut oil and palm oil, for example, saturated fat is blended in with other substances. Any food that is fried, baked, or otherwise combined with a vegetable oil high in saturated fat becomes itself a food high in saturated fat. For example, potatoes contain little fat; but when fried in a commercial oil high in palm oil that is used to make french fries, they become high in saturated fat. Other examples include fried chicken, fried fish, and cakes, pies, and cookies made with an oil high in saturated fat.

Most of the fatty acids in a saturated fat are saturated fatty acids. Imagine a hat rack with sixteen hooks, each of which can hold two hats (Figure 10-2, top). If all the available hooks are fully occupied

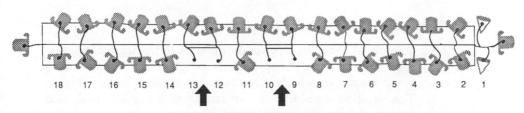

Saturated Fatty Acid (Palmitic Acid)

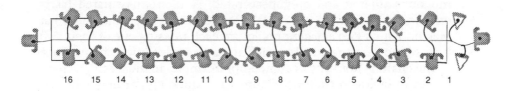

Monounsaturated Fatty Acid (Oleic Acid)

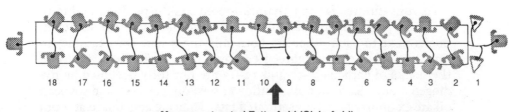

Polyunsaturated Fatty Acid (Linoleic Acid)

Fig 10-2. Chemical makeup of saturated, monounsaturated, and polyunsaturated fatty acids. The chain of carbon atoms is depicted by a straight line, to which are attached hydrogen atoms (shown as hats) or oxygen atoms (shown as white triangles). The carbons in the chain are numbered, by convention, from the acid end (far right), and the areas of unsaturation are indicated by arrows. The tail end (far left) contains the last, or omega, carbon.

with hats, the hat rack is "saturated." In this hat rack model, the hats represent hydrogen atoms, the hooks carbon atoms, and the number of hooks the chain length.

Can you eliminate saturated fat from your diet entirely? No. This is not possible since many foods that are low in fat still do contain some saturated fat. But you can select foods that are low in saturated fat, and cook with the proper oils as reviewed in Chapter 11. You will find some good low-fat meal plans in Chapter 14, and some delicious low-fat recipes at the back of the book.

Monounsaturated fat. There are two kinds of unsaturated fat, monounsaturated and polyunsaturated. A monounsaturated fat is one whose fatty acids are mostly monounsaturated. Imagine a hat rack on which two adjacent hooks are each missing one of their two hats. Monounsaturated fatty acids are fatty acids for which one place in the chain is not fully occupied; for example, in oleic acid, a chain length of eighteen carbons (Figure 10-2, middle), the hooks of carbons 9 and 10 are not fully occupied by hydrogen atoms. Olive oil and canola oil are high in monounsaturated fats. They are liquid at room temperature.

Polyunsaturated fat. In polyunsaturated fats the predominant fatty acids are polyunsaturated. At two or more places in the hat rack, hooks next to each other are both missing a hat. For example, in linoleic acid, a chain eighteen carbons long (Figure 10-2, bottom), the hooks of carbons 9–10 and 12–13 are not fully occupied by hydrogen atoms. Safflower oil, sunflower seed oil, corn oil, and soybean oil are examples of polyunsaturated fats. They are also liquid at room temperature.

Where the Fat in Your Diet Comes From

About 90 percent of the fat in your diet comes in the form of triglyceride, and the rest from phospholipids. Triglyceride consists of a backbone (glycerol) to which three fatty acids are attached (Figure 10-3). The relative amounts of saturated, monounsaturated, and polyunsaturated fatty acids contained in triglyceride can vary. For example, the triglyceride in lard is very high in saturated fatty acids, the triglyceride in olive oil contains mostly monounsaturated fatty acids, and that in corn oil contains a majority of polyunsaturated fatty acids.

Phospholipids usually contain two fatty acids and a phosphorus. As in triglyceride, the fatty acids, which can be saturated, monounsaturated, or polyunsaturated, are attached to two of the carbon at-

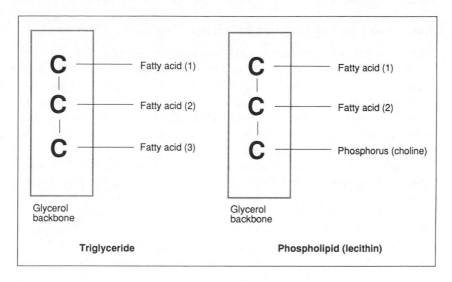

Fig. 10-3. Chemical makeup of triglyceride and a phospholipid.

oms in the glycerol backbone; but a phosphorus is attached to the third carbon, and one or another compound is then attached to the phosphorus. What this compound is determines the nature of the phospholipid. For example, in lecithin (Figure 10-3) a compound known as choline is attached to the phosphorus.

The total amount of fat in your diet is the total from saturated, monounsaturated, and polyunsaturated fats. If you eat a typical American diet, 15 to 20 percent of your calories come from saturated fat, 10 to 15 percent from monounsaturated fat, and about 5 percent from polyunsaturated fat. In the Action Plan diet of in the next chapter, the goal is to reduce the amount of total and saturated fat in your diet. Some of the saturated fat will be replaced with unsaturated fat; both polyunsaturated and monounsaturated fat can be used for this purpose.

Most of the foods you eat (with the exception of most fresh vegetables and fruits) contain all three kinds of fat. If you eat moderately and have no other risk factors, you need only select foods lower in saturated fat to achieve a lower blood cholesterol level. This principle holds for foods of both animal and vegetable origin. Chapter 11 will tell you what foods to select.

How Cholesterol and Dietary Fats Enter Your Blood

The foods you eat vary in the kind and amount of the nutrients they contain. Three major kinds of nutrients in food are fats, proteins, and carbohydrates. When you eat a meal, you must digest the various nutrients in the food. When nutrients are digested, they are broken down into their constituent parts, which the body then absorbs and uses for energy and for rebuilding its various cells.

The digestion of fats from your food takes place in your intestine. On a weight basis, the amount of saturated fats, monounsaturated fats, and polyunsaturated fats to be digested is over a hundred times greater than the amount of cholesterol.

In your intestine, many of the fatty acids attached to triglyceride, phospholipids, and cholesteryl esters are released by the process of digestion. The released fatty acids and the other byproducts of digestion, including cholesterol, are now ready to be taken up by the cells in the intestine. To facilitate this process, the body uses bile acids from your gall bladder to form complexes with these fats. After the fatty acids and cholesterol are taken up by the intestinal cells, triglyceride and phospholipids are re-formed and "packaged" along with cholesterol into lipoprotein particles called chylomicrons. The chylomicrons then leave the intestinal cell and eventually enter your bloodstream. Triglyceride is the major fat inside a chylomicron, making up about 90 percent of its weight.

Once the chylomicrons enter your bloodstream, the triglyceride is broken down by removing the fatty acids from the glycerol backbone. Smaller "chylomicron remnants" are formed, which contain much less triglyceride but relatively more cholesterol than the original chylomicrons. The chylomicron remnants are rapidly taken up by the liver, where cholesterol and other fats from the diet are processed.

How Dietary Cholesterol Affects Your Blood Cholesterol Level

As we noted in Chapter 7, most of the cholesterol in your diet ends up in your liver, where it causes a decrease in the production of a protein called the LDL receptor that is crucial to removing the cholesterol-rich LDL from blood. The more cholesterol you eat, the fewer the LDL receptors available and the higher the level of LDL cholesterol remaining in the blood. Reducing the amount of cholesterol you eat increases the number of LDL receptors, making the removal of LDL cholesterol from your blood more efficient.

When dietary cholesterol enters your liver, the liver decreases its own production of cholesterol. When this shutting off of cholesterol production in the liver is done efficiently, as it is in most people, an increase in your intake of dietary cholesterol will not lead to as great an increase in your blood cholesterol as it will in the one person in five whose feedback mechanism is not efficient. If your blood cholesterol is above 200 mg/dl, and especially if it is above 240 mg/dl, you may be that one person in five.

Why is this? Because your body will be making the same amount of cholesterol on a high-cholesterol diet as on a low-cholesterol diet. As the cholesterol in your diet increases, you have the additional burden of dietary cholesterol while still manufacturing the same amount of cholesterol in the liver. *This disturbs the cholesterol balance and your blood cholesterol level rises.* If your blood cholesterol is below 200 mg/dl, you are less likely to fit into this category.

Dietary cholesterol, particularly when present in large amounts, can also enter your arteries directly. Cholesterol in your diet normally moves from the chylomicrons to the chylomicron remnants, most of which are removed very quickly from the blood by your liver. But in some cases the chylomicron remnants are removed more slowly, and in others a heavy burden of dietary fat and cholesterol produces more chylomicron remnants than the liver can speedily process. In such cases the chylomicron remnants remain in the bloodstream longer, increasing the chance that a chylomicron remnant may directly enter the cells that line your arteries. Any such direct entry of chylomicron remnants, with their dietary cholesterol, will hasten the process of atherosclerosis. This is another reason, if one were needed, to decrease the amount of cholesterol in your diet.

How Much Can Decreasing Cholesterol Intake Change Your Blood Cholesterol Level?

Studies of the effects of special diets in which only the cholesterol content varied and all other nutritional factors were kept constant were performed in the mid-1960s and early 1970s by various groups headed by Dr. Ancel Keys, Dr. Mark Hegsted, Dr. William Connor, Dr. Fred Mattson, and others. Over the range of the usual American dietary cholesterol intake (100–600 mg a day), these studies all found a direct relation between the amount of cholesterol in the diet and the level of cholesterol in the blood. This relationship may be summarized by the following formula:

A decrease in cholesterol in the diet of 100 mg per 1,000 calories consumed produces a decrease in the blood cholesterol level of about 10 mg/dl.

This is of course an average. Some people will respond better, others less well, depending on their genetic makeup.

For example, if you are eating about 600 mg of cholesterol and 2,000 calories a day, you are taking in 300 mg of cholesterol for each 1,000 calories. If you follow the Action Plan diet of the next chapter, you will decrease the cholesterol in your diet from 600 mg per day to 200 mg per day (or from 300 mg to 100 mg per 1,000 calories). For each 1,000 calories you eat, you will decrease your dietary cholesterol 200 mg, which means that your blood cholesterol level will fall about 20 mg/dl.

That may not sound like much; and if you are one of the many Americans who have already decreased the amount of cholesterol in their diet, the improvement on this score from switching to the Action Plan diet will be even smaller. The average man consumes about 450 mg of cholesterol per day and the average woman about 300 mg of cholesterol per day. If you are such a person, you might expect only about a 10 mg/dl fall in your blood cholesterol level when you reduce your dietary cholesterol to 200 mg per day or less. But remember, so far we have considered only cholesterol. We have still to consider the effect on your cholesterol level of the saturated and unsaturated fats in your diet. The effect of saturated fat, *which is even greater than the effect of dietary cholesterol,* is our next subject.

How Saturated Fat Affects Your Cholesterol Level

Several studies have shown that three saturated fatty acids in particular—lauric acid, myristic acid, and palmitic acid—have a potent effect on blood cholesterol levels. One or more of the three are found in a number of commonly used fats and oils (Figure 10-4). Their effect on the blood cholesterol level can be summarized by the following formula:

Each 1 percent decrease in calories from saturated fatty acids in the diet produces a decrease in the blood cholesterol level of almost 3 mg/dl.

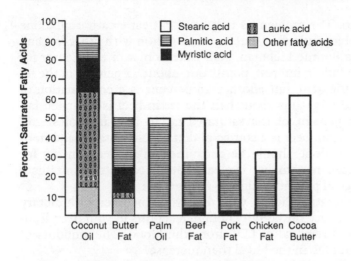

Fig. 10-4. Proportions of different saturated fatty acids in fats and oils.
Reproduced with permission from S. M. Grundy, *Newsletter: Cholesterol and Coronary Disease . . . Reducing the Risk* 1 (1987), no. 4, Science and Medicine, New York, N.Y.

For example, if your diet's saturated fat content decreases from 15 percent to 10 percent of total calories, you might see about a 15 mg/dl decrease in your blood cholesterol level. Again the figure is an average; individual results will vary.

Not all saturated fatty acids are the same. Stearic acid, a saturated fatty acid that contains eighteen carbons, is found in many fats and oils but is particularly prominent in beef fat and in cocoa butter, which is the fat in chocolate (Figure 10-4). Unlike such saturated fatty acids as lauric acid, myristic acid, and palmitic acid, which have potent cholesterol-raising properties, stearic acid does not raise the cholesterol level; indeed, a recent study suggests that it may actually decrease the cholesterol level.

Drs. Andrea Bonarome and Scott Grundy studied eleven men who were fed three different liquid diets for three weeks each. The diets were free of cholesterol and contained the same amount of total fat (40 percent of calories). The first diet had a high content of palmitic acid, the second of stearic acid, the third of oleic acid. Compared with the palmitic acid diet, the stearic acid and oleic acid diets lowered the blood cholesterol levels 14 percent and 10 percent, respectively.

Does this mean that it is all right to eat lots of red meat and chocolate? Alas, no. The problem is that we don't eat stearic acid alone (as in a special formula diet), but in combination with other fats and fatty acids. As Bonnie Liebman, staff nutritionist of the Center for Science in the Public Interest, points out, about 22 percent of the fat in beef is stearic acid, but another 29 percent is a combination of other saturated fats; thus about half the fat in beef is saturated fat, and about 60 percent of the saturated fat in beef is cholesterol-raising. In addition, beef is a source of dietary cholesterol, and from that standpoint alone should be consumed in moderation. As for chocolate, Figure 10-4 makes it clear that cocoa butter contains a high percentage of palmitic acid.

The saturated fatty acids in your diet work together with dietary cholesterol to reduce the activity of LDL receptors in your liver, leading to decreased removal of LDL from the blood. The amounts of cholesterol and LDL in the blood then increase.

There are many ways to lower the amount of saturated fatty acids in your diet. The Action Plan diet presented in the next chapter is an excellent start. In addition to the obvious sources of saturated fatty acids found in animal products, remember that saturated fatty acids are present in certain plant products, and that many hidden sources of saturated fatty acids are found in the typical American diet. If you are not sure about a given food, you can consult the Food Tables, which summarize the saturated fat content (in grams per serving) of many commonly eaten foods.

How Polyunsaturated Fat Affects Your Cholesterol Level

Unlike dietary cholesterol and saturated fatty acids, polyunsaturated fatty acids in your diet generally act to *decrease* your blood cholesterol level.

As Figure 10-2 shows, linoleic acid is a polyunsaturated fatty acid containing eighteen carbons and two areas of unsaturation. Because one area of unsaturation occurs at the *sixth* carbon atom from its tail end (also called omega for last carbon), linoleic acid is classed as a member of the omega-6 family of unsaturated fatty acids, a family discussed further in Chapter 13. Linoleic acid is very common in safflower oil, sunflower seed oil, and corn oil.

The classic studies of the effect of polyunsaturated fatty acids on blood cholesterol level were performed using linoleic acid. Their results are summarized by the following formula:

Each 1 percent increase in the calories from linoleic acid in the diet produces a decrease in the blood cholesterol level of about 1.5 mg/dl.

For example, if you increased the linoleic acid content of your diet from 5 percent to 10 percent of total calories, you might expect your blood cholesterol level to fall about 7.5 mg/dl. Once again, this is an average.

In the next chapter, you will learn how to increase the amount of linoleic acid in your diet. This increase will be a moderate one, since we now think that too much polyunsaturated fat in the diet may have possible long-term harmful effects, among them gall bladder disease, a decrease in the good HDL cholesterol, suppression of the immune system, and, just possibly, cancer of the intestines.

Fish oils are rich in polyunsaturated fatty acids that differ from linoleic acid. Because one of the areas of unsaturation in these fatty acids occurs at the *third* carbon atom from their omega (tail) end, they are called omega-3 fatty acids. Owing to the recent interest in omega-3 fatty acids and fish oils, Chapter 13 has been devoted to this subject.

How Monounsaturated Fat Affects Your Cholesterol Level

The most common monounsaturated fatty acid is oleic acid (Figure 10-2), which is plentiful in olive oil and canola oil. In earlier studies, monounsaturated fats seemingly had no effect on the blood cholesterol level, but recent studies reveal a more complex picture.

Drs. Mattson and Grundy studied twenty hospitalized men with an average blood cholesterol level of 263 mg/dl. They were fed three liquid diets in which the predominant fatty acids were either saturated (Sat), monounsaturated (Mono), or polyunsaturated (Poly); other nutrients were held constant. The fats in these diets made up 40 percent of total calories, and consisted of either palm oil (Sat), high-oleic safflower oil (Mono), or high-linoleic safflower oil (Poly).

As expected, the cholesterol levels were highest for the Sat diet (Figure 10-5), the first one administered. When the twelve men with normal triglyceride levels were changed to the Mono diet, their blood cholesterol and LDL cholesterol levels fell about 13 and 18 percent, respectively. When they were changed to the Poly diet, their blood cholesterol and LDL cholesterol levels measured 16 and 17 percent lower, respectively, than for the Sat diet. The Poly and Mono

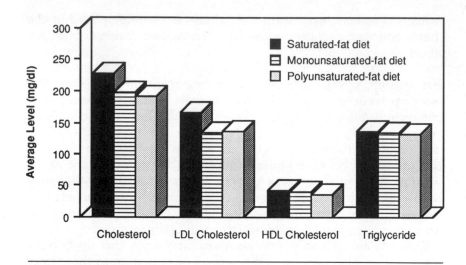

Fig. 10-5. Effects of three diets on blood lipid and lipoprotein levels.
Data plotted from F. Mattson and S. M. Grundy, *Journal of Lipid Research* 26 (1985): 194.

diets were about equally effective in lowering LDL cholesterol levels. The Poly diet's apparent superiority in lowering blood cholesterol masks the fact that it *lowered HDL cholesterol* almost 10 percent. The Mono diet did not produce this undesired fall in HDL.

Eight of the twenty men had a blood triglyceride problem. These eight experienced slightly lesser decreases in their blood cholesterol and LDL levels on average than the twelve men with normal triglyceride levels. Moreover, the eight varied considerably in their responses, with some showing no change and others even showing increases in their total and LDL cholesterol levels. *These findings emphasize a major theme of this book, namely the importance of genetic factors.* If under controlled conditions the same diet lowers one person's cholesterol levels and raises another's, genetic differences between the two persons must be responsible.

That is why it is important for you to have the levels of cholesterol, triglyceride, and lipoproteins in your blood measured as part of your general health assessment. If genetically transmitted abnormalities are found in your blood, the effect of dietary changes on these abnormalities must be determined and monitored by your doctor.

In another study in a hospital ward, Dr. Scott Grundy compared the effects of three different liquid diets on eleven patients with an average blood cholesterol level of 251 mg/dl. One was a Low-Fat diet (only 20 percent of calories as fat, even stricter than the Step Two diet in the next chapter); in this diet equal amounts (6.7 percent) of calories were from saturated, monounsaturated, and polyunsaturated fat, 63 percent from carbohydrate, and 17 percent from protein. The second was a High-Sat diet, with 40 percent of the calories from fat rich in saturated fatty acids; and the third was a High-Mono diet, with 40 percent of the calories from fat rich in monounsaturated fatty acids.

Compared to the High-Sat diet, both the High-Mono and Low-Fat diets resulted in considerable reductions in the average LDL cholesterol level (21 percent and 15 percent, respectively). The reduction in the average HDL cholesterol was about 6 percent on the High-Mono diet, compared to 24 percent on the strict Low-Fat diet. (The moderate low-fat diet recommended for you in the next chapter should not decrease your HDL level.) The triglyceride levels were higher on the Low-Fat diet than on the High-Sat or High-Mono diets.

The above study suggests that monounsaturated fatty acids are acceptable and even desirable sources of unsaturated fats. In this regard, several companies are developing oils that are higher in monounsaturated fats relative to polyunsaturated fats. For example, canola oil (Puritan®), which is a variety of rapeseed oil, contains about 58 percent monounsaturated fat, 35 percent polyunsaturated fat, and very little saturated fat. All the recipes presented on pp. 325–369 use canola oil as the source of unsaturated fat.

Other Dietary Influences on Your Cholesterol Level

Lecithin. You may have read that lecithin capsules will "clean the cholesterol from your system." Lecithin is a phospholipid commonly found in food. Dietary supplements of lecithin given to both animals and humans have produced conflicting reports. Since it is unclear at this time whether or not dietary lecithin will reduce the blood cholesterol level, dietary supplements of lecithin cannot be recommended.

Protein. In the next chapter you will learn how to cut down on cholesterol-containing foods from animal sources and to eat more cholesterol-free foods from plant sources. Less of your protein will come from animal foods and more from plant foods. The total amount of protein in your diet will remain the same, however, and you will eat a balanced diet containing all the essential amino acids you need.

Some doctors in the cholesterol field have reported that plant protein, particularly from soybeans, may help to lower the blood cholesterol level. However, soybeans contain other nutrients such as water-soluble fiber, and it has not yet been conclusively shown that plant protein *by itself* is effective in lowering blood cholesterol levels.

Carbohydrates. Fiber is found in certain kinds of carbohydrates. Some fibers of this sort are water-soluble and may help to lower your blood cholesterol level if taken in conjunction with a low-saturated-fat, low-cholesterol diet. Chapter 12 reviews the effect of water-soluble fibers such as oat bran on the blood cholesterol level and shows how you can increase the amount of water-soluble fiber in your diet.

Summary

1. A decrease in dietary cholesterol of 100 mg per 1,000 calories will produce, on average, a fall in the blood cholesterol level of about 10 mg/dl.

2. For each 1 percent decrease in calories from dietary saturated fats, there will be on average a fall in the blood cholesterol level of almost 3 mg/dl.

3. For each 1 percent increase in calories from dietary polyunsaturated fats, there will be on average a fall in the blood cholesterol level of about 1.5 mg/dl.

4. The effects of these three dietary changes are cumulative; a total decrease of about 10 to 15 percent in blood cholesterol is usually produced by a suitable low-fat, low-cholesterol diet. Thus is an average. Individual results will vary, depending on genetic constitution and former diet. Some people, particularly those with genetically determined blood lipid problems, respond very little or in unexpected ways to dietary changes.

5. Polyunsaturated fats tend to lower HDL cholesterol. Monounsaturated fats may be used in place of polyunsaturated fats and have no significant effect on HDL cholesterol.

6. The cholesterol, saturated fats, monounsaturated fats, and polyunsaturated fats in the foods you eat are often hidden. A working knowledge of the fat content of various foods is necessary if you are to make appropriate dietary changes.

Your Action Plan Diet

How can you enjoy eating and still lower your blood cholesterol level? Follow the Action Plan of this chapter for a healthful, nutritious, and well-balanced diet. Substitution is the key. Substitute foods low in total fat, saturated fat, and cholesterol for foods high in these fats. You will learn how to shop wisely, to read labels, to prepare delicious foods properly, and what to do when you eat in a restaurant. And, to top it all off, your diet will contain plenty of high-quality protein and will be higher in fiber than the standard American diet. Ample amounts of fresh fruits and vegetables will add zest and also supply minerals and vitamins that you need.

After you have read this chapter, if you have any questions about the amount of total fat, saturated fat, or cholesterol in any of your favorite foods, you can find the answers in the Food Tables at the back of the book. Beverages, candies, cereals, chips and snacks, entrees, frozen meals, dairy products, desserts, cookies, fast foods, pizza, margarines, salad dressings, crackers, rolls, vegetables, fruits, meat, fish and poultry, nuts, luncheon meats, soups, sauces and gravies, soybean products—most of the commonly eaten foods are listed there. If you have a question about some other food and cannot find the answer elsewhere, write me a letter and I'll try to help.

How much will this Action Plan lower your blood cholesterol? Depending on your current diet, your current cholesterol level, and your genetic makeup, you can expect an average fall of about 20 to 40 mg/dl, or about 10 to 15 percent. Remember that if you have one of the inherited conditions reviewed in Chapters 7, 8, and 9, or if you already have coronary heart disease, you may not respond the same way to this diet as most people; and that even if you do respond well, you may still need attention from your doctor, including the possible prescription of one or more drugs.

Table 11-1. Step One and Step Two Diets to Reduce Your
Blood Cholesterol Level

Nutrient	Step One diet	Step Two diet
Fat	Below 30%	Below 30%
Saturated	Below 10%	Below 7%
Polyunsaturated	10%	10%
Monounsaturated	10–15%	10–15%
Cholesterol (mg/day)	Below 300	Below 200
Carbohydrate	50–60%	50–60%
Protein	10–20%	10–20%

Source: Adult Treatment Panel, National Cholesterol Education Program,
National Heart, Lung, and Blood Institute, National Institutes of Health,
Arch. Intern. Med. 148 (1988): 36–69.
  Note: Percentages are percent of total calories.

Your Action Plan starts with a moderate low-fat diet, called the
Step One diet. The Step One diet is recommended by the National
Cholesterol Education Program's Expert Panel on Detection, Evaluation, and Treatment of High Blood Cholesterol in Adults (Adult
Treatment Panel), chaired by Dr. DeWitt Goodman of Columbia
University. As summarized in Table 11–1, it specifies an intake of
saturated fat of less than 10 percent of calories, total fat of less than
30 percent of calories, and dietary cholesterol of less than 300 milligrams per day. The American Heart Association's more recent rec-
ommendation for a low-fat diet is identical to that of the Adult Treatment Panel. As you adopt this Step One diet, you will find that many
of the suggestions made here for improving your nutrition are also
appropriate for your children, provided they are healthy and at least
two years old.

Millions of adult Americans (one in four) have a high blood cholesterol level (above 240 mg/dl). If you are such a person, you may require the Adult Treatment Panel's more restrictive Step Two diet
(Table 11-1), which further reduces saturated fat intake to less than
7 percent of calories and dietary cholesterol to less than 200 mg/day.
If your blood cholesterol level is still high after the Step One diet,
the Step Two diet is recommended. If you are overweight, weight loss
is promoted in both diets by eliminating excess calories.

Before modifying your diet, find out what your blood cholesterol
level is. If it is high (over 240 mg/dl) or borderline high (200–240 mg/
dl), discuss the matter with your personal physician. *In public
screening programs, the Adult Treatment Panel recommends that*

*all persons with a blood cholesterol level above 200 mg/dl be re-
ferred to their physician for remeasurement and evaluation.*

Your doctor will probably recommend a lipid profile, for which
you will need to fast overnight. This repeat blood test will measure
your total cholesterol, HDL cholesterol, and triglyceride levels, and
your LDL level can then be estimated by dividing the triglyceride
level by 5 to get your VLDL level, adding this number to your HDL
level, and subtracting the sum from your blood cholesterol level. Undesirable, borderline, and desirable ranges for these levels are discussed in Chapter 5; they are summarized in Table 11-2.

If some of your levels are in the undesirable range, a genetic condition may be the reason; or there could be some other underlying
health problem. Your doctor can determine whether you have another condition such as diabetes, thyroid disease, or liver or kidney
disease that may be contributing to (or even causing) your high cholesterol or triglyceride levels.

Your physician will also consider the other risk factors for coronary heart disease reviewed for you in Chapter 5. Briefly, these include male sex, a positive family history of premature (before age 55)
coronary heart disease, cigarette smoking, high blood pressure, diabetes, and obesity. As we have seen, the combination of a high or
borderline high blood cholesterol level with other risk factors can
double or even triple your risk of coronary heart disease. If you have
such a combination, the diet reviewed for you here will be a very
important first step to reduce your risk.

Your diet is vitally important to your health, and dietary requirements will vary from person to person. Thus it is important that you
speak with your doctor about your own individual needs before
starting the Step One diet. This is particularly true if you are already
under medical care for any illness, if you are over 65, or if the diet is
being considered for your child.

Table 11-2. Desirable, Borderline, and Undesirable Levels of
Cholesterol, LDL Cholesterol, HDL Cholesterol, and Triglyceride in
Adults (mg/dl)

Lipid	Desirable	Borderline	Undesirable
Cholesterol	Below 200	200–239	240 or higher
LDL cholesterol	Below 130	130–159	160 or higher
HDL cholesterol	Above 45	35–45	Below 35
Triglyceride	Below 150	150–249	250 or higher

ªThis figure may be too low. Some researchers consider up to 500 mg/dl to be borderline.

Goals of the Step One Diet

The Step One diet is a good idea for all healthy Americans above the age of two. If you have an LDL cholesterol level above 130 mg/dl (or some other undesirable or borderline lipid level, as shown in Table 11-2), it is an even better idea. Perhaps you have already modified your diet to some extent. If so, this chapter will help you determine how successful you have been. In any event, since the food products that are available to help you follow this diet are changing rapidly, I believe you will find this chapter's updated information useful.

Goal #1: Reduce your total dietary fat. Your first goal will be to decrease your average daily intake of total fat to less than 30 percent of calories. The average American consumes about 90 grams of fat per day; at nine calories per gram of fat, this is 810 calories from fat. Thus in an 1,800-calorie diet, 45 percent (810 divided by 1,800) of the total calories would come from fat. If you reduce the 90 grams of fat per day to 60, only 540 calories are from fat; divide by 1,800 and the percent of calories from fat is now decreased to 30 percent.

The formula that was used to make these calculations for you was:

Percent of calories from fat =
(Total grams of fat per day × 9 calories per gram) ÷
Total calories per day

The Food Tables list the grams of total fat and saturated fat in many of the foods that we commonly eat.

Goal #2: Reduce your dietary saturated fat. A decrease in total dietary fat is also achieved by decreasing saturated fat and replacing it, in part, with unsaturated fat. Many Americans eat about 15 to 20 percent of their total calories as saturated fat. A decrease in saturated fat intake to less than 10 percent of calories will produce an average fall of about 15 to 30 mg/dl in your blood cholesterol, depending on how much saturated fat you are now eating. For example, if you followed an 1,800-calorie Step One diet, you would eat about 60 grams of total fat. Saturated fat should be no more than 20 grams to meet the guidelines. Since the saturated fat allowance varies with caloric intake, here is a quick guide for you:

Total calories per day	Grams of saturated fat per day	Total calories per day	Grams of saturated fat per day
1,200	13	2,000	22
1,500	17	2,400	27
1,800	20	2,600	28

Goal #3: Increase your dietary polyunsaturated fat. On the Step One diet, the average consumption of polyunsaturated fat is increased from about 4.5 percent of total calories to no more than 10 percent of the total calories, providing, on average, an additional expected fall of about 5 mg/dl of blood cholesterol.

In earlier chapters and perhaps elsewhere you have seen references to "P/S ratio," a shorthand term for the ratio of polyunsaturated fat to saturated fat. On the Step One diet outlined below, it will not be necessary for you to compute the P/S ratio in your diet. By simply following my suggestions, you will end up with a suitable P/S ratio of about 1.0.

As noted in Chapter 10, recent evidence indicates that monounsaturated fats lower blood total and LDL cholesterol levels and do not decrease HDL cholesterol levels as much as polyunsaturated fats. Here you will learn what oils are high in monounsaturated fats, which make up about 10 to 15 percent of calories in the Step One diet. A balance of fats and oils that are enriched in monounsaturated fats or polyunsaturated fats is recommended.

Goal #4: Reduce your dietary cholesterol. Your goal will be to decrease the amount of cholesterol in your diet from the average consumed by most Americans (about 400–450 milligrams per day) to less than 300 mg per day. This will result in an additional fall of 5 to 10 mg/dl in your blood cholesterol. The stricter Step Two diet reduces your dietary cholesterol to less than 200 mg/day.

Goal #5: Increase the complex sugars and fiber in your diet. Americans generally eat too little fiber, and you will learn below how to double the amount of fiber in your diet. An increase in water-soluble fiber is particularly advantageous because it also lowers the blood cholesterol level. Part of the fat in your diet will be replaced with complex sugars (carbohydrates) found in fresh fruits, vegetables, and whole grain products.

Reading Labels

A good way to get started is to go through your refrigerator, freezer, and cupboards and gradually substitute foods that are low in total fat, saturated fat, and cholesterol for foods high in these nutrients. Practical hints for this operation are summarized for you in Tables 11-3, 11-4, and 11-5. You may have already made some of the more obvious changes. But there are many hidden sources of saturated fat and cholesterol in the foods you eat, particularly those made outside

Table 11-3. Practical Hints for Decreasing Saturated Fats in Your Diet

—Use skim or low-fat (1%) milk
—Replace butter with vegetable oil margarine
—Avoid food containing saturated vegetable oils such as palm oil and coconut oil
—Avoid solid cooking fats (usually hydrogenated soybean or cottonseed oil)
—Replace regular cheeses (Swiss, cheddar, American) with low-fat cheeses (part-skim mozzarella, low-fat American)
—Replace ice cream with ice milk, sherbet, or frozen low-fat yogurt
—Trim fat around meat, and use lean beef, pork, or veal
—Avoid meat products very high in fat (regular hamburger, hog dogs, bacon, sausage)
—Eat chicken and turkey (without skin) and fish more often
—Use turkey breast, lean roast beef, and lean ham in place of salami and bologna for luncheon meats
—Replace high-fat snacks (potato chips, peanuts, cashews, candy bars) with low-fat snacks (pretzels, home-made popcorn, carrots, fresh fruits)
—Have one meatless meal (pasta, fruit salad) at least once a week
—Avoid commercially made bakery products (doughnuts, cakes, cookies, pies)

Table 11-4. Practical Hints for Increasing Unsaturated Fats in Your Diet

—Use vegetable oils such as canola, sunflower, safflower, corn, soybean, and olive for cooking, frying, and baking
—Use vegetable oil margarine
—Use homemade salad dressing

Table 11-5. Practical Hints for Decreasing Cholesterol in Your Diet

—Decrease consumption of egg yolks to 1–2 per week
—Use egg whites or egg substitutes in cooking and baking
—Avoid commercially prepared cookies, cakes, and pies
—Limit portion sizes of lean meat, fish, and poultry to no more than six ounces per day
—Eliminate organ meats (liver, brain, kidney)

your home or commercially prepared, and some items in these tables may come as a surprise.

As you replace undesirable foods with nutritious, acceptable foods, it will be important for you *to read the labels carefully.* The label of a food product can provide a wealth of valuable and interesting information about the product. By order of the United States Food and Drug Administration (FDA), the label of every manufactured food must provide the following information: the product's name; the name and address of the manufacturer; the weight, measure, or count of the product package; and the ingredients, in descending order by weight.

When a food contains fat, the ingredient listing specifies what type of fat. If a predominantly saturated fat is listed, such as coconut or palm oil, avoid the food; when an unsaturated fat is listed, such as soybean oil, the food is probably a better choice.

You should also be on the lookout for foods that contain less total fat. Ingredients must be listed in decreasing order by weight. *When only ingredient information is provided, a general rule of thumb to help you select a low-fat item is to choose a product for which fat is one of the last of many ingredients listed.* If a saturated fat is one of the first three to five ingredients listed, or there are only two or three ingredients and one of them is fat, the product is probably not a good choice.

Flexi-labeling. One guideline that manufacturers may follow is called "flexi-labeling." By way of example, the label may state that "This product contains one or more of the following fats: corn oil, coconut oil, palm oil, lard." In such cases you do not really know which fat or fats are used in the product. When possible, avoid such products. When this is not possible, assume that the product contains the most saturated of the possible fats listed—in this case coconut oil (see Figure 11-1)—and proceed accordingly.

Labeling of health claim products. If a product makes any kind of health claim (such as low fat or low sodium), or if a nutrient has been added to the food, the label must provide the following information:

serving size

servings per container

calories per serving

protein per serving (in grams)

carbohydrate per serving (in grams)

fat per serving (in grams)

sodium per serving (in milligrams)

percentage of the US RDA (United States Recommended Daily Allowance) for protein, thiamine, niacin, riboflavin, Vitamin A, Vitamin C, calcium, and iron.

The US RDA is a standard level of nutrients that has been determined to cover the nutritional needs of a majority of the healthy

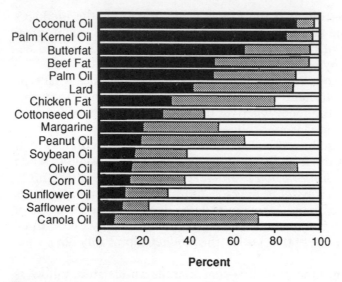

Fig. 11-1. Content in dietary fats of saturated fatty acids, monounsaturated fatty acids, and polyunsaturated fatty acids.

United States population. The manufacturer may also list additional nutrient information such as cholesterol or fiber content per serving, or the breakdown of polyunsaturated, saturated, and/or mono-unsaturated fats.

When nutrient information is listed, you have a much better idea of how much fat you will receive in one serving of food. Since 5 grams of fat is equivalent to 1 teaspoon of fat, you can visualize the quantity of fat you will be consuming when you eat one serving of that product.

Figure 11-2 offers a sample of the minimum information that must appear on a nutrition label for a product making a health claim. Since this particular label indicates that no fat is used in the product, you can safely assume that no saturated fat is present.

When looking at the label to see how much fat is listed, *look very carefully at the serving size.* For example, if the figures given are for a ½ cup serving but you usually eat one full cup, you must double

the amount of fat per serving to get the amount that you will actually consume.

Another item to consider is *what type of measure is used.* An
ounce of weight measure is not necessarily the same as an ounce of
fluid measure. For example, most cereal boxes list 1 ounce as the
serving size (in weight measure), but this ounce can be anything
from ⅓ cup (2½ fluid ounces) for a cereal like uncooked oatmeal to
1 cup (8 fluid ounces) of cornflakes.

Remember, not every package is required by the FDA to have a
nutrient listing on the label. A nutrient listing is not required on the
labels of foods that do not make a health claim; and manufacturers
of health claim products that follow certain standard federal guidelines or recipes (called "standards of identity") are also exempt.

Detailed labels. Some labels give even more specific details on the
amount of saturated fat and cholesterol in a serving. Figure 11-3
shows a label from a TV dinner that contains some of this optional
information.

When you eat this TV dinner you can expect to consume 6½ teaspoons of total fat (5 grams of fat per teaspoon), and about two teaspoons of this is from a saturated fat source. On an 1,800-calorie diet,

---

NUTRITION INFORMATION
(Per Serving)

Serving Size = 1 ounce
Servings per Container = 12

Calories	110	
Protein	2	grams
Carbohydrate	24	grams
Fat	0	grams
Sodium	140	milligrams

PERCENTAGE OF U.S. RECOMMENDED
DAILY ALLOWANCES (U.S. RDA)*

Protein	2
Thiamine	8
Niacin	2

*Contains less than 2 percent of US RDA for
Vitamin A, Vitamin C, Riboflavin, Calcium,
and Iron

Fig. 11-2. Sample nutrient listing for a health claim product.

NUTRITION INFORMATION
(Per Serving)

Serving Size = 8 ounces
Servings per Container = 1

Calories 560	Fat .... 33 gm	
Protein .... 23 gm	Polyunsaturated .... 2 gm	
Carbohydrate .... 43 gm	Saturated................ 9 gm	
	Cholesterol*	
	(20 mg/100 gm) mg/100 ... 40 mg	
	Sodium (365 mg/100 gm) ... 830 mg	

PERCENTAGE OF U.S. RECOMMENDED
DAILY ALLOWANCES (US RDA)

Protein 35	Riboflavin 15
Vitamin A 35	Niacin 25
Vitamin C (Ascorbic Acid) 10	Calcium 2
Thiamine (Vitamin B1) 15	Iron 25

*Information on Fat and Cholesterol content is provided for individuals who, on the advice of a physician, are modifying their total dietary intake of Fat and Cholesterol.

Fig. 11-3. Nutritional information for a TV dinner.

your daily allotment of saturated fat is 20 grams; and 9 grams, or almost half, would come from this TV dinner alone. *This is not a wise food choice when following a low-total-fat, low-saturated-fat diet.* In addition you will consume 40 mg of cholesterol.

Quick and helpful general guidelines for reading labels. The key words listed in Table 11-6 can guide you in determining whether a given food product is a good choice or not. When the nutrient information is listed, some general guidelines are as follows:

TOTAL FAT: For side dishes or snacks, look on the label for 2–3 grams of fat (or less) per serving; for entrées, 10 grams or less.

CHOLESTEROL: For side dishes, desserts, or snacks, look for 20 or fewer milligrams (mg) per serving. If a product is labeled "less cholesterol," look for 75 percent less cholesterol than the product it replaces.

SATURATED FAT: Look for less than one-third of the total fat to be from a saturated source. The lower the quantity of saturated fat in the product, the better.

CALORIES: If you are trying to lose weight, look for caloric information. A low-calorie product is one that contains 40 or fewer calories per serving. When purchasing a product that claims it is low in calories, aim at one-third fewer calories than the food it replaces.

SODIUM: A product labeled as "low sodium" will contain 140 milligrams (mg) or fewer per serving. A product labeled as "very low sodium" will contain 35 milligrams or fewer per serving.

FIBER: Look for 2 or more grams of fiber per serving (the label will not tell you whether the fiber is water-soluble or water-insoluble).

In addition, the American Heart Association has come up with guidelines to help you determine the acceptable amount of total fat for specific foods. These are listed in Table 11-7.

As you replenish your refrigerator, freezer, and cupboards with acceptable foods, you should increase the amount of fresh fruits and vegetables and other foods higher in fiber, notably certain cereals and grains such as oat bran. By substituting lean meat, fish, and poul-

Table 11-6. Key Words on Food Labels

Acceptable ingredients:

Canola oil	Olive oil
Carob powder	Safflower oil
Cocoa powder	Sesame oil
Corn oil	Skim milk
Diglycerides	Soybean oil
Hydrolyzed ingredients	Soybean oil, partially
Monoglycerides	hydrogenated
Nonfat dried milk solids	Sunflower oil

Unacceptable ingredients:

Bacon fat	Hardened fat
Beef fat	Hydrogenated fat or oil
Butter	Lard
Chicken fat	Meat fat
Chocolate, real	Milk chocolate
Chocolate, imitation	Palm or palm kernel oil
Cocoa butter	Shortening
Coconut	Turkey fat
Coconut oil	Vegetable fat (may be coconut
Cream and cream sauces	or palm)
Egg and egg-yolk solids	Vegetable shortening
	Whole milk solids

Table 11-7. Acceptable Amounts of Total Fat in Selected Foods

Food	Fat content (grams)	Food	Fat content (grams)
Cheese	2-3 per ounce (best choice)	Main dish	
		Canned	10 per 2 cups
	4-5 per ounce[a]	Frozen	10 per dinner
Crackers	3 per ounce	Pasta	1 per ½ cup
Desserts		Sauces	1 per serving
Cake or pie	4 per serving	Soups	3 per cup
Cookies	3 per ounce	Yogurt	0 per cup (best choice)
Frozen (dairy)	3 per ½ cup		
Pudding	1 per ½ cup		2–3 per cup

[a]6–10 grams per ounce if made with polyunsaturated oils.

try for fatter meals and substituting vegetable protein for some animal protein, you will get more than enough high-quality protein in your diet.

Changing the Fat Content of Your Diet

Your diet contains fats with various combinations of saturated fatty acids, polyunsaturated fatty acids, and monounsaturated fatty acids (Figure 11-1). In general, those rich in saturated fatty acids must be reduced and replaced by those low in saturated fatty acids and higher in monounsaturated and polyunsaturated fatty acids. Reducing saturated fat intake is probably the most important aspect of change in the American diet to lower blood cholesterol and LDL cholesterol levels.

Eating less saturated fat. How can you reduce the amount of saturated fat in your diet? Let's start with the useful hints listed in Table 11-3. Saturated fats are found mostly (but not exclusively) in animal products. Examples include the fat in and around beef, pork, lamb, and veal, and in dairy products such as butter, whole milk, cheese, and ice cream.

Three oils not of animal origin, palm oil, palm kernel oil, and coconut oil, are also important sources of saturated fats. These plant fats, which are just as saturated as animal fats, are commonly used in commercially available baked products (such as doughnuts, cakes, cookies, and pies), and as primary fats in nondairy products (such as whipped topping or cream substitutes). Cocoa butter and many solid cooking fats are other examples of saturated fat. Palm oil, palm kernel oil, and coconut oil can even be found in some commercially available cereals and crackers. These are oils to watch out for in reading labels.

As noted in Chapter 10, the saturated fatty acid called stearic acid does not appear to raise the blood cholesterol level and may even tend to lower it. Large amounts of stearic acid are found in cocoa butter, used to make chocolate, and in beef fat. Unfortunately, these fats also contain other saturated fats that do raise the blood cholesterol level, and beef contains cholesterol. The bottom line is that cocoa butter and beef fat are still restricted on your Action Plan diet.

Eating more unsaturated fat. Chapter 10 discusses the nature and chemical makeup of polyunsaturated and monounsaturated fats. Among the more common dietary fats, sunflower oil, safflower oil, corn oil, and soybean oils are polyunsaturated; olive oil and canola oil are monounsaturated.

There is now less emphasis on increasing polyunsaturated fats in a diet designed to lower the blood cholesterol level than there used to be. For one thing, we now know that people in countries such as Italy, Greece, and Israel, where the prevalence of coronary heart disease is half that in America, use polyunsaturated fats moderately rather than in large quantities. For another, as noted in Chapter 10, recent studies suggest that eating too much polyunsaturated fat may have certain detrimental effects, from decreasing your HDL cholesterol level to possibly causing intestinal cancer.

The emphasis now is on increasing both polyunsaturated and monounsaturated fats, the former only to about the level consumed in the Mediterranean countries. The best way to do this is to use appropriate vegetable oils for cooking, frying, and baking, and to use vegetable oil margarine and homemade salad dressing. Fats rich in monounsaturated fatty acids include olive oil, canola oil, and peanut oil (Figure 11-1); a sunflower oil that is high in monounsaturated fat is being developed.

One caution about peanut oil. Peanut oil does contain ample amounts of monounsaturated fats, but also contains more saturated fats than more acceptable vegetable oils. Peanut butter, peanuts, and peanut oil should be used in moderation.

Fish oils are high in polyunsaturated fats and contain two highly unsaturated fatty acids called eicosapentaenoic acid (or EPA) and docosahexaenoic acid (DHA). Because recent studies have shown benefits of fish oils on the incidence of coronary heart disease, I have written a separate chapter on this subject (Chapter 13). For reasons made clear in that chapter, I do not recommend that you take fish oil capsules. But eating fish caught in cold waters at least twice a week is a good nutritional way for you to get some fish oils in your diet.

Eating less cholesterol. Cholesterol is present in the cells of all animal products, but some foods of animal origin contain more cholesterol than others. One small egg yolk contains approximately 210 mg of cholesterol. This new figure was provided to me by Jacob Exler, Ph.D. of the Human Nutrition Information Services, United States Department of Agriculture. It is lower than the 270 mg heretofore used by most authorities, but alas, it is still too much cholesterol. Your consumption of eggs, either in a main dish such as scrambled eggs or in cooking and baking, needs to be reduced to one to two a week. In the Step One diet, your total daily cholesterol intake is reduced to less than 300 mg per day. If you eat one egg a day, you have already almost used up your daily allotment of dietary cholesterol. *It is therefore important for you to use egg whites or egg substitutes in cooking and baking.*

In recipes, two egg whites equal one whole egg. Many commercially prepared cookies, cakes, and pies are made with whole eggs, and these items will need to be replaced with homemade cookies, cakes, and pies in which egg whites or appropriate egg substitutes have been used. An appropriate vegetable oil will also need to be substituted for shortening. If you don't have the time to prepare homemade foods, you will need to read labels very carefully. A list of some acceptable commercial cookies, crackers, and baked goods is provided in Table 11-8.

Organ meats such as liver, brain, and kidney are exceedingly high in cholesterol. It's best to eliminate them from your diet. Did you know that lean meat, fish, and poultry all contain about the same amount of cholesterol (Figure 11-4)? Since that is quite a lot, you will need to limit your portion size to keep your total daily cholesterol intake less than 300 mg per day. For example, your combined breakfast, lunch, and dinner allotment for lean meat, fish, and poultry should not exceed six ounces cooked per day.

How can you determine how much "cooked meat" you are eating? *A deck of cards is the size of about three ounces of "cooked meat."* If you eat a six-ounce portion of lean meat, fish, or poultry for dinner, your lunch should be meatless. For increased protein, your lunch can include one-half cup of beans, perhaps in a soup. Or you may choose to eat three ounces of meat or fish at lunch and three ounces at dinner. In either case, you should eat a meatless breakfast, such as cereal and toast.

Table 11-8. Some Commercial Cookies, Crackers, and Baked Goods Containing 30 Percent or Less of Calories from Fat

COOKIES

Archway
  Old Fashioned Molasses
  Date Oatmeal
  Apple Oatmeal
  Oatmeal Rounds

Sunshine
  Animal Crackers
  Golden Fruit Raisin Biscuit
  Lemon Coolers
  Gingersnaps
  Honey Grahams

Nabisco
  Honey Maid Grahams
  Fig, Apple, Blueberry, Cherry,
    and other Newtons
  Gingersnaps
  Barnum's Animal Crackers
  Pantry Molasses
  Social Tea Biscuits
  Nilla Wafers
  Devils Food Cakes
  National Arrowroot Biscuit

Lance
  Fig Bar
  Choc-o-Lunch
  Van-o-Lunch
  Apple Cinnamon Cookie
  Strawberry Cookie
  Blueberry Cookie

FFV
  Devils Food Trolley Cake

Keebler
  Cinnamon Crisps

Health Valley
  Peanut Butter
  Oatmeal Jumbos

LU
  Les Petit-Beurre
  Milk Lunch Cookies

Rippin' Good
  Cookie Jar Assortment
  Lemon Crisp

CRACKERS

Sunshine
  Krispy Saltine
  Oyster Crackers

Lance
  Captains Wafers
  Rye Twins
  Sesame Twins
  Wheat Twins
  Wheatwafers
  Saltines
  Oyster Crackers
  Melba Toast: all flavors
    and brands

FFV
  Ocean Crisp
  Sesame Crisp
  Sesame Crisp Wafers

Hain
  Wheat Rye

Manischewitz
  All matzos except egg-type

OTC
  Oyster and Chowder

Pepperidge Farms
  English Water Biscuits
  Sesame Crackers
  Goldfish, pretzel-type
  Snack Sticks: Rye and
    Pumpernickel

Ry-Krisp
  Original
  Seasoned

Stella D'Oro Dietetic
  Bread Sticks

Waldorf
  Low Sodium Crackers

Finn Crisp
  All flavors

Kavli
  Thin Bread

Wasa
  Fiber

Table 11-8 (*continued*)

Nabisco	Golden Rye
Oysterettes	Hearty Rye
Premium Saltines	Light Rye
Triscuits	Rice Cakes: all flavors and
Uneeda Biscuits	brands
Zwieback Toast	

COMMERCIAL BAKED GOODS

SNACK CAKES	FROZEN CAKES
Hostess: Lil' Angels	*Weight Watchers*
FROZEN MUFFINS	Strawberry Cheesecake
Pepperidge Farms	Pound Cake with Blueberries
Carrot Walnut	*Betty Crocker*
Cinnamon Swirl	Applesauce Raisin
	Snackin' Cake

Sources. Cookies: *Nutrition Action Newsletter* 14, no. 10 (Dec. 1987), p. 10. Crackers: Giant Food Corp., *Eat for Health Food Guide* (1988). Cakes and muffins: *Nutrition Action Newsletter* 15, no. 5 (June/July 1988), p. 10.

The Six Food Groups

The Step One Diet contains the six basic food groups:

1. Vegetables and fruits
2. Bread, cereal, and starchy foods
3. Milk and cheese
4. Meat, poultry, and seafood
5. Fats and oils
6. Simple sugars and alcohol

A balanced and nutritious diet should contain foods from each of the first five. The sixth group, sugars and alcohol, supplies only calories and should be used in moderation. *Within each of these groups you can substitute delicious low-fat, low-cholesterol foods for those high in fat and cholesterol when you shop and cook, or when you eat out.*

Food Group # 1: Vegetables and Fruits

In general, on the Step One diet you should eat three or more servings of fruit per day and three or more servings of vegetables. A serving is approximately one-half cup. Fruit and vegetables are low in fat and calories and contain no cholesterol. This food group contains ample sources of both fat-soluble and water-soluble vitamins, and of trace minerals important for good health. Fruits and vegetables are also naturally low in sodium (except for canned vegetables), often high in potassium, and high in fiber. Table 11-9 lists foods from this group that are good sources of vitamin C and the fat-soluble vitamin, vitamin A.

Most vegetables and fruits are therefore excellent choices for your diet. *Coconut is an exception because of its high content of saturated fat.* Olives and avocados are quite high in total fat, and are

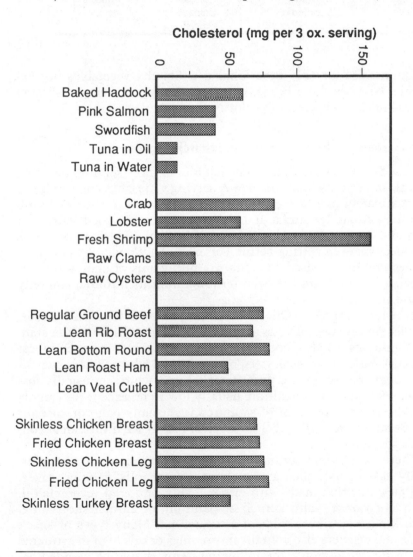

Fig. 11-4. Cholesterol content of fish, shellfish, meat, and poultry.

Table 11-9. Vegetables and Fruits High in Vitamins C and A

Vegetables	Fruits	Vegetables	Fruits
VITAMIN C		VITAMIN A	
Asparagus	Cantaloupe	Broccoli	Cantaloupe
Broccoli	Grapefruit	Carrots	Peaches
Cabbage	Oranges	Pumpkin	Apricots
Spinach	Strawberries	Spinach	
Tomatoes		Squash	

recommended for only occasional use. Starchy vegetables (for example, potatoes, lima beans, corn, green peas, winter squash, and pumpkin) are a bit higher in calories than many vegetables.

Food Group #2: Bread, Cereal, and Starchy Foods

On the Step One diet, you should eat four or more servings of bread, cereal, and starchy foods per day. A serving varies, but one serving is approximately one-half cup cooked, or one average slice of bread. These foods are low in fat and cholesterol, contain good sources of iron and B vitamins, and can be high in fiber (Table 11-10). Some products are even getting better. For example, Wonder Bread is now cholesterol-free (it used to contain 5 milligrams of cholesterol per slice); all animal lard has been removed from its formula, and only liquid vegetable oil is used.

In general, your Step One diet will contain more foods like breads, cereals, and pastas, such as spaghetti and macaroni, than the standard American diet. Good grain selections include cracked wheat (bulgur), barley, cornmeal, grits, oats, rice, and wheat. Breads such as whole wheat, rye, raisin, pumpernickel, and white are usually low in fat. Hot and cold cereals are usually low in fat except for granola cereals, which have a lot of saturated fat, usually palm or coconut oil. Be sure to read the label on a cereal box to see if the cereal contains coconut oil.

There are a number of *hidden sources of saturated fat*. Commercially baked goods such as doughnuts, sweet rolls, cookies, cakes, and pies are often made with either highly saturated vegetable oil, such as coconut, palm kernel, or palm oil, or animal shortening; both kinds contribute a lot of saturated fat. Many types of snack foods and crackers also contain shortenings or oils high in saturated fat. In the bread group, the following items should be *avoided* because of their high fat or high cholesterol content:

Bagels made with eggs or cheese (regular bagels are all right), butter rolls, cheese breads, commercial doughnuts, muffins, sweet rolls, biscuits, waffles and pancakes, croissants, and egg breads.

Granola-type cereals that contain coconut or coconut oil, chow mein noodles, fried vegetables (except for stir-fried vegetables prepared at home in unsaturated oils), and vegetables made with a non-modified "cream" sauce.

Crackers made with coconut or palm oil or with commercial cheese, and butter crackers.

Soups made with cream (the saturated fat content of a variety of commercial soups is listed in the Food Tables).

Desserts commercially made from unacceptable fats.

On this last point, however, there is good news for you. Some commercial companies, among them Lance, are no longer using palm oil or coconut oil in their crackers and cookies. Signs are beginning to appear in the supermarkets and in labels and ads: "No palm oil used."

The proper preparation or selection of foods in the bread, cereal, and starchy foods group is clearly important in decreasing the total amount of fat, saturated fat, and cholesterol in your diet. On the negative side, this group is frequently an offender because of the hidden sources of saturated fat and cholesterol used in the preparation of these foods. On the positive side, appropriate selections from this food group can provide ample sources of B vitamins and iron and also increase the fiber content of your diet. Many of my patients have lowered their blood cholesterol levels by using the delicious, quick recipes from the bread, cereal, and starchy food group that you will find at the back of the book.

Table 11-10. Some Nutritious, Low-Fat Breads, Cereals, and Starches

Cereals	Breads	Grains
All-Bran	Matzo	Rice
Corn flakes	Pumpernickel	Oats
Fiber One	Rye	Grits
Grape-Nuts	White	
Oat flakes	Whole wheat	
Product 19	*Starches*	
Rice Krispies	Spaghetti	
Special K	Enriched noodles	
Total	Macaroni	
Shredded Wheat		

Fiber in the First Two Food Groups

Foods in the fruit and vegetable and bread, cereal, and starch groups are high in carbohydrates. These carbohydrates are usually composed of simple sugars, such as glucose, linked together in a chain to produce a complex sugar or carbohydrate. Fibers are also complex carbohydrates. The part of fruits, vegetables, and whole grains that is not digested, and therefore not absorbed, is referred to as dietary fiber, or alternatively as "bulk" in the diet or "roughage." *Fiber is found in the cell walls of plants, including their seeds, leaves, stems, skin, and roots.*

Fiber passes unchanged from your stomach into your small intestine and finally into your large intestine. Fiber is often used to combat constipation and to promote regular bowel habits. But some water-soluble dietary fibers such as oat bran, pectin (found in apples, oranges, and grapefruit), and guar gum (found in beans, peas, and lentils) also have a cholesterol-lowering effect (see Chapter 12). Water-insoluble fibers, such as wheat bran, do *not* lower the blood cholesterol level.

The best way to increase fiber in your diet is to eat a variety of fiber-rich foods every day, including fruits, vegetables, whole grain cereals, and breads. Where possible, choose foods close to the natural state: for example, whole oranges instead of orange juice, whole wheat bread instead of white bread. Eat the skins on such fruits and vegetables as apples, carrots, potatoes, and tomatoes. For breakfast eat cereals with more fiber: for example, oat bran, oatmeal, Fiber One®, All-Bran®, and Shredded Wheat®. Avoid presweetened cereals, which are high in calories and simple sugars and are often low in fiber. Lentils or dried beans can be added to your meals. Finally, when you choose breads and cereals, select those that are in the whole grain category.

When you increase the fiber in your diet, drink more liquids, especially water, to avoid abdominal discomfort and gas. Try to increase your dietary fiber slowly up to 20 grams a day and gradually work up to as high as 40 grams a day.

In summary, increasing the fiber content of your diet will provide the following benefits:

1. You may lower your blood cholesterol level by eating more water-soluble fiber such as oat bran, guar gum from legumes, and pectin.

2. Fiber can also help you lose weight (if necessary), by increasing that feeling of fullness.

3. By slowing the absorption of foods, you will get less hungry between meals. Increasing the water-insoluble fiber such as wheat bran in your diet will relieve constipation and facilitate the development of normal bowel habits.

In the Recipes section, you will find foods high in fiber such as Bran Banana Bread, Bran Muffins, Whole Wheat Bran Pancakes, Bean Stew, Cinnamon Oat Bran Muffins, Golden Pilaf, Overnight Coleslaw, and Three Bean Salad.

Food Group #3: Milk and Cheese

Two or more servings of dairy foods are recommended because these foods are rich in animal protein, calcium, and phosphorus and other minerals; provide B vitamins, such as niacin and riboflavin; and can provide vitamin A and vitamin D in the form of fortifications, usually to milk. In the Step One diet, *dairy foods should not be eliminated, especially in children, teenagers, and pregnant or breast-feeding women; people in these categories need approximately 32 ounces of milk per day, or a milk substitute such as yogurt, low-fat cheese, or low-fat cottage cheese. The key here is substitution of low-fat dairy products, which contain adequate amounts of all the above nutrients, for high-fat dairy products.* On your Step One diet you can use skim or low-fat (1 percent) milk, low-fat cheeses, and skim or low-fat yogurt.

For ice cream lovers there are some cholesterol-free, low-fat ice cream substitutes available. A list of acceptable nonfat and low-fat yogurts (and of unacceptable higher-fat yogurts) is found in Table 11-11, along with a list of convenient low-fat frozen desserts. The tofu dessert Tofutti® is high in polyunsaturated fat (corn oil) but is too high in calories from total fat.

If you are a cheese lover, the best choice of low-fat cheese contains two grams of fat per ounce or less. Since regular cheese contains from seven to ten grams of total fat per ounce, any cheese with only four or five grams per ounce is an improvement; but the lower you can go, the less saturated fat you will consume. There are also some acceptable cheese substitutes that are made from polyunsaturated fat (Table 11-12). Two ounces a day of low-fat cheese (about two slices) is acceptable on your Step One diet.

Use the above low-fat products in place of butter, cream, sour cream, ice cream, regular cheese, and whole milk (4 percent butterfat). Select imitation dairy products carefully, since many contain

Table 11-11. Nonfat and Low-Fat Yogurts, and Low-Fat Frozen
Desserts

Nonfat yogurts	Low-fat frozen desserts
Columbo Light	Columbo Frozen Yogurt
Dannon	Crystal Light Bar
LaYogurt-25	Dannon Frozen Yogurt
Weight Watchers	Dole Fruit 'n Cream Bar
Yoplait 150	Dole Fruit 'n Juice Bar
Low-fat yogurts	Elan Frozen Yogurt
Dannon, low-fat types	Fruit and juice bars
Gaymont	Fudgesicle
Giant Brand	Ice milk
Kemp's	Jello Brand Fruit Bar
Light 'n Lively	Jello Brand Fruit and Cream Bar
New Country	Low-fat frozen tofu desserts
Nordica	Minute Maid fruit and juice bars
Old Home	Popsicle
Sweet-n-Low	Shamitoff's Fruit and Cream Bar
Higher-fat yogurts (not recommended)	Shamitoff's Fruit and Juice Bar
	Sherbet, all flavors and brands
Breyers	Sorbet, all flavors and brands
Columbo, original	Squeeze Pops
Whitneys	Weight Watchers Frozen Dietary
Yoplait, original, custard-	Dessert
style, breakfast-type	Weight Watchers Treats
	Yogurt Tree Frozen Yogurt
	Yoplait Squeeze

coconut oil, a highly saturated fat; look instead for imitation dairy products and nondairy liquid creamers made from polyunsaturated fat. You may use sherbet, frozen low-fat yogurt, sorbet, or ice milk in place of ice cream.

Food Group #4: Meat, Poultry, and Seafood

Quality of protein in your diet. Foods in the meat, poultry, and seafood group are important sources of protein for you. A protein is made up of a chain of building blocks called amino acids. Of the 23 known amino acids, nine are termed "essential" because your body needs them and cannot manufacture them; you must get them from your food. Proteins from meat, poultry, or seafood have been termed "complete proteins" because each of them supplies all the essential amino acids.

Most people get the essential amino acids from some form of animal protein. Vegetarians can and do get them from other sources, but the Step One diet does *not* call for the elimination of meat, poultry, or seafood.

It does call for replacing a certain amount of animal protein with plant protein: for example, from whole grains, vegetables, and legumes. Plant protein foods by themselves are usually less complete than animal protein food, since some lack one or more of the essential amino acids; wheat protein, for example, is deficient in lysine. One exception is plant protein from soybeans, which is a "complete" protein and contains all the essential amino acids, although its content of methionine is relatively low. In summary, use both plant and animal protein in your diet.

Quantity of protein in your diet. As noted above, you should eat no more than six ounces of meat, poultry, and seafood per day (cooked weight). Does that give you enough protein? The total amount of protein recommended in the Step One diet is 10 to 20 percent of total calories, more than enough for an average man (ap-

Table 11-12. Low-Fat Cheeses

Low-fat cheeses (2 grams of fat per ounce)
  Chef's Delight
  Cottage cheese uncreamed 1% and 2% (½ cup serving)
  Countdown (Fischer)
  Lite-Line (Borden)
  Parmesan, grated (1 tablespoon per serving)
  Romano, grated (1 tablespoon per serving)
  Weight Watchers Slices

Reduced-fat cheeses (3–5 grams of fat per ounce)
  Cottage cheese, creamed, small or large curd (½ cup serving)
  Farmer's cheese, part-skim
  Iceland Part-Skim Cheese
  Kraft Natural Light
  Laughing Cow, reduced calorie
  Light 'n Lively (Kraft)
  Mozzarella, part-skim
  Pot cheese
  Weight Watchers, natural block

Skim milk cheeses with polyunsaturated oils added (5–9 grams of fat per ounce)
  Cheezola (Fisher)
  Golden Image (Kraft)
  Lo-Chol Light (Dorman)

Soybean-based cheeses (9 grams of fat per ounce)
  Soyco Kaas: Cheddar, Monterey, and Monterey with Jalapeño

proximately 55 grams of protein per day) or a growing child (approximately 40 grams a day).

By way of confirmation, to determine how many grams of protein you eat per day, you can multiply the percentage of protein in your diet by your daily caloric intake and divide by 4, the number of calories per gram of protein.

Total grams of protein per day =
    (Percent protein in diet × Total calories)
                                        ÷ 4 calories per gram

For example, on an 1,800-calorie diet containing the Step One diet average of 15 percent of total calories as protein, you would consume 270 calories (1,800 calories × 15 percent) from protein; dividing this figure by 4 calories per gram gives 67.5 grams of protein, well above the adult daily requirement. A child consuming 1,200 total calories and 15 percent calories from protein would be eating about 45 grams of protein.

We turn next to some practical tips for decreasing the amount of total fat, saturated fat, and cholesterol derived from animal products in your diet.

Substitute poultry, fish, and shellfish for red meat. In the meat, poultry, and seafood group, about one ounce of flesh averages seven grams of protein. If you consume six ounces of meat, poultry, or seafood per day, you have already eaten 42 grams of protein. You will also get additional protein from vegetable sources and dairy products. In general, *fish, shellfish, and poultry are preferable to red meats as sources of animal protein because they have less total fat, less saturated fat, and fewer calories* (Figure 11-5). Seafood and poultry do contain cholesterol, however (Figure 11-4), which is why the portion sizes recommended are the same as for lean meat.

Poultry. When poultry is eaten, the skin should be removed *before cooking*, since skin is mostly fat and the yellow "globs" under the skin need to be removed. The poultry should be broiled or baked, not fried. If you must have fried chicken, use a polyunsaturated or monounsaturated oil or vegetable oil margarine. You will find some excellent recipes for poultry dishes in the Recipes section.

Shellfish. Shellfish, such as crabs, lobster, oysters, scallops, and clams, can be eaten on your Step One diet, again in limited quantities. For example, since hard-shell crabs are a favorite of Baltimoreans, we have learned that approximately five hard-shell crabs can be consumed as the total daily allotment of animal protein on

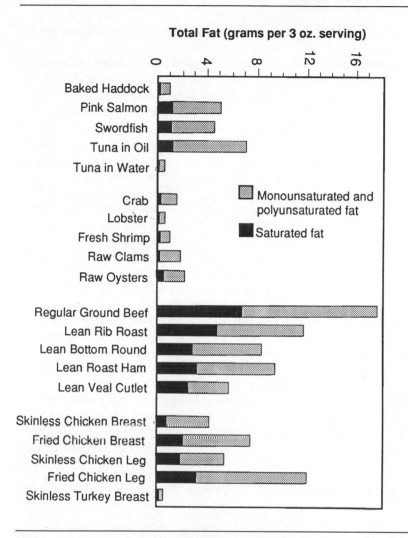

Total Fat (grams per 3 oz. serving)

Fig. 11-5. Fat content of fish, shellfish, meat, and poultry.

the Step One diet. Shrimp are higher in cholesterol than crab and lobster, and therefore should be used in smaller portions.

Beef. Your selection of beef is important. When buying beef that is *not* ground, "lean" on the label is supposed to indicate that the meat contains no more than 10 percent fat by weight, and "extra lean" that it contains no more than 5 percent fat by weight. These guidelines are from the U.S. Department of Agriculture, but not all stores follow this policy. Ask your butcher whether he follows these guidelines.

Important: the rules are completely different for ground beef or meat. According to the official policy of the USDA, ground beef can contain as much as 22.5 percent fat by weight and still be called lean or extra lean. Some labels specify the percentage. But probably the best thing to do is buy sirloin or round steak and have your butcher trim the fat and then grind it. This may give you a little more cholesterol than regular ground beef (Figure 11-4), but will give you much less saturated fat and total fat and is thus on the whole a much better choice.

Proper preparation of poultry, fish, and red meats. The proper cooking of animal proteins is very important to your intake of fat and cholesterol. Broiling or baking with a rack so that the juices fall away is preferable to frying. Before adding meat juices to stews, gravies, or soups, skim the fat off. To do this, leave the meat juices in the refrigerator; the fat will rise to the top and solidify, and then can be easily removed.

Luncheon meats and hot dogs. A special warning is necessary about luncheon meats and high-fat processed meat products, such as bologna, salami, corned beef, pastrami, frankfurters, and bacon. The fat content of various frankfurters is summarized for you in Table 11-13; these figures speak for themselves. If you use cold meats in sandwiches, use very lean ham, roast beef, or turkey breast. For example, Louis Rich® lean ham contains 2 grams of fat per ounce compared with bologna (8) and salami (6).

Sandwich fillings such as peanut butter (limit portion to one

Table 11-13. Fats and Calories in Frankfurters

Type of frankfurter	Serving size (ounces)	Calories per serving	Total fat per serving (grams)	Percent of calories from fat
Weight Watchers turkey	1.5	84	6.0	64%
Louis Rich turkey	1.5	103	8.5	74%
Louis Rich turkey-cheese	1.5	108	8.5	71%
Perdue chicken	2.0	140	11.0	71%
John Morrell beef	1.5	138	12.5	82%
Kirschner Extra Mild	1.5	142	12.5	79%
Oscar Mayer Wiener	1.5	144	13.5	84%
Oscar Mayer Bacon & Cheese	1.5	143	12.5	79%
Ball Park	2.0	174	16.5	85%

Source: *Tufts University Diet & Nutrition Letter* 4, no. 5 (July 1986).

tablespoon), tuna salad, chicken salad, and turkey salad are a good substitute for meat fillings. The mayonnaise in salad mixes does contain a small amount of cholesterol and saturated fat, but is high in unsaturated fats. The light versions of mayonnaise are just as good, especially for weight-conscious people and those who like a bit more mayonnaise in their salads.

Meat cuts and types to be avoided. Avoid:

—organ meats such as liver, kidney, heart, tongue, brains, sweet-breads, chitterlings, and gizzards

—cuts of beef that are graded prime, heavily marbled, or untrimmed; regular ground meat; rib roast; and spareribs

—pork spareribs; ground pork; shoulder, arm, or blade pork roast; bacon; canned deviled ham; smoked pork; and pork sausage of all kinds

—ground lamb and mutton

—breast riblets of veal

—commercially fried fish or shellfish; caviar

—poultry skin, domestic game such as goose or duck

—luncheon meats with more than 10% fat

If you need to limit further your consumption of total fat, saturated fat, and cholesterol (for example, in a Step Two diet), you can arrange to have meatless lunches or dinners starting with once a week at first and increasing to three times a week or more. Alternatives to meat include low-fat cheese, peanut butter (limit the serving to one tablespoon), and legumes (dried beans, peas, lentils, and soybean curd). Tofu is one example of soybean curd; tofu is different from Tofutti®. Such meat substitutes can be used effectively as a substitute for animal proteins. To ensure that you get all the essential amino acids you can include a small amount of some form of animal protein with the meatless meal, such as egg white or skim milk.

Food Group #5: Fats and Oils

The Step One diet calls for six to eight servings per day from the fats and oils group. One serving equals one teaspoon of fat or oil. The percentage of saturated, monounsaturated, and polyunsaturated fats in various types of fats and oils was summarized for you in Figure 11-1.

Use an acceptable vegetable oil margarine as your substitute for butter. The margarine should be made with a liquid oil such as safflower, sunflower, corn, or soybean oil as the first ingredient on the label. You can then use either the stick type, the tub type, or the liquid type. This simple step will decrease the amount of saturated fat and increase the unsaturated fat in your diet.

Since margarines are made from vegetable oil, they do not contain any cholesterol. In a butter/margarine blend, cholesterol is present owing to the butterfat content. *It is important to read the labels on the margarines and avoid those made with butterfat or lard.* For cooking, canola, corn, safflower, soybean, sunflower, or olive oil can be used. One caution, however, is that oils high in unsaturated fats should not be re-used. With repeated heating there is greater danger that the fats may become oxidized, and oxidized fats may cause damage to your blood vessels.

Avoid lard and solid cooking fats. Make your salad dressings with the unsaturated oils. You can also use many commercial salad dressings, but be sure to read the labels first.

Nuts are part of the fats and oils food group. Are they good or bad for you? On the whole, not wonderful, since they are very high in fat (Table 11-14). Cashews, macadamia nuts, and Brazil nuts are particularly high in saturated fat, and should be avoided. Walnuts are high in polyunsaturated fat, and peanuts contain an approximately equal amount of saturated and polyunsaturated fat. Commonly eaten nuts such as peanuts, walnuts, almonds, and pecans should be consumed in limited amounts, since they are high in both total fat and calories. How many can you eat? One tablespoon of chopped nuts equals one serving in the fats and oils group. For example, if you ate two tablespoons of chopped nuts, you would need to decrease your consumption of other fats or oils by two servings.

Food Group #6: Simple Sugars and Alcohol

In general, your Step One diet includes a decrease in the percent of calories from simple sugars, and an increase in calories from complex carbohydrates (Table 11-1). Simple sugars provide a source of energy for you, namely, four calories per gram, but little else in the way of food value. In contrast, complex carbohydrates can provide the same amount of energy but also can provide minerals, vitamins, and fiber.

Since the body can change simple sugars into fats called triglycer-

Table 11-14. Saturated Fat and Calorie Content of
Common Nuts

Type of nut	Saturated fat content (gm/oz)	Calories per ounce
Chestnuts, roasted	<1	70
Soybean kernels, roasted	<1	129
Almonds	1–2	167
Hazelnuts, dried	1–2	179
Peanuts, oil roasted	1–2	165
Pecans, dried	1–2	190
Pistachio nuts, dry roasted	1–2	172
Walnuts, English	1–2	182
Brazil nuts	>2	186
Cashews, dry roasted	>2	163
Macadamia nuts, oil roasted	>2	204

ide, a diet high in carbohydrates can increase the blood level of triglyceride. Therefore simple sugars such as table sugar, jams, jellies, syrups, honey, and candy should be consumed in moderation. Some companies such as Polaner and Smuckers have made available low-sugar jams that contain one-half the sugar of regular jams and that have no artificial sweeteners.

Alcohol that you drink is ultimately processed in your liver. Alcohol can be converted into triglyceride and especially needs to be consumed sparingly by people with a blood triglyceride problem (see Chapter 8). If you do not have a blood triglyceride problem, and are not trying to lose weight, moderate ingestion of alcohol (a can of beer, a glass of wine, or a mixed drink several times a week) is acceptable on the Step One diet. Alcohol apparently does raise your HDL cholesterol level (see Chapter 4), but this advantage is offset by its many disadvantages to those who drink a lot.

The calories in sweet snack foods add up fast, and these foods can also be hidden sources of total fat. For example, a doughnut contains 150 calories and is quite high in saturated fat and simple sugars. A 1½-ounce chocolate candy bar has 150 calories, and contains a significant amount of saturated fat and simple sugars. One 12-ounce can of a regular soft drink provides 150 calories from simple sugars, but no fat.

Recommended daily allowances from the six food groups are summarized in Table 11-15.

Table 11-15. Daily Allowances from the Six Food Groups in the Step One Diet

Food Group	Serving Size	Portion per Day
1. Vegetables and fruits	½ cup	3 or more servings each
2. Breads, cereals, and starchy foods	½ cup cooked, or 1 slice bread	4 or more servings
3. Milk and cheese	1 cup of milk or 1½ ounces of cheese	2 or more servings
4. Meat, poultry, and sea-food	—	at most 6 ounces cooked weight
5. Fats and oils	1 teaspoon	6–8 servings, minimizing saturated fats
6. Sugars and alcohol	—	in moderation only

Making Good Snack Food Choices

Snacks that are low in calories and fat include any number of raw vegetables such as celery, carrots, cauliflower, broccoli, mushrooms, zucchini, and fresh fruits such as oranges, apples, bananas, pears, melons, grapes, and pineapples. Popcorn made in an air popper contains few calories, and makes a nice snack food when judiciously combined with a vegetable oil margarine to provide some unsaturated fat. Pretzels and low-fat crackers such as matzos are good snack food choices. Unsweetened fruit juices and coffee or tea with no sugar are other acceptable alternatives. Skim milk, nonfat yogurt, and cereal with skim milk are also good choices. There are a wide variety of low-fat frozen desserts that can also be used as snacks (Table 11-11).

Hidden sources of calories and saturated fat are important to identify. For example, two ounces of peanuts (less than a handful) contains 322 calories, a cup of ice cream 270 calories, and both are also high in saturated fat. You can check out snacks on both counts in the Food Tables, not only in the section "Chips and Snacks," but also in some of the other sections.

Several products that are meant to be fat substitutes have been developed. One called Simplesse® is made by the NutraSweet Company, which also manufactures aspartame, an artificial sweetener. Simplesse is a "fake fat" made from protein derived from milk and egg whites. Billions of minute spheres are found in an ounce of Simplesse, giving the product the texture of fat. It feels smooth and rich to the tastebuds, but contains only 1⅓ calories per gram (fat contains 9). If approved by the Food and Drug Administration (FDA), Simplesse could be used to make artificial milk and dairy products such as butter, cheese, ice cream, and yogurt. One drawback of Simplesse is that it cannot be used in cooking and frying.

Another fat substitute, called Olestra®, *can* be used for frying and for baked products. Made by Procter and Gamble, Olestra contains about two-thirds "sucrose polyester," a large complex of sugar bound to oil that is not taken up by the intestine, and about one-third liquid vegetable oil. Like Simplesse, Olestra has not yet been approved by the FDA for general use. Unlike Simplesse, it contains calories, about one-third the number found in regular oils.

Should you use artificial fat products if and when they become available? The major drawback of many of them is that they have *no nutritional value.* In my view, you are better off changing your diet naturally by substituting regular low-fat foods for high-fat foods. Artificial foods might satisfy your tastebuds and lower your blood cholesterol level; but regular low-fat foods can do both these things and also satisfy your body's nutritional requirements. The choice seems clear to me.

Eating in Restaurants

More and more Americans these days are eating outside the home. If you eat in restaurants often, you will need to use extra care to minimize your consumption of saturated fat and cholesterol. Planning ahead—where you will eat, when you will eat, and especially what you will eat—is very important in following the diet.

In addition, you should feel free to ask what a dish consists of and how it is prepared, and to request reasonable substitutes for ingredients high in saturated fat and cholesterol. In Table 11-16 you will find some practical suggestions for ordering in a restaurant.

Fast food restaurants. Fast food restaurants usually offer a reasonable price with quick service for standardized items such as hamburgers, fried chicken, pizza, roast beef sandwiches, or fried fish. Fast food restaurants get about 40 percent of all money spent in restaurants (about $2.00 out of every $5.00 spent). Most fast foods are high in calories and saturated fat; many are also high in sugar, meaning more calories unaccompanied by other nutrients, and in sodium (a major component of salt).

The good news about fast food restaurants is that they are changing. Many now offer salad bars, baked potatoes, and sugar-free soft

Table 11-16. Practical Tips for Ordering Foods in a Restaurant

1. Better choices for preparing meat and fish:

Au jus	Boiled	Poached
Baked	Char-broiled	Roasted
Barbecued	Marinated	Steamed

Poor choices:

Au gratin	Casserole	Gravy
Bacon	Coconut	Hollandaise
Bearnaise	Creamed	Prime
Buttered	Escalloped	Sausage

Terms to question:

"Breaded": Is it fried? What type of fat is used?

"Broiled": Often butter is used in broiling; ask for fat to be left off

"Fried": What type of fat is used?

"Grilled": What type of fat is used?

"Seasoned": What type of fat is used?

"Specially prepared": What exactly does this mean?

2. Order salad dressings, sauces, and gravies served on the side.

3. Divide the meat portion into two servings instead of one large serving. Eat one and ask for a "doggie bag" to take the other home.

4. Ask for margarine instead of butter.

5. Ask for skim or low-fat milk to drink or use in coffee or tea.

6. Avoid rich cheese dishes and foods that are obviously high in egg, such as Quiche.

7. Ask for sherbet or fruit for dessert instead of rich pastries or ice cream.

drinks. A tossed salad consisting primarily of vegetables and pinto beans, or a plain baked potato, adds complex carbohydrate and fiber to your diet; a moderate amount of mayonnaise-based salad dressing and a pat of margarine on the potato are permitted.

Fast food menus often contain items that, if properly selected, make up a meal adequate in protein and some vitamins and minerals. An occasional meal at a fast food restaurant will not upset an otherwise balanced low-fat, low-cholesterol diet. But don't eat frequently at such restaurants. And when you do eat at one, choose your food carefully. The following guidelines should be helpful:

1. Know your diet and how much fat you are allowed. Think about the food choices you will make the rest of the day.

2. Know the nutritional value (calories, carbohydrate, protein, and fat) of fast food items. Many fast food chains offer a nutrition analysis of their foods. These foods change frequently. Keep up to date

with the information. Fat, listed in grams, is a key in comparing various foods.

3. Avoid items high in fat and saturated fat. Many restaurants use beef tallow (fat trimmed from meat cuts and rendered into shortening) for frying meat, french fries, chicken, and fish. This is high in saturated fat and cholesterol.

4. Go easy on the salt. Salt does not affect blood cholesterol, but because of its effect on blood pressure you would do well to reduce the amount you consume. Not only are many fast foods high in salt content by themselves, but condiments such as pickles, mustard, ketchup, and tartar sauce are also high in salt content.

5. Shakes, apple pies, soft-serve ice cream, and regular soft drinks are high in empty calories. Avoid dessert at fast food restaurants.

6. Avoid biscuits and croissant sandwiches. Croissant sandwiches average 400–600 calories each, and are high in fat. Biscuit sandwiches typically contain 500–700 calories.

7. Avoid stuffed potatoes. A plain potato contains about 200–250 calories. Add bacon and cheese and the calories jump to 520–570, many of them from saturated fat.

8. Beware of large or double-decker burgers, and burgers with cheese and other toppings. These average between 525 and 980 calories.

Fast food guide. The Food Tables at the back of the book list the total fat, calorie, and cholesterol content of many popular items served at various fast food chains. The information in this part of the Food Tables was obtained from the food companies and is subject to change.

The Center for Science in the Public Interest (CSPI) in Washington, D.C., has obtained data from many restaurant chains and has documented the type of fat used in preparing the food. Many use beef tallow (a saturated animal fat). Some use vegetable oil, but "all vegetable" does not guarantee that saturated fat is not present, since coconut oil or palm oil may be used. It is usually difficult to obtain information on the breakdown of types of fat. As an example, we do know that french-fried potatoes fried in beef tallow contain approximately 41 percent of their total fat from a saturated source. But some fast food items, such as burgers, include mayonnaise in total fat, and this is primarily a polyunsaturated fat. Others "butter" the roll or bun, and the spread used may or may not be a saturated type.

When choosing foods at a fast food restaurant, look for items that contain less than 15 grams of fat and remember that adding "extras" increases the fat and calories. An example from McDonald's is a comparison between the plain Hamburger and the Cheeseburger:

Food item	Calories	Protein (gm)	Fat (gm)
Hamburger	263	12	11
Cheeseburger	318	15	16

As a guide, consider the increase in calories and fat that the following additions can provide:

Food item	Calories	Protein (gm)	Fat (gm)
Cheese (1 slice)	70	4	6
Bacon (1 slice)	37	2	3
Sausage (1 ounce)	50	3	4

Summary

1. Know your blood cholesterol level. If it is above 200 mg/dl, have your blood levels of LDL cholesterol, HDL cholesterol, and triglyceride measured.

2. Know whether you have other risk factors for cardiovascular disease, such as high blood pressure, cigarette smoking, obesity, diabetes, and a positive family history of premature coronary heart disease.

3. Eat a balanced diet, with appropriate choices from each of the six food groups.

4. Consume enough calories to maintain ideal body weight or reduce calories to achieve ideal body weight (see Figure 5-2).

5. Follow a diet reduced in total fat, saturated fat, and cholesterol and moderately enriched in unsaturated fat; both polyunsaturated fat and monounsaturated fat can be used to replace some of the saturated fat.

6. Go through your refrigerator, freezer, and cupboards and substitute nutritious low-fat, low-cholesterol foods for foods high in fat and cholesterol.

7. Eat fish caught in cold waters at least twice a week.

8. When you eat out, choose restaurants that offer you choices compatible with your Step One diet.

9. If you have a blood cholesterol problem, have it followed by your personal physician. Some people, particularly those with coronary heart disease or other cardiovascular risk factors, may need the addition of a drug to their diet program.

CHAPTER 12

Can Increased Fiber Benefit?

The effects of dietary cholesterol, saturated fats, monounsaturated fats, and polyunsaturated fats on your blood cholesterol level are the most important part of your diet. However, other nutrients such as fiber can also have an effect. How much can dietary fiber affect your cholesterol level? What kind of fiber should you eat? How much fiber should you eat? In this chapter you will find the answers to these questions.

Dietary fiber is vegetable material that is resistant to digestion. In the past fifteen years, interest in dietary fiber has increased thanks to the finding by Burkitt, Trowell, and others that populations with a diet high in fiber had a low incidence of coronary heart disease, diabetes, and diseases of the intestines such as cancer of the colon and appendicitis. In contrast, Western countries such as the United States, where the diet is low in fiber, have a high incidence of such diseases.

The results from two studies support the conclusion that diets high in fiber decrease coronary heart disease. In both studies, one of Irish brothers in Boston and Ireland and the other of Seventh Day Adventists in California, people matched in other respects were followed for over twenty years. It was found that those whose diets were high in fiber had a significantly lower rate of coronary heart disease.

Populations with diets naturally high in fiber frequently also eat relatively little total fat, saturated fat, and cholesterol, whereas populations with diets low in fiber usually eat a lot of total fat, saturated fat, and cholesterol. The American diet is particularly deficient in fiber. Over the last hundred years, the average daily intake of fiber in the United States has decreased by about 80 percent. Two things caused this decrease. One was that more and more fiber was removed from the diet by the refinement of food products, such as the ex-

Table 12-1. Water-Insoluble Fiber

Type	Plant source	Food source	Action
Cellulose	Chief part of cell wall of plant	Wheat bran and 25% of plant fiber	Speeds up gastrointestinal transit and fecal bulk
Lignin	With cellulose makes up cell wall of plant and the cementing material between cell wall and cell	Vegetables and fruits	May bind bile acids and other materials
Hemicellulose	Part of cell wall, less complex than cellulose and easily changed to simple sugar	50–70% of plant fiber of grains and vegetables	Helps relieve constipation

traction of bran from flour. The other was an increase in the consumption of meat and fats, with a concomitant decrease in the consumption of cereals and vegetables.

Types of Food Fiber

Food fibers are generally divided into two types: those that are insoluble in water (Table 12-1) and those that are soluble in water (Table 12-2). Food from plants can contain both types of fiber, although many types of food have much more of one than of the other.

Water-insoluble fibers. Water-insoluble fibers (Table 12-1) are found in the cell walls of plants. Wheat bran, vegetables, and whole grain cereals such as oats are good sources of water-insoluble fibers. These fibers add bulk to the diet, absorb water in the intestines, and decrease the time it takes food to pass through your digestive system. They help to prevent constipation and are also useful dietary adjuncts in conditions such as diverticulitis and other problems of an irritable bowel or colon.

One of the best-known sources of water-insoluble fibers is wheat bran. (Bran refers to the skin or husk of grains from wheat, rye, oats, etc., which can be separated from the flour by sifting.) It was once thought that wheat bran might lower blood cholesterol levels, but a number of studies have not shown that it does not.

Water-soluble fibers. Water-soluble fibers (Table 12-2) are found in fruits, gums from legumes, and oat grain. Like water-insoluble fibers, they are useful in increasing bulk and facilitating laxation. However, water-soluble fibers have an additional property: *they can lower your blood cholesterol level.*

Oat Bran

Unlike wheat bran, oat bran is rich in water-soluble fiber and has been shown to have a modest cholesterol-lowering effect. Dr. James Anderson and co-workers added oat bran to the regular diet of twenty hospitalized men with blood cholesterol levels above 260 mg/dl. The oat bran, provided by the Quaker Oats Company, was served as a bowl of hot cereal and five oat bran muffins every day for 21 days, a total of 100 grams daily. The addition of this amount of oat bran to the diet lowered the men's blood cholesterol level an average of 19 percent and their LDL cholesterol level 23 percent.

What effect might you expect if you added water-soluble fiber from oat grain to the Action Plan diet of Chapter 11? Dr. Linda Van Horn and colleagues studied 208 healthy men and women from 30 to 65 years old who were recruited from the Merchandise Mart in Chicago. All had normal levels of blood total and LDL cholesterol. All participants were first put on a diet similar to the Step One diet of Chapter 11. After six weeks on this diet (no oat products were consumed), the average total cholesterol fell from 208 mg/dl to 197 mg/dl.

The participants were then assigned to one of three groups, all of whom remained on the diet. Group 1 added two ounces of oat bran (⅔ cup) daily. Group 2 substituted two ounces of oatmeal for other foods high in carbohydrate. Group 3 simply remained on the low-fat diet, adding no oat products.

Table 12-2. Water-Soluble Fibers

Type	Plant source	Food source	Action
Pectin	Binds cell wall in plant tissue, giving a gel	Gel in fruit; some vegetables and legumes	Holds water and can bind bile acids
Plant gum	Sticky material at point of plant injury	Fruits and vegetables	Water binding capacity; used as emulsifier
Mucilages	Gelatinous substance similar to plant gum	Guar gum (legumes); plant seeds; part of fruits and vegetables	Influences plasma glucose and insulin levels

About half the oat bran or oatmeal was eaten as hot cereal; the remainder was eaten in the form of muffins and the like. After six weeks, both group 1 and group 2 experienced further average reductions in their blood cholesterol levels of about 6 mg/dl; group 3 experienced no further reduction.

Clearly, then, the addition of only *two ounces a day of oat bran or oatmeal* to your low-fat diet is likely to produce a further small decline in your blood cholesterol level. The amount of water-soluble fiber contained in two ounces of oat grain products is modest: thus group 1, on oat bran, ingested eleven grams of total fiber, of which five grams was water-soluble; group 2, on oatmeal, ingested only six grams of total fiber, of which three grams was water-soluble. Other studies have shown that eating larger amounts of oat bran or oatmeal can produce even greater decreases in your blood cholesterol level.

In addition to water-soluble fiber, oats contain more protein than any other grain. They are also rich in minerals and vitamins, and as plant products they contain no cholesterol.

Here are some practical hints for increasing the amount of oat grain in your diet:

1. Increase your consumption of oatmeal or oat bran in hot cereal or oats in cold cereal.
2. Substitute ground oat flour for one-third of the all-purpose flour in muffins, breads, pastry, cookies, and cakes.
3. Use oats as an ingredient in toppings for coffee cakes, fruit cobblers, and crisps.
4. Use oats instead of bread crumbs as a meat extender or in stuffings and fillings.

In addition, the Recipes section contains delicious recipes for bran banana bread, bran muffins, and cinnamon oat bran muffins.

As the good word about oat bran has got out, more and more commercial oat bran products are finding their way into supermarkets. Alternatively, one of my patients recommends a good, inexpensive source of oat bran, where in 1989 you could buy a six-pound bag for $8.95, a three-pound bag for $4.65, or a one-pound bag for $1.85:

> Nutrition Headquarters
> 104 West Jackson Street
> Carbondale, Ill. 62901
> Outside Illinois (1-800-851-3551, toll free)
> Inside Illinois (1-800-642-3536, toll-free)

Pectin

Another water-soluble fiber, pectin, is concentrated in the white in-
ner rind of apples, citrus, and various other fruits. Pectin from apples
has been used as a jelling agent in the preparation of jams for centu-
ries. In the studies described below, concentrated pectin, usually in
a powdered form, was added to a liquid and taken with meals.

Keys and co-workers were among the first to show that pectin lowered blood cholesterol levels. When they fed fifteen grams per day of
pectin to 48 male mental patients, the average blood cholesterol
level decreased 5 percent. More recently, in a short-term British
study in London, Jenkins and co-workers added a high dose of pectin,
36 grams per day, to the diet of twelve healthy volunteers for two
weeks. The average blood cholesterol level fell about 12 percent
(from 236 mg/dl to 207 mg/dl). Durrington and co-workers, using a
smaller dose of pectin, five grams three times a day, found an average
decrease in the blood cholesterol of 8 percent. Using a similar dose,
Kay and Truswell found a decrease of 13 percent in the blood cholesterol.

Durrington estimated that to ingest an amount of pectin in a natural diet equivalent to 15 grams per day, you would need to eat
approximately two and one-half pounds of apples, or about five
medium-sized apples. Jenkins has estimated that the minimum dose
of a purified pectin preparation required to produce some lowering of
blood cholesterol is about six grams per day.

Miettinen and Tarpila found that pectin was more effective in lowering total blood cholesterol and LDL cholesterol in people with
higher blood cholesterol levels than in those with perfectly normal
cholesterol levels. Hillman found little decrease in blood cholesterol
level in ten healthy volunteers fed ten grams of pectin per day.

Legumes

Legumes are vegetables like beans, with pods that enclose seeds.
Legumes, and particularly their seeds, contain the water-soluble fiber guar gum. In several studies of the effect of guar gum on blood
cholesterol level, the guar gum was obtained from the seeds of the
Indian cluster bean, *Cyanopisis tetragonolobus.*

Boscello and associates fed sixteen grams of guar gum per day for
60 days to twelve patients with high blood cholesterol and triglyceride levels. These patients, who were otherwise on their ordinary

diet, had an average decrease in cholesterol of 13.7 percent and in triglyceride of 32.1 percent. There was no change in the HDL cholesterol level.

In a British study, Jenkins administered guar gum from the cluster bean, in powdered form mixed with water, in a dose of 36 grams per day; the average total cholesterol fell 16.3 percent. In an Italian study, Penagini and co-workers administered 5.7 grams of guar gum twice a day in the form of a fine powder baked into crisp bread; the average blood cholesterol level fell 16 percent, about the same as in the Jenkins study.

Anderson and co-workers used a different approach. They administered a "bean diet" by giving subjects 115 grams of dried beans per day, as either pinto beans or navy beans, some provided as cooked beans and the rest in bean soup. The blood cholesterol and LDL cholesterol levels of these subjects fell an average of 19 percent and 24 percent, respectively.

Psyllium

Psyllium is a water-soluble fiber that comes from the seed of a plant related to the common weed plantain. The widely used bulk laxative Metamucil® is high in psyllium. In a recent well-designed study, researchers from the University of Kentucky gave one teaspoon of Metamucil three times a day to thirteen men with an average cholesterol of 250 mg/dl. At the end of eight weeks, their average blood cholesterol had fallen by 35 mg/dl, or 14 percent. Thirteen other men who were fed the water-insoluble fiber cellulose, which was made to resemble Metamucil, had no significant change in their average cholesterol level.

Psyllium works by binding the bile acids in the intestine, initiating a series of events that leads to lowering LDL in your blood. The prescription drugs cholestyramine (Questran and Cholybar) and colestipol (Colestid), discussed in Chapter 16, also work this way. Psyllium seems to have less annoying side effects than these drugs sometimes have, the most common complaint being mild cramping in the abdomen.

Metamucil is not a substitute for your low-cholesterol, low-saturated-fat diet. If after diet and oat bran your cholesterol level is still borderline high (200–240 mg/dl) or high (over 240 mg/dl), you and your doctor can consider adding one teaspoon of Metamucil three times a day to achieve an additional modest reduction. But if you need more than a modest further reduction, as many people do, you will probably require the addition of a lipid-lowering drug to your diet program.

Water-Soluble Fiber in Diabetes

Dr. James Anderson and co-workers also studied the effects of a high-fiber diet in patients with diabetes. Fourteen lean diabetic men being treated with insulin were switched from a control diet to a diet high in carbohydrate and high in fiber. The average insulin dose required by these subjects decreased from 27 units to 12 units per day. Their average fasting blood sugar decreased by 26 mg/dl. Their average total cholesterol level fell 32 percent.

In eleven other diabetic men, the high-carbohydrate, high-fiber diet was compared with a high-carbohydrate, low-fiber diet to determine the separate effects of high carbohydrate and high fiber. Both diets decreased the need for insulin, but the high-fiber diet prevented the increase in the blood triglyceride levels that occurred in those on the low-fiber diet. These doctors concluded that the high-carbohydrate, low-fat component of the diet played a major role in improving the processing of glucose in these diabetic men. The high-plant-fiber component of the diet played a minor role in improving the processing of glucose, but appeared to play a more important role in helping to control the levels of blood lipids in these men.

This study helps to emphasize one of the major points of this book, namely, *that a diet low in total fat, saturated fat, and cholesterol is the cornerstone of therapy.* The addition of water-soluble fibers is a good way to lower the blood cholesterol level still further by natural, nutritional means; but the basic diet comes first.

How Fiber Works on Cholesterol

We do not yet know exactly how water-soluble fibers lower the blood cholesterol level. For one thing, not all water-soluble fibers act the same way. For example, Anderson and associates found that oat bran increased the removal of bile acids from the body, whereas the addition of beans to the diet had the opposite effect. Yet, both these water-soluble fibers lowered the blood total cholesterol by about the same amount (19 percent).

The effect of water-soluble fibers may also depend on how much fat a person is eating. Dr. David Kritchevsky from the Wistar Institute in Philadelphia, in discussing a study by Antonis and Bersohn, points out that an increase in fiber content from 4 to 15 percent, when combined with a diet low in total fat, saturated fat, and cholesterol, increased the removal of both bile acids and other derivatives of cholesterol from the body. Miettinen and Tarpila, using pectin in a high dose (40 to 50 grams per day), also found an increased removal of bile acids and derivatives of cholesterol from the body. However, pectin was only about one-fourth as effective as a bile acid binding medicine.

Sometimes increased fiber does not lower the blood cholesterol level. A study by Dr. William Connor and associates indicates that simply adding a diverse source of fiber (which usually contains a lot of water-insoluble fiber) to a good low-saturated-fat, low-cholesterol diet does not have any significant effect on the blood cholesterol level. In that study, about 16 grams of crude fiber derived from corn, beans, bran, protein, and purified cellulose was added to a cholesterol-free diet and the blood cholesterol levels did not change. To be effective, you must add a large amount of water-soluble fiber to your diet; oat bran or oatmeal is the most practical way to do this. Pectin and guar gum capsules or powder are inconvenient to use and expensive.

Other Effects of Increased Fiber

In addition to your low-fat diet, you may need to reduce your weight to lower your blood cholesterol level and improve your risk profile. Increasing the fiber content of your diet can help you lose weight, as Dr. James Anderson and co-workers have found. Here is how:

1. It takes longer to eat fiber-rich foods than highly refined foods.
2. You will have a greater feeling of fullness and less between-meals hunger.
3. The absorption of nutrients in your meal will be slower and more "smoothed out," sustaining the energy level of your body and thereby also reducing hunger.

Some other effects of increased fiber may be less benign. Dr. David Kritchevsky has pointed out that a diet very high in fiber might inhibit the absorption of essential trace minerals. Heaton and Pomare found decreased calcium levels in the blood in subjects fed 38 grams per day of unprocessed wheat bran for one to two months. In a Danish study, Persson and co-workers, feeding ten to twenty grams of unprocessed bran daily to 27 elderly men, found a decrease in the levels of iron and calcium (in its ionized form) in the blood. It is

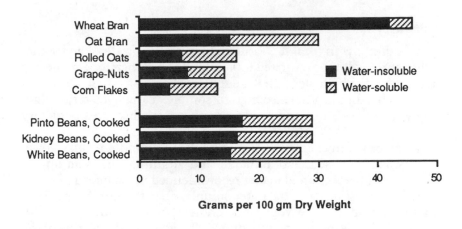

Fig. 12-1. Fiber content of various commercial cereals and types of beans.
Data from W. J. Chen and J. W. Anderson, in *American Journal of Clinical Nutrition* 34 (1981): 1080.

probably not a good idea to add very large amounts of fiber to the diet of people over 75.

How Much Fiber Should You Eat?

The average American consumes only some 10 to 20 grams of dietary fiber per day, clearly an insufficient amount. Many nutrition experts recommend 30 to 35 grams a day. The increase in fiber must be accomplished gradually to avoid intestinal discomfort and flatus. Drink plenty of fluids.

Here are some practical hints to help you increase the fiber in your diet:

1. Leave the skin on fruits and vegetables.
2. Use brown rice instead of white rice.
3. Sprinkle whole grain cereals on vegetable dishes and casseroles.
4. Eat whole baked or boiled potatoes, including skins.
5. Use whole grain rather than white breads.
6. Increase your consumption of whole beans, such as kidney beans, pinto beans, and navy beans.

The fiber content of various foods is provided for you in Figure 12-1. In addition, you will find a number of recipes high in fiber in the Recipes section.

Summary

1. A diet low in total fat, saturated fat, and cholesterol and somewhat enriched in unsaturated fat remains the cornerstone of dietary treatment of a high blood cholesterol level.

2. Such a diet is often also high in complex carbohydrates, including vegetables, fruits, and grains, which are good sources of dietary fiber.

3. Increased fiber in your diet is likely to promote regular bowel habits, is a good source of minerals and vitamins, and is an important part of the Action Plan diet recommended in Chapter 11.

4. The addition of extra water-soluble fiber to your Action Plan diet may help to lower your blood cholesterol level further without the use of cholesterol-lowering drugs. The additional lowering of the blood cholesterol level is likely to be modest, about 5 to 10 percent.

5. Oat grain is an effective and natural dietary component that can be easily and practically added to your diet, either as oatmeal or as oat bran in cereals and in muffins.

6. Fresh fruits and vegetables such as legumes are a desirable part of your diet. However, if the fruit fiber pectin or the vegetable fiber guar gum is to lower your blood cholesterol level significantly, it may need to be taken in the form of concentrated powder; and this can be inconvenient and expensive.

7. Metamucil®, a bulk laxative, is rich in psyllium, a water-soluble fiber. In a dose of one teaspoon three times a day, Metamucil may lower your blood cholesterol level 10 to 15 percent.

CHAPTER 13

Fish Oils:
Fact and Fiction

Eskimos are known for their ability to catch and eat fish, whales, and polar bears. Despite eating a diet high in fat and cholesterol, Eskimos have very little coronary heart disease. How can this be?

A clue may be found in another characteristic of the Eskimos, their marked tendency to nosebleeds and other bleeding problems. Here you will learn more about the importance of *the nature of the fat that you eat* and about *the important role that clotting can play in coronary heart disease.* Finally, practical tips are provided to help you get more fish oils into your diet without the expensive, unnecessary, and possibly unsafe addition of fish oil capsules.

How much fish should you eat? How often? What type of fish is best for you to eat? Will fish oils lower your blood cholesterol and prevent coronary heart disease? Are there any possible harmful effects of fish oils? This chapter is devoted to answering these questions.

EPA and Arachidonic Acid

Fish oils are the fats contained in fish and shellfish, either from their flesh and fatty tissue or from certain organs such as the liver. These fats are different from the fats in animals. Of the wide variety of fatty acids in fish oils, two are especially rich: EPA (eicosapentaenoic acid) and DHA (docosahexaenoic acid). EPA and DHA are both polyunsaturated fatty acids. Using the hat rack model, you can visualize EPA (Figure 13-1). In EPA there are five places in the hat rack where hooks next to each other are both missing a hat; EPA consists of a chain of 20 carbons. DHA is similar to EPA except that it has six areas of unsaturation and is a chain of 22 carbons.

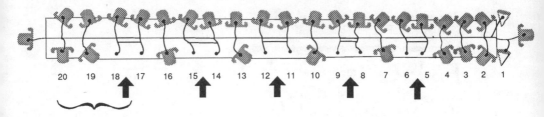

Omega-3 Fatty Acid (EPA)

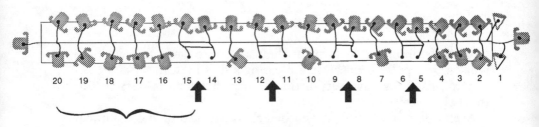

Omega-6 Fatty Acid (Arachidonic Acid)

Fig. 13-1. Schematic drawings of an omega-3 fatty acid (EPA) and an omega 6 fatty acid (arachidonic acid). The chain of carbon atoms is depicted by a straight line, to which are attached hydrogen atoms (shown as hats) or oxygen atoms (shown as white triangles). The carbons in the chain are numbered, by convention, from the acid end (far right), and the areas of unsaturation are indicated by arrows. The tail end (far left) contains the last, or omega, carbon.

Fish oils become so enriched in EPA and DHA because the minute plant life in water (phytoplankton) is high in these fatty acids. Through consumption of these plants by smaller fish, and then of the smaller fish by larger fish, these fatty acids are transferred up through the food chain. This phenomenon occurs primarily in fish caught in cold waters.

One place in EPA that is "missing two hats" is found at the third position from the tail end of the fatty acid: it is thus termed an omega-3 fatty acid. In contrast, this position is saturated in linoleic acid and arachidonic acid, which are polyunsaturated fatty acids found in vegetable oils; the last unsaturated area in these fatty acids occurs at the sixth position from their tail end, and they are thus termed omega-6 fatty acids. As Figure 13-1 makes clear, the only difference between EPA and arachidonic acid is that EPA has one more unsaturated area, at the third position from its tail end. But what a difference that difference makes in regard to their effects in your body!

As noted above, EPA is plentiful in fish oils and arachidonic acid is found in vegetable oils; the body can also use linoleic acid to make arachidonic acid. After a meal, fats such as triglyceride are broken down in the intestine, liberating EPA or arachidonic acid. These fatty acids are taken into the intestine and reincorporated into triglyceride, which is then packaged inside chylomicrons for transport into the blood. As the triglyceride is broken down in the blood, these fatty acids are released and are taken up by various cells.

Arachidonic acid and EPA differ in their effect on the balance between clotting and bleeding. Ordinarily, when you bleed, the natural reaction of your body is to clot so that the bleeding will stop. *The processes of bleeding and clotting actually reflect the balanced effect of factors in your blood, of which some promote clotting and others inhibit clotting.*

Arachidonic acid is converted in your blood into two products: thromboxane A_2, which causes your blood vessels to become narrower and also promotes clotting by causing the platelets to clump in your blood; and prostaglandin I_2, which has the opposite effect, dilating your blood vessels and inhibiting the clumping of platelets in your blood (Figure 13-2).

As the content of EPA in your system increases, the balance is shifted toward an inhibition of clotting. This happens because your body converts EPA into two products that differ in a small but significant way from those produced by arachidonic acid: thromboxane A_3, which is biologically *inactive* and does not cause your blood vessels to narrow or your platelets to clump together; and prostaglandin I_3, which dilates your blood vessels and inhibits clumping of your platelets (Figure 13-2).

Another effect of EPA is the decreased production of triglyceride in the liver. Much of the EPA from the fish oil in your diet ends up in your liver. When EPA is present, your liver produces triglyceride more slowly. VLDL, the major carrier of triglyceride, is also made at a decreased rate, and less VLDL and triglyceride are released from the liver into the bloodstream. The blood triglyceride level falls.

Fish Oils and Coronary Heart Disease

Eskimos. About fifteen years ago it was recognized by two Danes, Drs. Bang and Dyerberg, that Greenland Eskimos had a significantly

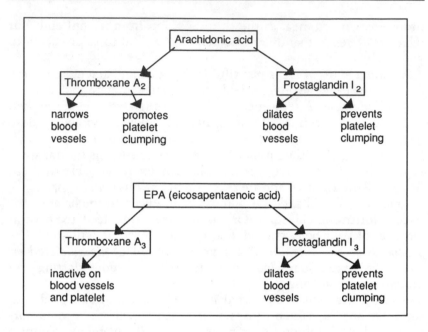

Fig. 13-2. The effects of arachidonic acid and EPA on the blood vessels and on platelet clumping.

lower rate of coronary heart disease than Eskimos who lived in Denmark. The diet of the Greenland Eskimos consisted almost entirely of marine products: the average adult Eskimo consumed 16 ounces of fish per day. (In contrast, Americans average only about half an ounce.) A favorite delicacy of the Eskimos was "muktuk," made by cutting the skin and top layer of fat from a whale into strips. Since their diet was high in total fat, it appeared paradoxical that the Eskimos had a low incidence of coronary heart disease. However, upon closer scrutiny, this diet was found to be high in polyunsaturated fats and monounsaturated fats but *low in saturated fats.*

Japanese. The beneficial effect of fish consumption on heart disease does not appear to be limited to Eskimos. For example, Japanese living on fishermen's islands, who ate an average of four ounces of fish per day, were found to have lower rates of coronary heart disease than Japanese in urban areas.

Netherlands. More recently, an interesting study was reported in the *New England Journal of Medicine* by Kronhout and co-workers from Zutphen, Netherlands. As part of the original Coronory Heart Disease in Seven Countries Study reviewed for you in Chapter 2, some 852 middle-aged men were followed for twenty years. In 1960, 20 percent of these men ate no fish at all, and the group's average consumption was between one-half and one ounce of fish per day. After twenty years, death from coronary heart disease was 50 percent lower in those men who averaged at least one ounce of fish per day. Those who ate no fish had the highest rate of death from coronary heart disease, those who ate the most fish had the lowest rate, and those who ate an intermediate amount had an intermediate rate. This correlation persisted after all other risk factors for coronary heart disease were considered. Finally, the fish consumption of the Zutphen men consisted of two-thirds lean fish and one-third fatty fish. Consumption of lean fish was also of apparent benefit.

The Zutphen study does not prove that the EPA and DHA prevented death from coronary heart disease. Perhaps it was some other constituent in the fish, or simply the fish eaters' decreased intake of saturated fat. Nevertheless, this study, when combined with the other information that we will discuss in this chapter, raises the intriguing possibility that eating fish oils may help prevent coronary heart disease.

The Action Plan to lower your blood cholesterol level found in Chapter 11 includes the consumption of fish caught in cold waters at least twice a week. Not only are fish and shellfish low in saturated fat, but, in view of the above observations, the EPA and DHA they provide may be a further benefit for you.

Fish Oils and Blood Clotting

Recently, Dr. Weiner and co-workers at the University of Massachusetts Medical Center studied the effect of cod liver oil on the development of atherosclerosis. Eighteen young pigs were placed on a diet high in cholesterol and saturated fat that raised their blood cholesterol level from about 150 mg/dl to over 500 mg/dl. Three weeks later, all the animals had the lining on the inside of one of their three major coronary arteries disrupted with a balloon to induce an area susceptible to atherosclerosis. Seven of the pigs then had about one ounce of cod liver oil added to their high-fat diet; the other eleven had no cod liver oil added.

Eight months later the pigs were sacrificed and their coronary arteries examined. The results were striking (see Figure 13-3). The

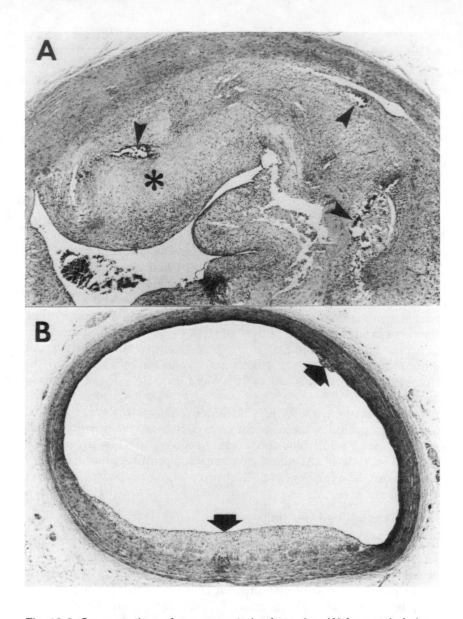

Fig. 13-3. Cross-sections of coronary arteries from pigs: (A) from a pig fed a
high-fat diet and cod liver oil; (B) from a pig fed the same high-fat diet but no
cod liver oil. In panel A there is severe thickening of the lining of the coronary
artery; areas of calcium deposits are indicated by the arrows and an area of
dead tissue by the asterisk. In panel B there is only a small degree of thickening of the blood vessel, indicated by the arrows.

Reproduced with permission of B. H. Weiner et al., *New England Journal of Medicine* 315
(1986): 841–846.

seven pigs who received cod liver oil had minimal atherosclerosis; most of the other eleven had marked atherosclerosis not just in the one disrupted artery but in all three major coronary arteries.

The cod liver oil did not lower the elevated cholesterol levels of the seven pigs that received it. Rather, its preventive effect on atherosclerosis in these pigs seems to have come from inhibiting the clotting of their blood. The process of clotting in the blood involves platelets and "clotting factors," a family of specialized proteins. In this study, EPA was present in significantly increased amounts in the platelets from the blood of the animals treated with cod liver oil; also some of the clotting factors were decreased in this group.

The history of the Greenland Eskimos provided a clue to the effects of fish oil on clotting. These Eskimos were famous for their tendency to bleed. Drs. Bang and Dyerberg quoted from a fifteenth-century Norwegian history: "When they (Eskimos) are hit by weapons . . . their wounds will stay white and without blood, but if they die the blood will almost not stop flowing." Did this tendency to bleed come from the effect of fish oils on clotting?

To study this effect, Dr. Knapp and co-workers from Vanderbilt University administered high doses of MaxEPA (roughly equivalent to the amount of fish oil in the Eskimo diet) to six patients with atherosclerosis in their legs and to seven healthy people. The MaxEPA, in the form of capsules, was added to their regular diet and given daily for a month.

What happened? There was a significant increase in the amount of EPA in the phospholipids of the platelets from the blood of those receiving EPA. Ordinarily arachidonic acid is the most common fatty acid in platelets, but now the balance was shifted and there were about equal amounts of EPA and arachidonic acid. The patients treated with MaxEPA had developed a fatty acid profile in their platelets *similar to that found in the Eskimos*. This shift toward an EPA-enriched platelet was accompanied by all the other changes expected when arachidonic acid is replaced with EPA (Figure 13-2).

If you have poor circulation and atherosclerosis, should you take fish oil capsules? My patients often ask me this question, and I say No. Studies of more people and for a longer period of time are needed to determine whether EPA in such high doses (10 grams a day) should be routinely used to inhibit clotting in patients with hardening of the arteries. Also, as we shall see below, fish oils have some possible adverse effects that need to be considered.

Your body has a built-in mechanism to ensure a balance between clotting and bleeding. It can be dangerous to disturb this balance toward either extreme. However, some people have a greater tendency to form clots than others, and this can be dangerous, especially to people whose coronary arteries are significantly blocked with atherosclerosis. A clot can form on top of these blockages, causing a heart attack; or a similar process in the blood vessels of the brain can lead to a stroke. If you have coronary heart disease or known atherosclerosis, you should ask your doctor whether you need medication to decrease the tendency of your blood to clot.

If you don't have coronary heart disease, what should you do? A recent study in Boston of 20,000 doctors found that those doctors who took one buffered aspirin or one enteric coated aspirin (such as Ecotrin) every other day *had one-half as many heart attacks as those doctors who took an inactive medicine (placebo)*. But those on aspirin had slightly more strokes. Discuss this study with your doctor and both of you can decide what is best for you, depending on your age and general health status.

What do I do? I take one enteric coated aspirin every other day. I do not take fish oil capsules, but I try to eat fish or shellfish at least twice a week. If you and your doctor decide to decrease the tendency of your blood to clot, everything I have read and heard indicates that one aspirin every other day can do the job just as efficiently as taking fish oil capsules. It is also less expensive and less time-consuming.

Fish Oils and Lipid Levels

The initial studies of Eskimos also indicated that fish oils had beneficial effects on the profile of lipids and lipoproteins in the blood. For example, Greenland Eskimos generally have lower levels of blood cholesterol and triglyceride but higher levels of HDL cholesterol, leading to a more optimal LDL/HDL ratio. Of course, this healthy lipid profile may also have been influenced by their hardy lifestyle, and by genetic factors.

Over a dozen studies have now been performed on the effect of fish oils on humans. Among those studied have been healthy adults, diabetics, people with cardiovascular disease or high blood cholesterol or triglyceride levels, and even patients undergoing hemodialysis for severe kidney disease. The results of these trials, in general, are related to the amount of fish oils consumed.

Fish oils affect the triglyceride level far more than the cholesterol level. When people were fed eight ounces of fish several times a week, the total triglyceride level decreased 5 to 10 percent, compared to a drop of almost 50 percent when they were fed eight ounces of a fatty fish each day. The cholesterol level did not fall at all in some studies; in others some decrease in blood cholesterol was found, but only when relatively high doses of MaxEPA were used. In one interesting study in the Netherlands, five ounces of cheese was simply replaced each day in the diet with seven ounces of a fatty fish, mackerel. This single substitution produced a decrease in both the blood cholesterol and triglyceride levels.

How does fish oil produce its effect on blood triglyceride and cholesterol levels? Several studies have consistently found that fish oil decreases the amount of VLDL that is made in liver. Less VLDL, which is rich in triglyceride and also contains smaller amounts of cholesterol, is released from the liver into the bloodstream. The level of VLDL in the blood falls, accompanied by a decrease in triglyceride and (sometimes) in cholesterol.

The effects of fish oil vary from person to person. In some people the fall in VLDL is accompanied by an increase in LDL. In diabetics, fish oil may actually increase the blood sugar and raise the triglyceride level. In one study a high MaxEPA diet led to a significant increase in HDL cholesterol, but with time the HDL cholesterol level tended to return to baseline. The effects of fish oil can be tricky, another reason why the casual use of fish oil capsules is not recommended.

Some Other Effects of Fish Oils

Your body has a natural defense against foreign materials. When you have an infection by bacteria, the white blood cells, with the help of antibodies, ingest the bacteria and help ward off the infection. One type of white blood cell is called a "monocyte." Monocytes can leave your bloodstream and enter your artery walls, where they become "Pac-Men" or macrophages. Macrophages "eat up" foreign materials, including damaged LDL particles from your blood. Macrophages can become "full" of LDL and its cholesterol, causing them to release substances that adversely affect the muscle cells inside the wall of the artery. These events are believed to be involved in the earliest stages of atherosclerosis. The less LDL cholesterol you have in your blood, the less will become damaged, and the less will be ingested by the macrophages.

Lee and co-workers published a study in 1985 in the *New England Journal of Medicine* in which they found that monocytes from patients who were fed EPA did not adhere to the surface of test tubes as readily as monocytes from patients who were not fed EPA. These researchers speculated that these "non-sticky" monocytes will not be turned into macrophages as easily as "sticky" monocytes that adhere to the blood vessel wall more readily. Further studies are necessary to clarify the meaning of these findings.

Studies of rats indicate that fish oils may decrease the rise in blood pressure often induced under experimental conditions. Other polyunsaturated fats such as linoleic acid have been previously shown to be associated with lower blood pressure levels in humans. Thus the EPA and DHA in your diet may help to lower your blood pressure.

You may have heard the old saying that fish is "brain food." In fact, from 60 to 70 percent of the gray matter in your brain is made of fats, and DHA is one of the most important fatty acids in brain fats. Fish oils may also be important in the function of the part of your eye called the retina. In one study of infant nonhuman primates, Dr. William Connor and co-workers found that depriving these animals of omega-3 fatty acids led to problems with vision and mental function. These results indicate that the omega-3 fatty acids have a specific role in the normal development of the eye and the brain.

In addition to being lower in total fat and saturated fat than beef, pork, or veal, and being enriched in EPA and DHA, fish and shellfish have other desirable nutritional characteristics. Fish is generally a rich source of B vitamins, especially niacin (B_3) and B_6. Seafoods are an abundant source of minerals, such as phosphorus, potassium, and iron. Salt water fish provide iodine and selenium. Shellfish such as oysters are among nature's best sources of zinc. Shrimp, clams, oysters, sardines, and salmon are high in calcium.

Sources of Omega-3 Fatty Acids

Fin fish. Table 13-1 lists the fin fish that are the richest sources of EPA and DHA. These fish are caught in cold waters and contain at least 1 percent by weight of these two omega-3 fatty acids. The fish on this list are usually referred to as "fatty fish," but this is somewhat of a misnomer, since on average only 7.6 percent of their weight comes from fat; they are all acceptable on the low-saturated-fat diet outlined for you in Chapter 11. The portion size is limited to five or six ounces because fish do contain cholesterol. Of the fatty fish, pink salmon is the lowest in total fat (3.4 percent); Pacific herring and Atlantic mackerel are the highest (13.9 percent).

The fin fish in the second list of Table 13-1 are less rich, but still acceptable, sources of EPA and DHA. These "lean fish" contain at least 0.2 percent by weight of the two fatty acids, and on average 1.7

Table 13-1. Good Fin Fish Sources of Omega-3
Fatty Acids

Richer Sources	Less Rich Sources
Anchovy	Bass, fresh water
Bluefish	Bass, striped
Herring, Atlantic	Cod, Atlantic
Herring, Pacific	Flounder
Herring, rand	Haddock
Mackerel, Atlantic	Halibut, Pacific
Salmon, Atlantic	Perch, yellow
Salmon, Chinook	Rockfish
Salmon, pink	Shark
Trout, lake	Snapper, red
Tuna, albacore	Swordfish
Tuna, bluefin	Trout, rainbow
Whitefish, lake	Tuna, unspecified

Source: United States Department of Agriculture, Human Nutrition
Information Services, Provisional Table on the Content of Omega-3
Fatty Acids and Other Fat Components in Selected Foods (Revised
May 1986).

percent of their weight comes from fat. They are excellent substitutes for meats high in fat. Atlantic cod and haddock are the lowest in total fat (0.7 percent); the highest is rainbow trout (3.4 percent). Tuna lovers should note that albacore and bluefin tuna contain about three times as much EPA and DHA as tuna whose type is unspecified on the can.

Some fish that did not contain enough EPA and DHA to make the second list were dolphin, Atlantic hake, northern pike, scrod, and sole. Although acceptable as low-fat entrées, they contain relatively little EPA and DHA.

Shellfish. Table 13-2 lists commonly eaten shellfish that contain at least 0.2 percent EPA and DHA by weight. Both the crustaceans and the mollusks were low in total fat (0.8 percent to 2.5 percent by weight), and both contained from 0.2 percent (lobster) to 0.5 percent (prawn shrimp, mussel, oyster) EPA and DHA by weight. The content of omega-3 fatty acids in the shellfish was therefore similar to that in the lean fish in Table 13-1. Shellfish too low in EPA and DHA to make the list include crayfish, hard-shell clam, and little neck clam.

Commercial fish oils. There are a number of commercial fish oil preparations, among them cod liver oil, once widely fed to children as a source of fat-soluble vitamins. Commercial fish oil capsules such as GNC mega-EPA-1,000, Royal Oak epaPlus, and Solgan

Table 13-2. Good Shellfish Sources of Omega-3
Fatty Acids

Crustaceans	Mollusks
Crab, Alaskan king	Clam, soft-shell
Crab, blue	Mussel, blue
Lobster	Oyster
Shrimp, Atlantic brown	Scallop
Shrimp, Atlantic white	Squid
Shrimp, Japanese (Kuruma) prawn	

Source: United States Department of Agriculture, Human Nutrition
Information Services, Provisional Table on the Content of Omega-3
Fatty Acids and Other Fat Components in Selected Foods (Revised
May 1986).

MaxEPA generally contain about 300 mg of EPA and DHA per capsule. How many capsules would you need to take to get the equivalent amount of the EPA and DHA found in four ounces of pink
salmon? Seven.

Other sources of omega-3 fatty acids. Vegetable oils contain primarily omega-6 fatty acids such as linoleic acid and arachidonic
acid. But some vegetables and vegetable oils such as soybeans and
soybean oil, green leafy vegetables, wheat germ, walnuts, and lin-
seed, canola, and rapeseed oils contain an omega-3 fatty acid called
linolenic acid. It is not yet known whether dietary linolenic acid has
the same effects as EPA and DHA.

Possible Adverse Effects of Fish Oils

Calories. If the minimum dose of fish oils required to achieve a
significant effect on clotting and lipid levels is quite high—for example, 30–40 grams/day—this will add excessive calories to your
diet (nine calories per gram, or 270–360 calories per day).

Excess of fat-soluble vitamins. One ounce of cod liver oil contains
six times the recommended dietary allowance of vitamins A and D.
Since these fat-soluble vitamins are stored in the liver, hypervitami-
nosis (an abnormal condition requiring medical treatment) might be
produced when too much cod liver oil is used as the source of fish
oils.

Vitamin E deficiency. Fish oils are high in EPA and DHA, both
polyunsaturated fatty acids; and the excessive ingestion of polyunsaturated fatty acids increases a process called oxidation. Since your

body uses vitamin E to combat oxidation, large amounts of fish oil may deplete your body of vitamin E.

Pesticide contaminants. Fat-soluble pesticides such as PCB and DDT may be concentrated in the liver and fatty tissues of fish caught in contaminated waters. Fish oils derived from such sources will contain increased amounts of these contaminants.

Cholesterol in fish oils. Some fish oil capsules such as MaxEPA contain about five milligrams of cholesterol per capsule. Taking six capsules a day would not provide excessive cholesterol to the diet; but taking fifteen capsules a day would provide about 75 mg of cholesterol a day—an unacceptably high amount, especially if your dietary cholesterol from natural food sources remains at the same level as before. Newer, more highly concentrated formulations such as Promega (Parke Davis) are essentially cholesterol-free.

Future Research on Fish Oils

Fish oils seem to have two major effects: decreasing the tendency to clot, and decreasing the levels of VLDL and triglyceride in the blood. These effects are important, particularly if either, or both, are responsible for the beneficial effect of fish consumption on the rate of coronary heart disease seen in the Zutphen study.

Several questions remain. What is the minimum amount of fish oil (specifically EPA and DHA) necessary to achieve the desired effect on clotting and lipid levels? Is the minimum amount also a safe amount? Is the effect of fish oils on clotting more important to preventing atherosclerosis than their effect on lipid levels? Is the minimum dose of fish oils required to achieve a desired effect on clotting different from that required to affect lipid levels? Is it possible to develop highly purified preparations of EPA and DHA that contain no cholesterol, no contaminants, and no vitamins A and D?

Summary

1. Omega-3 fatty acids, EPA and DHA, are polyunsaturated fatty acids that are enriched in fish oils. Omega-3 fatty acids appear to decrease the tendency of the blood to clot and to decrease the levels of VLDL and triglyceride in the blood. Increased consumption of fish may decrease the rate of coronary heart disease.

2. A diet low in total fat, saturated fat, and cholesterol remains the cornerstone of dietary treatment; but you would do well to increase

your consumption of fish caught in cold waters to at least twice a week. Limit your portions to five or six ounces.

3. It is the medical consensus at the present time that supplementing your daily diet with large amounts of fish oils is not a good idea.

CHAPTER 14

Delicious, Quick Menus
for Your Action Plan Diet

Many people want to make the dietary changes outlined in the previous chapters but find that putting it all together into meal planning is an overwhelming task. A two-week series of menus is offered in this chapter as a planning aid. Following each day's menu you will find the content of that menu in total fat (grams and percent of total calories), saturated fat (also grams and percent of total calories), cholesterol (milligrams), calories, carbohydrate (grams), and protein (grams). The ranges for these nutrients are as follows: total fat, 25.9–50.4 gm, 17–27%; saturated fat, 5.1–10.7 gm, 3–6%; cholesterol, 64–225 mg; calories, 1,257–1,956; carbohydrate, 174–274 gm; and protein, 59–115 gm.

If you followed these menus exactly, your Action Plan diet would be even stricter than the Step Two diet of Table 11-1. In practice, however, additional calories and other nutrients from snacks can make the entire day's intake quite variable. Also you will be eating out and occasionally indulging in high-fat treats; so you will end up closer to a Step One diet.

These menus draw heavily on the Recipes section (pp. 325–369), a mini-cookbook of some 90-odd delicious recipes submitted by my friends and patients as their favorites. Many menus featuring recipes require quite a bit of planning and time in the beginning. Before starting with the menus offered here, it is recommended that you choose only one new recipe at a meal and stick with the basics for the other menu options. Then, when your new eating lifestyle has become a part of your everyday routine, you can try some of the featured menus.

Some basic steps can help ensure a balanced diet reduced in saturated fat and cholesterol. For adults there are key food groups that should be included every day to achieve this balance. Your first step in meal planning, then, is to check to see if you are eating the correct number of servings from each of these food groups every day.

To start, see how many of the foods in Table 14-1 you currently eat each week. The key to a successful diet is sticking, so far as possible, to the recommended types of food and numbers of servings. There is no real harm in going under or over these recommendations in a single day, but to ensure good nutrition this should not be your standard routine. In general, the smaller number of servings will add up to about 1,200 calories each day, the larger number to about 1,600 calories. The optional food group does not contribute any essential nutrients; it fits into the diet strictly according to preference and individual caloric needs.

Since people vary greatly in their caloric needs, it is important to consider what your goal of daily calories should be, especially if you are trying to lose weight. The amount of fuel the body needs varies at different stages of life and usually decreases with age. Your sex, body size, and frame as well as your physical activity also need to be

Table 14-1. Approximate Daily Allowances of Various Foods in Your Action Plan Diet

Food group	Number of servings per day	Approximate size of 1 serving
	KEY GROUPS	
1. Vegetables and fruits		
Vegetables	3 or more	½ to ⅔ cup
Fruits	3 or more	½ cup cut-up fruit
2. Breads, cereals, and starchy foods	4 or more	1 slice bread ½ cup cooked starch 1 ounce ready-to-eat cereal
3. Milk and cheese	2 or more	1 cup skim or low-fat milk or yogurt 1½ ounces low-fat cheese
4. Meat, poultry, and seafood or	1 or more	2–3 ounces cooked lean meat, fish, or poultry without skin[a]
Low-fat meat substitutes	1 or more	1 cup dry beans, cooked 3 ounces tofu ½ cup egg substitute
5. Fats and oils	at most 6–8 (including for cooking)	1 teaspoon oil or margarine 2 teaspoons diet margarine or regular mayonnaise
	OPTIONAL GROUP	
6. Sugars and alcohol		
Sugars	not required	as appropriate for caloric needs
Alcohol	not required	in moderation only

[a]No more than 6 ounces a day of lean meat, fish, or poultry.

Table 14-2. Number of Servings per Day from the Basic
Food Groups to Achieve Various Caloric Levels

Caloric level	Food group	Number of servings per day
1,200	Skim or low-fat dairy	2
	Lean meat, fish, or poultry	5 oz.
	Vegetables	3
	Fruits	3
	Breads, cereals, and starches	6
	Fats	5
1,500	Skim or low-fat dairy	2
	Lean meat, fish, or poultry	5 oz.
	Vegetables	3
	Fruits	4
	Breads, cereals, and starches	8
	Fats	6
1,800	Skim or low-fat dairy	2
	Lean meat, fish, or poultry	5
	Vegetables	5 oz.
	Fruits	6
	Breads, cereals, and starches	9
	Fats	8
	Sugar (1 tablespoon pure sugar)	1
2,000	Skim or low-fat dairy	3
	Lean meat, fish, or poultry	6
	Vegetables	6 oz.
	Fruits	6
	Breads, cereals, and starches	9
	Fats	8
	Sugar (1 tablespoon pure sugar)	1

considered. It is not a good idea to eat less than 1,000 calories a day unless you are under a doctor's supervision; most weight loss diets average between 1,200 and 1,500 calories a day. The average adult eats from 1,500 to 2,400 calories a day. Children, teenagers, athletes, and pregnant or lactating women have additional nutrient and caloric needs. Table 14-2 gives you a general idea of how to achieve four different daily caloric levels by choosing basic foods from the six food groups.

Snacks may include low-calorie, low-fat foods of all sorts, but often they run to high-calorie, high-fat foods such as chips or cookies. When this happens, the fat composition changes and the total calories increase quickly. When you are trying to lose weight, be sure to choose your snacks carefully. Some suggestions, for which the recommended portion contains less than three grams of saturated fat and less than five milligrams of cholesterol, are as follows:

Angel food cake (1 small slice)
Animal crackers (10)
Bran muffin (1 average)
Fig bars (2)
Frozen fruit bar (1 bar)
Frozen yogurt (½ cup)
Gelatin (½ cup)

Gingerbread (a 3-inch square)
Gingersnaps (2)
Popsicle (1 bar)
Pudding made with skim milk
   (½ cup)
Sherbet (½ cup)
Sorbet (½ cup)

Snacks, dessert items, sweets, and alcohol are extras that people eat or drink for enjoyment and when extra calories are needed. The sample menus concentrate on the three basic meals only. Snacks are suggested for each day to give you a sense of the possibilities; but basically when it comes to allocating your snack allowance between snacks, desserts, sweets, and alcohol, you're on your own.

TWO WEEKS OF MENUS FOR YOUR ACTION PLAN DIET

The following two weeks' worth of menus feature recipes from this book; the page numbers are provided. Where a quantity is not specified, "one serving" is the quantity.

Monday

Breakfast
   ½ cup sliced strawberries
   ½ cup low-fat cottage cheese
   1 Always Ready Bran Muffin (p. 325)
   1 tsp. margarine
   Coffee

Lunch
   Sandwich:
      2 slices whole wheat bread
      2 oz. sliced turkey breast
      1 tsp. mayonnaise
      lettuce and sliced tomato
   1 peach
   8 oz. skim milk

Dinner
   Spaghetti with Turkey Tomato
      Sauce (p. 351)
   Tossed salad
   2 Tb. Italian salad dressing
   1 slice Italian bread
   1 tsp. margarine
   1 cup fresh fruit cup
   8 oz. skim milk

Snack
   ¾ cup Total cereal
   4 oz. skim milk

total fat....... 43.4 gm (26%)	cholesterol...... 84 mg	carbohydrate...206 gm
saturated fat ... 7.7 gm (5%)	calories..........1,525	protein..........88 gm

Tuesday

Breakfast
¼ honeydew melon
½ cup low-fat cottage cheese
½ bagel
1 tsp. margarine
Coffee

Lunch
Sandwich:
   2 oz. Lite Line cheese
   2 slices whole wheat toast
   Lettuce and tomato
   1 tsp. mayonnaise
1 cup tomato soup
1 nectarine
Iced tea

Dinner
Sirloin steak, trimmed, 3 oz.
½ cup white rice
½ cup string beans
Cucumber-Radish Salad (p. 362)
1 cup grapes
8 oz. skim milk

Snack
1 Apple Cinnamon Muffin (p. 326)

total fat....... 43.0 gm (26%)	cholesterol ..... 108 mg	carbohydrate... 200 gm
saturated fat .. 10.6 gm (6%)	calories 1,479	protein.......... 82 gm

Wednesday

Breakfast
1 whole English muffin
2 tsp. margarine
½ cup orange juice
1 cup low-fat plain yogurt
Coffee

Lunch
Meatless Bean and Corn Stew
   (p. 347)
6 saltines
¾ cup fresh fruit cup
Iced tea

Dinner
4 oz. roast turkey breast
¼ cup cranberry sauce
½ cup cooked carrots
1 tsp. margarine
Nutted Wild Rice (p. 357)
Fruit Ambrosia (p. 363)
8 oz. skim milk

Snack
3 cups air-popped popcorn

total fat....... 31.2 gm (17%)	cholesterol ..... 101 mg	carbohydrate... 256 gm
saturated fat ... 7.0 gm (4%)	calories 1,611	protein.......... 82 gm

Thursday

Breakfast
½ cup orange juice
1 sv. Apple Raisin Coffee Cake
(p. 327)
Coffee

Lunch
1 cup low-fat plain yogurt
1 cup fresh fruit
Tossed salad
2 Tb. low-calorie French
dressing
Apricot Oat Bread (p. 327)
Coffee

Dinner
Chicken Nuggets (p. 343)
Cold Pasta Salad Vinaigrette (p.
361)
1 slice French bread
1 tsp. margarine
½ cup low-fat frozen yogurt
8 oz. skim milk

Snack
1 apple

total fat .... *48.5 gm (26%)*	*cholesterol* ..... *105 mg*	*carbohydrate* ... *246 gm*
saturated fat ... *8.4 gm (5%)*	*calories* *1,679*	*protein* .... *74 gm*

Friday

Breakfast
½ cup peaches
1 whole bagel
2 tsp. margarine
1 cup low-fat plain yogurt
Coffee

Lunch
Submarine sandwich:
  Sub roll
  1.5 oz. turkey breast
  1.5 oz. ham
  Lettuce leaf
  2 slices tomato
  2 tsp. mustard
1 apple
8 oz. skim milk

Dinner
Pita Pizza (p. 348)
Tossed salad
1 Tb. Thousand Island dressing
½ cup sherbet
Coffee

Snack
1 Oat Bran Muffin (p. 331)

total fat .... *38.8 gm (20%)*	*cholesterol* ...... *88 mg*	*carbohydrate* ... *274 gm*
saturated fat .. *10.7 gm (6%)*	*calories* *1,750*	*protein* .... *79 gm*

Saturday

Breakfast
½ grapefruit
1 sv. Omelet (p. 332)
1 slice whole wheat toast
1 tsp. margarine
Coffee

Lunch
Sandwich:
2 slices whole wheat bread
2 oz. chicken breast
1 tsp. mayonnaise
1 banana
8 oz. skim milk

Dinner
Shrimp and Vegetable Pasta (p. 350)
Sliced tomato
1 Apple Cinnamon Muffin (p. 326)
1 tsp. margarine
½ cup sorbet
8 oz. skim milk

Snack
1 cup grapes

total fat .... *48.3 gm (27%)*   *cholesterol* ..... *203 mg*   *carbohydrate* ... *207 gm*
saturated fat .. *10.7 gm (6%)*   *calories* .... *1,633*   *protein* .... *102 gm*

Sunday

Breakfast
½ grapefruit
1 sv. Michele's Pancakes (p. 331)
2 Tb. pancake syrup
2 tsp. margarine
Coffee

Lunch
Chef's salad:
Lettuce and tomato
1 oz. turkey breast
1 oz. ham
4 Tb. low-calorie Italian dressing
2 melba toast crackers
1 pear
8 oz. skim milk

Dinner
Grilled Tuna Steak with Dill Sauce (p. 346)
Baked potato
1 tsp. margarine
½ cup broccoli
1 cup watermelon
Coffee

Snack
8 oz. nonfat flavored yogurt

total fat .... *32.9 gm (21%)*   *cholesterol* ...... *84 mg*   *carbohydrate* ... *211 gm*
saturated fat ... *5.5 gm (4%)*   *calories* .... *1,412*   *protein* .... *74 gm*

Monday

Breakfast
½ cup tomato juice
¾ cup Nutrigrain cereal
4 oz. skim milk
Coffee

Lunch
Golden Harvest Soup (p. 366)
Tossed salad
2 Tb. low-calorie Italian
   dressing
1 bread stick
1 banana
Coffee

Dinner
Rice Balls (p. 349)
1 slice French bread
1 tsp. margarine
½ cup green beans
Tossed salad
2 Tb. low-calorie French
   dressing
1 orange
8 oz. skim milk

Snack
1 apple

total fat . . . . *29.4 gm (20%)*	*cholesterol* . . . . . . *82 mg*	*carbohydrate* . . . *215 gm*
saturated fat . . . *8.1 gm (6%)*	*calories* *1,318*	*protein* . . . .*59 gm*

Tuesday

Breakfast
½ cup orange juice
¾ cup Raisin Bran cereal
4 oz. skim milk
1 slice whole wheat toast
1 tsp. margarine
Coffee

Lunch
Sandwich:
   2 slices whole wheat bread
   ½ cup tuna salad
½ cup carrot sticks
1 apple
8 oz. skim milk

Dinner
Sante Fe Chicken (p. 350)
½ cup white rice
½ cup steamed vegetables:
   zucchini, cauliflower, and
   carrots
2 slices tomato
1 tsp. light mayonnaise
1 plum
Coffee

Snack
8 oz. skim milk
2 graham crackers

total fat . . . . *25.9 gm (18%)*	*cholesterol* . . . . .*115 mg*	*carbohydrate* . . .*201 gm*
saturated fat . . . *5.1 gm (3%)*	*calories* *1,322*	*protein* . . . .*79 gm*

Wednesday

Breakfast
4 oz. orange juice
¾ cup Product 19 cereal
4 oz. skim milk
½ English muffin
1 tsp. margarine
Coffee

Lunch
Tabouli on lettuce (p. 365)
1 Kaiser roll
1 tsp. margarine
½ cup low-fat frozen yogurt
Iced tea

Dinner
4 oz. flank steak
1 slice French bread
2 tsp. margarine
Broccoli Salad (p. 361)
Stuffed Tomato Halves (p. 359)
½ cup butterscotch pudding
  (made with skim milk)
Coffee

Snack
1 pear

total fat....... 50.4 gm (27%)	cholesterol.....105 mg	carbohydrate...235 gm
saturated fat .. 10.1 gm (6%)	calories..........1,655	protein..........72 gm

Thursday

Breakfast
½ cup sliced strawberries
1½ cups Shredded Wheat cereal
4 oz. skim milk
Coffee

Lunch
1 pita bread
½ cup tuna salad
1 tomato
1 pear
8 oz. skim milk

Dinner
Turkey Chili (p. 355)
½ cup white rice
Lettuce wedge
2 Tb. Italian salad dressing
½ cup gelatin dessert
Iced tea

Snack
1 Oat Bran Muffin (p. 331)

total fat....... 35.9 gm (22%)	cholesterol......92 mg	carbohydrate...217 gm
saturated fat ... 6.2 gm (4%)	calories..........1,462	protein..........75 gm

Friday

Breakfast
½ grapefruit
1 whole bagel, toasted
1 tsp. margarine
1 oz. Lite Line cheese
Coffee

Lunch
Curry Chicken Salad (p. 363)
4 slices tomato
1 pan roll
1 tsp. margarine
2 graham crackers
8 oz. skim milk

Dinner
Baked Fish Fillet (p. 341)
1 cup noodles with 1 Tb.
    Parmesan cheese and 2 tsp.
    margarine
½ cup steamed zucchini
2 slices tomato
1 peach
Coffee

Snack
1 cup grapes

total fat .... *33.2 gm (24%)* *cholesterol* ..... *156 mg* *carbohydrate* ... *174 gm*
saturated fat ... *7.2 gm (5%)* *calories* .... *1,257* *protein* .... *67 gm*

Saturday

Breakfast
4 oz. grapefruit juice
1 sv. French Toast (p. 329)
2 tsp. margarine
2 Tb. pancake syrup
Coffee

Lunch
Sandwich:
    2 slices whole wheat bread
    2 oz. lean roast beef
    1 tsp. mustard
Pickled Beets (p. 358)
½ cup melon balls
8 oz. skim milk

Dinner
Hearty Pea Soup (p. 367)
Tossed salad
1 Tb. Thousand Island dressing
1 slice homemade cornbread
1 tsp. margarine
Strawberries and "Cream" (p.
    339)
Iced tea

Snack
¾ cup Cheerios cereal
4 oz. skim milk

total fat .... *41.4 gm (25%)* *cholesterol* ...... *64 mg* *carbohydrate* ... *215 gm*
saturated fat ... *7.3 gm (4%)* *calories* .... *1,465* *protein* .... *65 gm*

Sunday

Breakfast
½ cup blueberries
1 sv. Breakfast Waffle (p. 328)
2 tsp. margarine
2 Tb. pancake syrup
Coffee

Lunch
Seafood Chowder (p. 369)
6 saltines
½ cup cole slaw
½ cup grapes
8 oz. skim milk

Dinner
Stir Fry Chicken (p. 352)
½ cup rice
Tossed salad
2 Tb. French salad dressing
Frozen Fruit Dessert (p. 336)
Iced tea

Snack
8 oz. nonfat flavored yogurt

---

total fat . . . . *48.8 gm (22%)*   *cholesterol* . . . . . *225 mg*   *carbohydrate* . . . *268 gm*
saturated fat . . . *9.3 gm (4%)*   *calories* . . . . *1,956*   *protein* . . . . *115 gm*

If you are accustomed to fried foods, fast foods, big desserts, and the like, this sort of menu may at first seem strange. But after only a month or two of such meals, some wonderful things begin to happen. Your extra pounds melt away, your cholesterol level falls, and more often than not—if my patients are representative—you feel better all over, better about yourself and better about the world. This is especially likely to happen when you accompany your diet with a program of adequate aerobic exercise, as recommended in the next chapter.

PART FOUR

Exercise, Drugs, and Cholesterol

CHAPTER 15

Exercise:
How Much Can It Help?

Runners and joggers. Aerobics on TV, or by Jane Fonda, or in a health spa. The interest in exercise now is much greater than fifteen years ago. Why are so many people exercising? Because exercise makes them feel better physically and mentally, gives them a feeling of accomplishment and discipline, helps with weight control, and generally improves their health. That's a hard combination to beat.

Is physical activity related to the development of coronary heart disease? *Yes.* We now know for certain that those who are more physically active have a lower rate of cardiovascular disease, whereas those who are inactive have a higher rate. It is also important for you to understand the effect of exercise on other cardiovascular risk factors such as obesity, hypertension, and blood levels of total cholesterol, HDL cholesterol, and triglyceride.

Not all types of exercise can be recommended: some may be too strenuous, some not strenuous enough. Generally speaking, aerobic exercise is the key for you. In this chapter you will learn what aerobic exercise is, how to assess your ability to perform aerobic exercise, what type of exercise is appropriate for you, how many times a week you need to exercise and for how long, and finally what benefits you may expect. You will also learn about certain precautions that should be taken before you begin an exercise program.

Aerobic Exercise

The word *aerobic* is derived from the Greek *aer*, air, and *bios*, life; it means something like "living in air." Processes in your body that can work only when oxygen is present are collectively referred to as "aerobic metabolism." Alternatively, "anaerobic metabolism" refers to processes that do not depend on oxygen.

When you exercise, energy is required. This energy can be derived from aerobic or anaerobic metabolism. Within the first few minutes of exercise, you produce more energy from anaerobic processes than from aerobic processes; but energy from anaerobic sources is primarily for high-intensity, very brief efforts. After the initial burst of energy, you can continue exercising only by taking in oxygen from the atmosphere. This oxygen is necessary to produce the further energy that comes from burning calories and to stimulate the cardiovascular system.

Repetitive, rhythmic exercises such as brisk walking, running, swimming, cycling, rowing, jumping rope, and skating, even for ten or fifteen minutes, are aerobic exercises because you need oxygen from the atmosphere to continue to contract your muscles. In contrast, quick, short-term exercises such as sprinting, weight lifting, push-ups, sit-ups, hand grip, and isometrics are less beneficial because most of the energy in these anaerobic exercises is from stored energy sources. These exercises end too quickly to benefit the cardiovascular system, and they burn very few calories.

The oxygen consumed by your body during aerobic exercise can be measured. "Maximal oxygen uptake," or VO_2 max for short, refers to the greatest amount of oxygen that you can take up from the air as you exercise. The higher your VO_2 max, the more work you can do.

VO_2 max differs for various ages and for males and females. Before puberty, boys and girls have about the same VO_2 max. After puberty, females have somewhat lower levels because they generally have a higher percent of fat and less muscle capable of using oxygen. The VO_2 max of both sexes reaches a peak between the ages of eighteen and twenty, after which there is a gradual decline. However, such differences can be *very much influenced by your exercise habits.* The more fit you are, the greater your VO_2 max will be. In fact, although a 65-year-old typically has only about 70 percent of the VO_2 max of a 25-year-old, a *fit* 65-year-old can have as high a VO_2 max as a nonexercising 25-year-old.

Usually the VO_2 max is measured in a special laboratory while you are exercising: for example, walking on a treadmill or riding a stationary bicycle. But you don't really need to know exactly what your VO_2 max is, nor do you need to exercise to your maximum capacity when you work out. In fact, to improve your cardiovascular endurance you need only exceed 50 percent of your VO_2 max, a level sufficient to produce a significant training effect. If you follow the aerobic exercise program outlined for you in this chapter, you will achieve this goal.

During exercise the oxygen uptake increases gradually over the first few minutes and then reaches a plateau. At the end of exercise, the oxygen uptake returns to the pre-exercise level but does so only gradually. This means that even after you finish exercising, you continue for a while to take up more oxygen and burn more calories.

Beneficial Effects of Exercise

Your potential for achieving a high level of fitness is established at birth. To develop this potential, you need to engage in a regular routine of physical activity. Regular aerobic exercise will also produce the following beneficial changes for you:

1. Your VO_2 max will be greater, and you will be able to do greater amounts of physical work.

2. Any given level of work will feel much easier to perform, and you will be able to perform for a longer period of time.

3. You will notice a decrease in your heart rate (pulse rate) and your breathing rate for the same amount of exercise.

4. Your coronary risk profile will improve: that is, you will likely have lower blood lipid levels, lower blood pressure, and lower relative body fat, but a higher blood HDL cholesterol level (see below).

5. Your body's cells will be more responsive (sensitive) to the normal effects of insulin, handling your blood sugar more efficiently.

6. You will feel and look better, producing a positive change in your attitude about yourself.

If you have atherosclerosis, exercise may allow some compensation for the reduced flow of blood and oxygen through your coronary arteries. Your collateral circulation may be improved, and the oxygen demands of your heart muscle may be reduced by a lower heart rate, lower blood pressure, and other beneficial changes of your heart muscle that enable your heart to perform more efficiently. For example, the volume of blood that your heart pumps each time it beats will be greater, thereby decreasing the number of beats needed per minute to pump a given amount of blood. The skeletal muscles in the arms and legs of a trained person use oxygen more efficiently and impose less demand on an already compromised heart for a given amount of work.

Exercise is now prescribed regularly for patients with coronary

Table 15-1. Calories Expended by Various Types of Aerobic Exercise

Activity	Calories expended per 1 pound per minute	Activity	Calories expended per 1 pound per minute
Aerobic dance (vigorous)	.062	Rowing (vigorous)	.097
Basketball (vigorous, full-court)	.097	Running (8 mph)	.104
Bicycling (13 mph)	.071	Snowshoeing (2.5 mph)	.060
Canoeing (flat water, 4 mph)	.045	Soccer (vigorous)	.097
Cross-country skiing (8 mph)	.104	Swimming (55 yd/min)	.088
Golf (twosome carrying clubs)	.045	Table tennis (skilled)	.045
Handball (skilled, singles)	.078	Tennis (beginner)	.032
Jogging (5 mph)	.060	Walking (4.5 mph)	.048

Source: Modified from Peter D. Wood, "The Science of Successful Weight Loss," *Encyclopedia Britannica Health and Medical Annual*, 1984, pp. 1–138.

heart disease. Medically supervised programs that enroll patients two months after they have had a heart attack or coronary artery bypass surgery are widely available, and some programs even accept patients within two weeks of hospital discharge. Such persons under proper medical supervision can generally demonstrate the same type of cardiovascular conditioning as persons who have not had clinical evidence of coronary heart disease.

Exercise and Weight Control

Exercise consumes calories; if your energy intake remains the same and you exercise more, your weight will fall. The number of calories expended by various types of exercise is summarized for you in Table 15-1. The more strenuous and longer the exercise, the greater the number of calories you burn. For any type of exercise, a heavy person will expend more calories than a thin person. To determine how many calories you will expend in a certain type of exercise, simply multiply the exercise time in minutes by your weight in pounds, and then multiply that figure by the factor in the righthand column of Table 15-1.

Your ability to lose weight is influenced in part by your basal metabolic rate, or BMR, a measure of the energy you require when you are at complete rest. One-third to one-half of your total daily energy expenditure is needed to maintain your BMR. Such energy is used by your cells to process fats, carbohydrates, and proteins, and to maintain your body temperature. The BMR may vary from 1,300 to 1,900 calories per day, but the average BMR is about one calorie per minute for an average-sized person, or 1,440 calories per day. The remaining differences between individuals in their daily caloric expenditure are related to energy expenditure.

A balance, or imbalance, in calories determines your total body weight, and more importantly your total body fat. When calories eaten are *equal to* calories burned (BMR plus energy expended), your weight is stable. When calories eaten are *less than* calories burned, you lose weight; fat is stored energy and used to make up the calorie deficit. When calories eaten are *greater than* calories burned, you gain weight; the energy from the excess calories is stored as fat.

Exercise helps you to lose weight by increasing the amount of energy you expend. As we shall see below, exercise also increases your BMR. To lose one pound, you must burn 3,500 calories more than you eat.

A common misconception among some laymen and their doctors is that obese people eat more and consume more calories than lean people. This is not true. *Obese, inactive people actually consume, on average, a lower number of calories than lean, active people.* The major difference between the two groups is that lean, active people expend more calories through exercise than obese people. Over the last 80 years American per capita food consumption has actually decreased, but the population has become heavier because it is less active. Doctors hope that the recent interest in exercise will help to reverse this trend.

Exercise can make a big difference in your weight. Did you gain weight after you graduated from high school ten, twenty, or thirty years ago? Are you ten or twenty pounds overweight? It doesn't take much to get that way. *To gain a pound and a half of fat per year, you need only eat 14.4 calories per day more than you expend.* That's one-quarter of a slice of bread.

Conversely, regular aerobic exercise expends a certain number of calories per day, on average, and when spread out over a year or longer translates into a considerably large number of pounds lost. For example, if you exercise for 30 minutes four times a week, you will burn approximately 1,200 *extra* calories a week, about 4,800 calories a month, and 62,400 calories a year. If you continue to eat the same number of calories as before, you will lose approximately 18 pounds in that year.

Reducing your calories is not enough. An overweight person is usually advised to eat less; but *eating less without exercising more decreases your BMR.* Dr. Peter Wood points out that if you eat 600 fewer calories per day, your BMR will fall from 1,400 to 1,000 calories per day; thus you will lose weight at the rate of only 200 calories a day *if you don't exercise.* No wonder many people experience a disappointingly small weight loss when they simply eat less.

By contrast, if you are active you may actually eat more, and many of the extra calories will be burned by an increase in your BMR rather than converted to fat. As noted above, there is now evidence that your BMR remains elevated for at least several hours after you finish exercising, so that you burn calories over and above those burned in performing the exercise itself.

Another benefit of exercise is that the distribution of your weight changes. Compared with a sedentary person, if you exercise regularly, you will carry a greater proportion of your body mass as energy-burning muscle and a smaller proportion as heat-insulating fat. This shift in the balance is toward expending more energy and storing less as fat.

Exercise and Your Cholesterol Level

How is regular aerobic exercise likely to affect your blood lipid and lipoprotein levels? Dr. Seals and co-workers from the Washington University School of Medicine in St. Louis studied five subject groups of men that varied in age, training, and body weight. The mean HDL cholesterol level in these groups varied considerably as follows: older (masters) athletes, 66 mg/dl; young athletes, 55 mg/dl; young untrained men, 50 mg/dl; older untrained men, lean, 45 mg/dl; and older untrained men, not lean, 42 mg/dl. The ratios of total cholesterol to HDL cholesterol were similarly low (2.8 to 3.4) for the athletes and the young untrained men, compared with the older untrained men (4.0 to 5.6). On the basis of their HDL cholesterol levels alone, the masters athletes might be expected to incur coronary heart disease at a rate of 25 per 1,000, whereas the sedentary men are at three times that risk, or approximately 75 per 1,000.

In this study, the VO_2 max of the subjects was determined during exercise on a treadmill, and the masters athletes had markedly higher levels. The researchers also compared young athletes with young nonathletes. The young athletes had a higher average HDL cholesterol level (55 mg/dl) and a lower ratio of total cholesterol to HDL cholesterol (2.8) than the young untrained men (50 mg/dl and 3.4, respectively). Since the differences on both counts increased with age, it could be inferred—as many people believe—that exercise helps you stay young!

Exercise and HDL cholesterol levels in those with coronary heart disease. Dr. George Cowan from the Queen Elizabeth Military Hospital in London, England, studied the effects of an intensive rehabilitation program on HDL cholesterol levels in 40 men between 29 and 56 years old who had experienced heart attacks, coronary artery bypass surgery, or angina pectoris. The exercise program involved aerobic activities that increased the heart rate to 80 percent of maximum. The exercise was performed five days a week, three times a day, for twenty-minute periods and lasted three weeks. The average HDL cholesterol increased from a low of 32 to 35 mg/dl, and the ratio of total cholesterol to HDL cholesterol decreased significantly. *Those who continued to smoke during the exercise program had virtually no change at all in their HDL cholesterol levels.* In another study, Dr. Stubbe and his co-workers in Lund, Sweden, found that subjects who stopped smoking cigarettes experienced a 29 percent increase in HDL cholesterol levels *in only two weeks.*

The above studies and others indicate that men with coronary heart disease can exercise regularly and relatively vigorously, provided appropriate care is taken and supervision is provided, and can attain improvements in their coronary risk factors in a manner similar to men without coronary heart disease.

Exercise, HDL cholesterol, and lipids in women. Hartung and co-workers from the Baylor College of Medicine found that the HDL cholesterol level was higher in 44 long-distance female runners (78 mg/dl) and in 47 female joggers (70 mg/dl) than in 45 inactive females (62 mg/dl). The active women also had lower ratios of total cholesterol to HDL cholesterol. When the women were divided into premenopausal and postmenopausal, these trends persisted. Apparently, then, exercise can help prevent the decrease in HDL cholesterol, and the increase in the ratio of total cholesterol to HDL cholesterol, that occurs in many women following menopause.

How much exercise is required to increase your HDL cholesterol level? Dr. Leclerc and co-workers at the Physical Activity Sciences Laboratory of Laval University, in Quebec, estimated that the minimum amount of exercise required to raise the HDL cholesterol level was fifteen minutes every three days. But for a significant increase, you need more than this minimum: I recommend regular aerobic exercise, lasting at least 30 minutes, three or four times a week. If you are a runner, both Dr. Peter Wood and associates in 1983 and Dr.

Hartung in 1980 estimated the threshold to be eight to eleven miles a week.

How long will it take before your HDL cholesterol level increases significantly? It depends. Dr. Wood found that California men who were initially sedentary required a supervised running program of twelve miles a week for approximately one year before meaningful changes in their HDL cholesterol levels occurred; but he built up their weekly mileage very slowly to minimize injuries. The current medical literature suggests that a significant cardiovascular response to conditioning requires at least six to eight weeks.

The same probably applies to deconditioning. Thompson and co-workers from the Department of Health, Physical Education, and Recreation in Seattle found that cessation of exercise for six weeks in endurance-trained men between 18 and 45 years old led to no significant changes in HDL cholesterol, percent of body fat, or VO_2 max. Ordinary people have not been studied in this regard; but doctors tend to agree that if you go without exercise for longer than six weeks, you will probably begin to lose its benefits.

Exercise and Other Cardiovascular Risk Factors

High blood pressure. Dr. Kerry Stewart and co-workers at the Francis Scott Key Medical Center in Baltimore recently completed a study of the effect of an exercise program of jogging and circuit weight training on blood pressure in hypertensive men with an average diastolic blood pressure of 96 off medication. (In circuit weight training, the subject moves from weight machine to weight machine, performing for 30 seconds at 40 percent of maximum capacity, with 30 seconds of rest between exercises, for a total of twenty minutes.)

Fifty-one men from 29 to 59 years old exercised one hour three times a week for ten weeks. Before beginning this program the men were assigned by chance into one of three groups: placebo, propranolol (240 mg/day), or diltiazem (360 mg/day), propranolol and diltiazem being drugs commonly used to treat high blood pressure. By the seventh week of exercise, the average diastolic blood pressure of these men had fallen from 96 to 84 and there were no differences among the three groups.

The results suggest that exercise alone was as effective as exercise combined with drugs in controlling blood pressure. To top it off, exercise increased the men's average HDL cholesterol level by 10 percent and decreased their LDL cholesterol levels by 8 percent without a low-fat diet or weight loss.

Risk factors in women. Coronary heart disease is the leading cause of death in American women; almost 250,000 deaths in 1986, a higher rate than women in other countries. Dr. Kenneth Cooper, of the Cooper Clinic and Institute for Aerobics Research in Dallas, studied the association between coronary heart disease risk factors and physical fitness in about 1,700 healthy adult women. After considering the effects of age and body weight, he found physical fitness to be independently associated with the blood levels of triglyceride and HDL cholesterol, the ratio of total cholesterol to HDL cholesterol, blood pressure levels, and cigarette smoking. Women who were physically fit had risk factor profiles that placed them at lower risk of coronary heart disease than women who were not physically fit.

Exercise and Coronary Heart Disease

Results from many population studies indicate strongly that exercise decreases the risk of coronary heart disease. The greater the level of physical activity, the lower the death rate from coronary heart disease. This effect is present even after other cardiovascular risk factors are considered.

In the Framingham Heart Study, resting heart rate, relative weight, and vital capacity of the lungs were used as indicators of physical activity. Those subjects classified as physically inactive had one or more of the following characteristics:

1. Their resting heart rate was rapid, above 85 beats per minute.
2. They were at least 20 percent overweight.
3. Their vital capacity (lung capacity) was low: men less than three liters, women less than two.

After twelve years of follow-up annual examinations of men and women 30 to 62 years old, *those subjects with two or more of these three indicators of poor fitness had about five times as high a death rate from coronary heart disease as those with no indicators of poor fitness* (Figure 15-1). For those with only one indicator of poor fitness, the death rate was in between that of the most fit and least fit groups.

Even a simple measure of heart (pulse) rate on a resting EKG (electrocardiogram) was a potent predictor of sudden death in the Fra-

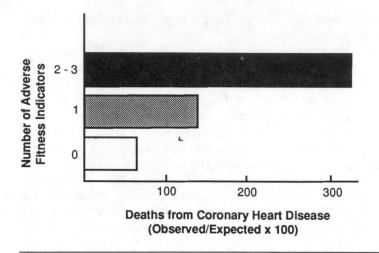

Fig. 15-1. Relative risk of coronary heart disease by number of fitness indicators. The fitness indicators are rapid pulse, obesity, and low vital capacity. Reproduced with permission from the twelve-year follow-up of men and women aged 30–62 in the Framingham Study, W. B. Kannel, P. Wilson, and S. N. Blair, *American Heart Journal* 109 (1985): 879.

mingham Heart Study over a 26-year follow-up of men and women 35 to 84 years of age. As Figure 15-2 shows, men with a rapid heart rate (above 87) had a rate of sudden death almost six times as high as those with a slow heart rate (below 64), and those men with a heart rate between these two extremes had intermediate rates of sudden death. In women, the relation between sudden death and heart rate was less striking.

In 1988 investigators from the Lipid Research Clinics Mortality Follow-Up Study used stress exercise tests to assess the relation between physical fitness and death from cardiovascular disease. They found that a lower level of physical fitness was associated with a higher risk of death from coronary heart disease in healthy men, independent of other coronary risk factors.

Regular physical training also appears to have a positive effect on blood coagulation: that is, fit people appear to be less prone to form clots or thrombosis in their coronary arteries.

How much physical activity is necessary to ward off coronary artery disease? Estimates, based on population studies, vary from a rather intense effort, 30 minutes of vigorous physical activity every day, to as little as 20 minutes of walking per day. Dr. Paffenberger and associates, from their study of 17,000 Harvard alumni followed for about twenty years, concluded that the expenditure of between 500 and 2,000 calories a week from exercise was sufficient; about 2,000 calories a week was ideal, with no further benefit beyond this level.

To define these calories in exercise terms, simply multiply the number of minutes that you exercise by your weight in pounds, and then multiply that number by the factor in Table 15-1. For example, let's say that you decide to burn 1,200 extra calories per week. You weigh 170 pounds and you have a chosen a stationary bike as your exercise. If you ride the bike at 13 mph, you will expend the following number of calories per minute:

170 pounds × .071 calories per pound per minute
= 12 calories per minute

To burn 1,200 extra calories per week, you will need to ride the bike the following number of minutes:

1,200 calories ÷ 12 calories = 100 minutes

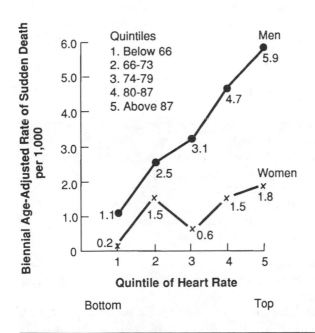

Fig. 15-2. Risk of sudden death by heart rate on EKG.
Reproduced with permission from the 26-year follow-up of men aged 35–84 in the Framingham Study, W. B. Kannel, P. Wilson, and S. N. Blair, *American Heart Journal* 109 (1985): 878.

If you exercise four times a week, you would need to spend 25 minutes per session.

In a study by Morris and co-workers in 1973, men who exercised vigorously on weekends were only one-third as likely to have a first heart attack as inactive men over a four-year follow-up. There is probably a gradation of effect. If you undertake regular aerobic exercise, 30 to 40 minutes three to four times a week is likely to reduce your risk of coronary heart disease.

Is increased physical activity associated with less coronary heart disease in older people as well? In the Framingham Study, this relationship held for those 55–64 years old as well as for younger people. Of course, greater precautions must be taken with older people, especially those with risk factors such as a high blood cholesterol level, high blood pressure, and obesity (see below).

A word of caution. Although there is substantial evidence that increased physical activity leads to lower rates of coronary heart disease, this has not been shown conclusively in a large, prospective, well-controlled clinical trial. Nevertheless, the beneficial effects of exercise for you appear substantial. There can be no doubt that physical fitness plays an important part in any overall program designed to prevent coronary heart disease by controlling and modifying cardiovascular disease risk factors.

Your Exercise Program

Precautions concerning exercise. Before you undertake any type of exercise, certain precautions will be necessary. The older you are, the greater the precautions. If you have not exercised regularly in years, you will need to plan out your exercise program carefully. *It is important that you have a general physical examination, and that you and your doctor discuss what kind of exercise program makes sense for you.* In particular, a stress electrocardiogram should be considered if:

1. You are older than 35.
2. You have a positive family history of premature (under 55 years) coronary heart disease.
3. You are male and have another risk factor for coronary heart disease such as high blood cholesterol, high blood pressure, or cigarette smoking.
4. You are female and have two risk factors for coronary heart disease.

If you have coronary heart disease or diabetes, or are obese, or have been inactive for a number of years, you will need to use even greater caution before beginning an exercise program. If you are pregnant, you should plan your exercise program with your obstetrician.

Take it easy to begin with. For example, start by walking 10 to 15 minutes a day for two or three weeks, then increase gradually to brisk walking for up to 30 minutes at least four times a week. You may then wish to alternate jogging and walking, and later build up to jogging and finally to running. If you prefer bicycling, swimming, or an exercise machine such as a stationary bike or a rowing machine, start with 10- or 15-minute workouts and gradually work up to 30-minute workouts over a period of several months.

As a rule of thumb, stay at the same number of minutes for at least one week and do not increase more than 10 percent at a time. Remember also to warm up before exercise. Take about five minutes to stretch your muscles and to loosen up before starting your exercise. Wear comfortable, loose-fitting clothes that are appropriate for the weather and the exercise you have chosen. Pay special attention to the proper selection of footwear.

Deciding how much to exercise. How much exercise should you do? Enough to make a *DIF*ference. Your exercise should be of sufficient *D*uration, *I*ntensity, and *F*requency to produce a significant training effect:

*D*uration—how long you exercise

*I*ntensity—how fast or hard you exercise

*F*requency—how often you exercise

The bottom line is that your aerobic exercise program should be sufficient to expend at least 1,200 calories a week. If the exercise you choose is less intense, that is, expends fewer calorics, you will need to do it for a longer time. Conversely, if you choose more intensive exercise (for example, running rather than jogging), you will need less exercise time to expend the same number of calories. You can determine the proper length of your workouts by a calculation of the sort shown on pp. 259–60.

Remember, an expenditure of 1,200 calories a week is the *minimum*. This level of exercise should enable you to exceed 50 percent of your VO$_2$ max, and thus should have a significant training effect. But all indications are that a little more would be even better. If you wish to do more, you may want to work toward a goal of 2,000 calories a week.

Let's take another example. A 60-year-old man weighs 180 pounds and selects walking (4.5 mph) as his exercise. Table 15-1 indicates that this exercise expends 0.048 calories per pound per minute. For each minute of walking, this man will expend 8.64 calories (180 × 0.048). Since he needs to burn at least 1,200 calories a week, he will need to walk 138.8 minutes (1,200 calories divided by 8.64 calories per minute). If he walks four times a week, he will need to walk about 35 minutes each time.

You can see from this example that walking can be an acceptable aerobic exercise. A long, low-intensity workout is equivalent to a short, high-intensity workout if the same number of calories is expended.

Achieving sufficient intensity. Roughly, your intensity is sufficient if you are slightly out of breath during the entire course of exercise. Alternatively, you can determine your *target heart rate* and see if you achieve it with exercise.

First, you need to know how to measure your heart rate. Take the second and third fingers of your left hand and place them on the edge of your right wrist below your thumb. You will feel your pulse with each beat of your heart. Count the number of pulses for 15 seconds and multiple them by 4; this is your heart rate.

Doctors who specialize in exercise frequently use the following formula to arrive at a rough prediction of maximum heart rate: 220 minus your age. At the beginning, your target heart rate during exercise should be about 70 percent of your maximum heart rate. For example, if you are 40 years old, your maximum heart rate is 220 minus 40, or 180. Seventy percent of 180 gives you a target heart rate of 126.

As you become a more experienced exerciser, you can increase your target heart rate to 80–85 percent of your maximum rate. This greater intensity will allow you to reach 70 percent of your predicted VO_2 max. To help you determine your target heart rate, you can find your "target zone" in Figure 15-3.

Cooling down. Because about half of your circulating blood can pool in your lower extremities after aerobic exercise, it is very important that you walk around (do not sit or lie down) for at least five minutes after you exercise. Otherwise your blood pressure may fall, decreasing the amount of blood circulating to your brain and heart. This can result in fainting, dizziness, nausea, abnormal heartbeats (arrhythmias), and an insufficient supply of oxygen to the heart (ischemia).

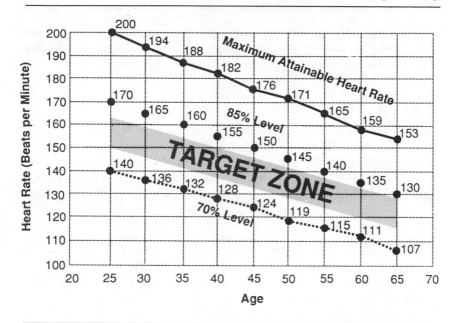

Fig. 15-3. Maximum attainable heart rate for men and women. The "target zone" for your target heart rate depends on your age and whether you are at a beginning exercise level (70%) or a more experienced exercise level (85%). Note: These values are average and do not apply to one-third of the population. Modified from L. Zohman, M.D., *Beyond Diet: Exercise Your Way to Fitness and Heart Health* (Englewood Cliffs, N.J.: CPC International).

Eating and Exercise

What should you eat to achieve maximal physical performance? A well-balanced low-fat, low-cholesterol diet of the sort presented in Chapter 11 contains an adequate amount of protein, including all the essential amino acids; use lean meat, fish, and poultry, low-fat milk, and high-quality vegetable proteins such as soybean protein. You do not need supplementary protein over and above what is furnished by the diet.

In exercise taking less than one hour, your available supplies of stored energy, namely, fat in your adipose tissue and glycogen in your liver and muscle, are generally ample. *No meal should be taken less than one hour prior to exercise.* In particular, don't consume large quantities of carbohydrates right before exercise; this can stimulate the release of insulin by your body, which decreases its ability to use free fatty acids as energy sources from the fatty tissue.

For longer athletic events, those lasting over an hour, carbohydrate loading for several days before will help to fill up the deposits of glycogen in your muscles.

Can Exercise Be Bad for You?

In his book *Running Without Fear*, Dr. Kenneth H. Cooper discusses the untimely death of Jim Fixx. Dr. Cooper describes persons who have what he calls "The Jim Fixx Syndrome," the belief that in one way or another exercise is the "ultimate antidote against coronary heart disease and sudden death." As part of this syndrome, these exercisers put their faith in one or more of the following four "myths of invulnerability":

1. "I couldn't have heart disease and run the way I run without symptoms." (You saw in Chapter 2 that collateral arteries can form, supplying oxygen to the heart muscle despite significant blockages in the coronary arteries.)
2. "People who run marathons don't die of heart attacks." (They can if they have hidden or undiagnosed coronary heart disease.)
3. "Stress tests are worthless because they produce too many false readings [false positives and false negatives]. Also, physicians don't know how to interpret the stress electrocardiogram of an athlete." (Although it is true that a negative stress EKG is not an absolute guarantee of safety, you saw in Chapter 2 that repeated stress EKGs over time can help to identify a hidden problem with coronary heart disease.)
4. "If you are a highly conditioned long-distance runner, you can forget your heredity." (Wrong. Inherited cholesterol or triglyceride disorders or problems in HDL processing cannot be cured by running.)

As the death of Jim Fixx makes clear, aerobic exercise can be unwise when undertaken in ignorance (or defiance) of a proper evaluation of your lipid profile, your blood pressure, and other cardiovascular risk factors, especially if you have a personal or family history of coronary heart disease. On the other hand, if you are one of the many people whose physical condition permits exercise, an aerobic exercise program that fits your lifestyle and risk profile will provide the many advantages reviewed in this chapter and will help you to live a longer, healthier life.

Summary

1. A low level of fitness and physical activity is associated with a higher rate of death from coronary heart disease.

2. Regular aerobic exercise performed with sufficient duration, intensity, and frequency can make a *DIF*ference for you.

3. Before you undertake any type of aerobic exercise, your doctor should give you a physical examination. The two of you should then discuss the proposed exercise program in the light of what your examination discloses.

4. Regular aerobic exercise may lower your blood pressure; lower your levels of total and LDL cholesterol, triglyceride, and blood sugar; and increase your HDL cholesterol.

5. Regular aerobic exercise can play a vital role in a program for losing weight or for maintaining ideal or appropriate body weight.

6. People with coronary heart disease can exercise regularly and relatively vigorously in a medically prescribed program.

7. People who continue to smoke during an aerobic exercise program appear to have little change in their HDL cholesterol level.

8. Good habits of aerobic exercise, once established, must be maintained over a lifetime for the beneficial effects of exercise to continue.

9. Although it has not been proved conclusively that increasing physical activity decreases the rate of coronary heart disease, physical fitness plays an important part in an integrated, comprehensive program designed to prevent coronary heart disease by controlling and modifying cardiovascular disease risk factors.

10. An exercise program should be complemented with a diet low in total fat, saturated fat, and cholesterol. For periods of strenuous exercise lasting longer than an hour, such as athletic events, it is now thought that carbohydrate loading over the preceding days is more helpful than fat or protein loading.

11. It is not wise to institute a low-fat, low-cholesterol diet and an aerobic exercise program *without a proper prior evaluation of other cardiovascular risk factors*, notably blood pressure, blood levels of cholesterol, triglyceride, and LDL and HDL cholesterol, and family history of premature coronary heart disease. A diet low in fat and cholesterol makes sense for most people; so does a good exercise program. But precisely because this is so, someone whose specific condition requires something more than diet and exercise, such as drugs, can be misled into thinking that diet and exercise by themselves are enough to minimize the risk of coronary heart disease. Sometimes this just isn't so.

Can Drugs Help Make Up for What You Inherited?

This chapter provides guidelines to help you and your doctor decide when drug treatment might be indicated for your blood lipid problem, and reviews the drugs that are commonly used to treat either blood cholesterol or triglyceride problems. The information given for each drug includes its usual dose, its major effect on levels of blood cholesterol, LDL cholesterol, HDL cholesterol, and triglyceride, its major side effects, what special precautions it requires, and its cost.

When Is Drug Treatment Advisable for a Cholesterol Problem?

To determine whether you need drug treatment for a blood cholesterol problem, you must first have your blood cholesterol level measured. If it is over 200 mg/dl, your doctor will probably want to repeat the test after an overnight fast to confirm the blood cholesterol level and to measure your levels of HDL cholesterol, LDL cholesterol, and triglyceride.

At the same visit, your doctor can review with you as necessary some of the other risk factors for coronary heart disease discussed in Chapter 5: male sex, family history of premature coronary heart disease, cigarette smoking, high blood pressure, low blood level of HDL cholesterol (under 35 mg/dl), diabetes, personal history of stroke or poor circulation, and obesity.

Your doctor will also want to determine whether your high blood cholesterol level may be aggravated (or even caused) by some other condition, such as a thyroid, liver, or kidney problem, or by a medication that you are taking. Some medications that can raise cholesterol or triglyceride levels include oral contraceptives, steroids, diuretics such as the thiazides, and drugs for hypertension such as beta blockers.

The cornerstone of treatment is diet. Before considering drug therapy for your blood lipid problem, you must first change to a low-saturated-fat, low-cholesterol diet. If you are eating the usual American diet, which is high in total fat, saturated fat, and cholesterol, you can change to a Step One diet (Table 11-1), which contains fewer than 30 percent of calories as fat, fewer than 10 percent of calories as saturated fat, and less than 300 mg of cholesterol per day. This diet is discussed at length in Chapter 11, some sample menus for it are presented in Chapter 14, and some excellent low-fat, low-cholesterol recipes will be found on pp. 325–369. The actual amounts of saturated fat and cholesterol in the foods that you usually eat are summarized in the Food Tables, pp. 296–324.

It is also important for you to work toward achieving optimum body weight. If you are overweight and are able to lose ten or twenty pounds, the weight loss will help you to lower your blood cholesterol, LDL cholesterol, and triglyceride levels, and may also increase your HDL cholesterol level. (An increase in HDL cholesterol often accompanies the decrease in blood triglyceride that occurs with weight reduction.) An exercise program appropriate for your age, general state of health, and physical conditioning can help you to lose weight and may in itself help to lower your cholesterol level.

If you are on a weight reduction diet, or if you have a blood triglyceride problem, you will need to restrict your alcohol intake to two or three drinks a week. An average mixed drink has one and one-half ounces of 80-proof liquor, or 105 calories; a four-ounce glass of wine comes to 100 calories, and 12 ounces of regular beer to 150 calories.

The goals for lowering your blood cholesterol and LDL cholesterol levels through diet, weight control, and exercise are summarized in Table 16-1. If you are otherwise healthy and do not have any risk factors for coronary heart disease, an LDL cholesterol level less than 160 mg/dl (corresponding to a blood cholesterol level of less than 240 mg/dl) is your *minimum* goal. If you already have coronary heart disease, or have two or more risk factors for coronary heart disease, your goal will be an LDL cholesterol less than 130 mg/dl (blood cholesterol less than 200 mg/dl).

If you have not achieved these goals after three months, the stricter Step Two diet is recommended by the Adult Treatment Panel. The Step Two diet (Table 11-1) is even more restricted in saturated fat (less than 7 percent of total calories) and cholesterol (under

Table 16-1. Goals for Lowering Your Blood Cholesterol and
LDL Cholesterol Levels by Dietary Treatment

	Goals (mg/dl)	
Category	Blood cholesterol	LDL cholesterol
No coronary heart disease and fewer than two risk factors	Below 240	Below 160
Coronary heart disease or two or more risk factors	Below 200	Below 130

Source: Recommendations of the Adult Treatment Panel, National Cholesterol Education Program, National Heart, Lung, and Blood Institute, National Institutes of Health, *Arch. Intern. Med.* 148 (1988): 36–69.

200 mg/day). The two-week menu plan in Chapter 14 is essentially for a Step Two diet. Ideally, you should discuss the Step Two diet with a registered dietician. If after further tightening of your diet for three months, you have not achieved the goals in Table 16-1, it is time for you and your doctor to consider a cholesterol-lowering drug. *But you should do your best to make diet and weight control work before you begin any drug treatment.*

Table 16-2 shows the values of blood cholesterol and LDL cholesterol at which treatment with cholesterol-lowering drugs may be initiated. If you are without coronary heart disease and have fewer than two risk factors, you are a candidate for drug treatment if your LDL cholesterol after diet is 190 mg/dl or higher (blood cholesterol 265 mg/dl or higher). If you already have coronary heart disease or have two or more risk factors for coronary heart disease, drug therapy should be considered if your LDL cholesterol after diet is 160 mg/dl or higher (blood cholesterol 240 mg/dl or higher). Remember that male sex is a risk factor. If you are male and your blood cholesterol is 240 mg/dl or higher after diet, you need only one other risk factor to be considered for drug treatment.

How does HDL cholesterol fit into this scheme? The Adult Treatment Panel considered a low HDL cholesterol (less than 35 mg/dl) to be one of the risk factors for coronary heart disease. If your HDL cholesterol is low and you have one other risk factor (including being male), your levels for initiating drug treatment are those shown in Table 16-2.

Chapter 4 discusses the LDL/HDL ratio, which is another way to assess your risk of coronary heart disease. An LDL/HDL ratio of 3.0 is considered average risk, 4.0 above-average risk, and 5.0 or more high risk. If your LDL cholesterol is above 160 mg/dl and your HDL cholesterol below 35 mg/dl, your LDL/HDL ratio will be at least 4.7.

The recommendations in Table 16-2 are conservative. For example, if I have a patient with premature coronary heart disease, I often recommend a cholesterol-lowering drug to get the blood cholesterol level below 200 mg/dl, especially if the HDL cholesterol level is below 35 mg/dl. The presence of other risk factors in such patients, such as high blood pressure or a positive family history of premature coronary heart disease, also makes me quicker to prescribe a drug.

This approach is supported by the results of CLAS (the Cholesterol-Lowering Atherosclerosis Study), in which the use of colestipol and nicotinic acid successfully slowed the progression of atherosclerosis in the bypass grafts and coronary arteries of patients with marked coronary heart disease. If you have coronary heart disease, you have a life-threatening illness, one that may well warrant aggressive treatment of your blood lipid problem and other modifiable risk factors that you may have.

When Is Drug Treatment Advisable for a Triglyceride Problem?

According to the NIH Consensus Development Conference on Treatment of Hypertriglyceridemia (reviewed in Chapter 5), drug treatment is advisable if after suitable diet and weight control measures your blood triglyceride level is above 500 mg/dl (very high). The dietary measures for a high blood triglyceride level are the same as those for a high blood cholesterol level; but weight loss, maintenance of ideal body weight, and alcohol restriction are *even more important* in managing a high blood triglyceride problem than in managing a high blood cholesterol problem.

Table 16-2. Levels of Blood Cholesterol and LDL Cholesterol at Which Treatment with Cholesterol-Lowering Drugs May Be Initiated

	Levels (mg/dl)	
Category	Blood cholesterol	LDL cholesterol
No coronary heart disease and fewer than two risk factors	265 or higher	190 or higher
Coronary heart disease or two or more risk factors	240 or higher	160 or higher

Source: Recommendations of the Adult Treatment Panel, National Cholesterol Education Program, National Heart, Lung, and Blood Institute, National Institutes of Health, *Arch. Intern. Med.* 148 (1988): 36–69.

Table 16-3. Drugs for Treatment of Blood Lipid Problems

Type of drug	Names of drugs
Bile acid sequestrant	Cholestyramine (Questran®, Cholybar®)
	Colestipol (Colestid®)
Niacin	Nicotinic acid
(vitamin B₃)	
HMG CoA reductase	Lovastatin (Mevacor®)
inhibitor	Simvastatin (Zocor®)*
	Pravastatin (Pravachol®)*
	Fluvastatin (LoChol®)*
Fibric acid	Gemfibrozil (Lopid®)
	Clofibrate (Atromid-S®)
	Fenofibrate (Lipidil®)*
Butylphenol	Probucol (Lorelco®)

*Not yet approved by the Food and Drug Administration for prescription use.

What if your blood triglyceride level is less than 500 mg/dl after diet and weight control but still in the high range (250–500 mg/dl)? If your blood cholesterol and LDL levels are below those set forth in Table 16-2, you are probably not a candidate for drug therapy, although drug treatment should be considered if you have premature coronary heart disease or other risk factors in addition to your high triglyceride level. Some medications such as nicotinic acid, discussed below, lower both the blood cholesterol and triglyceride levels.

What Drugs Help?

The drugs used for treatment of a blood cholesterol or triglyceride problem are listed in Table 16-3 according to type. The Adult Treatment Panel considers the bile acid sequestrants and nicotinic acid the drugs of first choice for two reasons: both have been shown to decrease heart attacks and deaths from heart attacks, and both, having now been used for about fifteen years, have a long track record of safety. Although both have side effects (Tables 16-4, 16-5), they are comparatively minor.

The HMG CoA reductase inhibitors are a newer class of drugs. One of these, lovastatin (Mevacor®), has been approved by the Food and Drug Administration for prescription use, though it has been used for only about five years and its long-term safety has not yet been established. Several studies are in progress to document the effect of lovastatin on coronary atherosclerosis and the incidence of heart attacks.

At this writing, all indications are that the HMG CoA reductase inhibitors will work at least as well as the bile acid sequestrants and nicotinic acid in preventing coronary heart disease. Several other HMG CoA reductase inhibitors that will become available in the future include simvastatin (Zocor®), pravastatin (Pravachol®), and fluvastatin (LoChol®).

Two derivatives of a compound called fibric acid are also available: gemfibrozil (Lopid®) and clofibrate (Atromid-S®). Both are primarily used for blood triglyceride problems; but also both, particularly gemfibrozil, tend to increase HDL cholesterol. Another drug in this class, fenofibrate (Lipidil®), will also soon be available in the United States, after thirteen years on the European market.

As noted in Chapter 3, gemfibrozil was found in the Helsinki Heart Study to cause a significant (34 percent) reduction in heart attacks. It produced about a 10 percent lowering of LDL cholesterol in addition to lowering triglyceride and increasing HDL cholesterol; all these effects were of benefit in preventing heart disease. In contrast, clofibrate (Atromid-S) is not routinely recommended for prescription use. Although it was shown in the World Health Organization study to reduce the incidence of heart attacks, it was associated also with a higher than predicted number of deaths from other causes.

Another drug, probucol, lowers blood cholesterol and LDL cholesterol to a modest degree, but also lowers HDL cholesterol considerably. I do not usually prescribe probucol for this reason. But it is currently the subject of much research, and there are signs that it may help to prevent deposits of cholesterol in arteries that are not simply related to the blood levels of LDL cholesterol and HDL cholesterol.

Next, each of these classes of drugs will be reviewed for you in detail. The pertinent facts about them are summarized in Tables 16-4 through 16-8.

Bile Acid Sequestrants

There are two drugs that bind bile acids: cholestyramine (Questran® or Questran® Light and Cholybar®) and colestipol (Colestid®). Information about both is given in summary form in Table 16-4.

Usual dose. These medicines are in a powder form and are taken

Table 16-4. Facts about Bile Acid Sequestrants

Names of drugs:	Cholestyramine (Questran® or Questran® Light) Colestipol (Colestid®) Cholestyramine (Cholybar®)
Supplied as:	Cholestyramine powder 　Carton of 60 nine-gram packets 　Can of 378 grams Colestipol granules 　Box of 30 five-gram packets 　Bottle of 500 grams Cholestyramine bars
Usual dose:	One to two packets, scoops, or bars twice daily (1 packet = 1 scoop = 1 bar)
Major effect:	Lowers total and LDL cholesterol
Mechanism of action:	Binds bile acids in intestine; induces LDL receptors in liver
Side effects:	Constipation; abdominal fullness; discomfort
Precautions:	Can interfere with absorption of most other medications and of folic acid and iron; can raise triglyceride levels
Costs:[a]	Questran 　$55.68 per carton of 60 packets 　$22.87 per can (378 grams, 42 scoops) Colestid 　$20.11 per box of 30 packets 　$45.63 per bottle (500 grams, 100 scoops) Cholybar (caramel and raspberry flavors) 　$27.00 per box of 25 bars

[a]Source of costs in this and subsequent tables: Medi-span, *Hospital Formulary Pricing Guide*, May 1989. The cost reflects the *average acquisition price* paid by pharmacies for the drug.

mixed with water or some other liquid, such as orange juice or grape-fruit juice. Both cholestyramine and colestipol come either in pack-ets or in bulk form with a plastic scoop, where one "scoop" is the equivalent of one packet. The usual dose is one to two packets (or scoops) twice daily. Cholestyramine is also available in the form of an edible bar (Cholybar); the bars come in different flavors, and one bar equals one dose. A pill form of cholestyramine is also being de-veloped.

Cholestyramine and colestipol are equally effective in lowering LDL cholesterol. Colestipol has less bulk per dose than cholestyra-mine; but cholestyramine contains ingredients such as citric acid, natural and artificial flavor, sucrose, and a filler, polysorbate 80, that give the resin a better texture, taste, and smell. And cholestyramine is now also available as Questran Light, which provides four grams of the resin, only one gram of filler, and only 1.6 calories per dose at no extra cost.

The bile acid resins are most effective if taken at least two times daily, either just before, during, or after meals. This is because the food you eat forces your gall bladder to contract, spilling out bile from the gall bladder into the intestine. If you take this drug at mealtime, more bile acids are available to be bound and their removal is facilitated. Patients on a low dose (one or two packets a day) often lower their LDL cholesterol sufficiently by taking the entire dose with dinner.

Major effect. In many patients on an average dose of four packets a day, the bile acid resins reduce the LDL cholesterol level from 15 to 25 percent. As noted in Chapter 3, one of the Coronary Primary Prevention Trial participants, Charles Maddox, lowered his LDL cholesterol from 189 mg/dl to 118 mg/dl, a reduction of almost 40 percent, by taking a high dose of cholestyramine, six packets a day, without a missed dose for seven years.

In general, the higher the LDL cholesterol level, the greater the daily dose required to lower it into a satisfactory range. If your LDL cholesterol level is between 160 and 200 mg/dl, you will require at least one dose twice a day; if it is above 200 mg/dl, you will require two doses twice a day, or more. The fall in LDL cholesterol begins within three to four days and reaches its maximum after several weeks of treatment. If treatment is discontinued, the LDL cholesterol promptly rises to its pretreatment level.

Mechanism of action. Bile acids are normally reabsorbed from your intestine and returned to the liver for future use (see Figure 7-3). When a bile acid sequestrant is used, the bile acids are "bound" to the resin and leave the body in the bowel movement (Figure 7-3, middle). When the normal recycling of the bile acids back to the liver is interfered with, the processing of cholesterol within the liver is changed dramatically and much more cholesterol is used to make bile acids. The amount of cholesterol inside the liver consequently decreases, sending a signal to the cell to make more LDL receptors. As the number of LDL receptors on the surface of the liver cell increases, more cholesterol-rich LDL is removed from your blood and the cholesterol level falls.

The use of bile acid resins also produces a small increase in the "protective" HDL; this is a further benefit of this drug.

Side effects. The most common side effect of these drugs is constipation, which occurs in about two out of three adults who take them. This side effect is dose-dependent; the incidence of constipation is much lower on two doses per day. Moreover, the constipation often passes after several weeks of treatment or responds to an increase in bulk or fiber in the diet. (Guidelines for increasing the fiber in your diet were reviewed for you in Chapter 12.) The use at bedtime of a stool softener, Colace®, or a bulk laxative such as Metamucil® can also alleviate constipation. Because of the cholesterol-lowering properties of Metamucil, it is preferable to Colace.

Occasionally a patient will be unable to tolerate a bile acid sequestrant because of persistent and severe constipation. Some experience a feeling of fullness or some heartburn when taking the drug. Although the texture of the powder is somewhat gritty, most patients have no trouble swallowing the mixture.

Precautions. If your doctor prescribes a bile acid sequestrant and you are on one or more other medications, you and your doctor will need to review the dose schedules for your other drugs. Bile acid binding resins can bind a variety of medications, notably thiazides (taken for high blood pressure), blood thinners (or anticoagulants) such as one of the coumarin derivatives, a heart medicine called digitalis, and thyroid preparations. Other drugs should be taken at least one hour before the bile acid binding resin, or, if this is not possible, four hours afterward.

A potential side effect of the resins is interference with the absorption of fat-soluble vitamins (such as vitamins A, D, and K) from the diet by the intestinal cells. When the doses discussed here are used, this is not a problem. The body's absorption of one of the water-soluble vitamins, folic acid, can also be decreased by the resins, but this decrease is not associated with any significant problems such as anemia. Finally, the level of iron in blood can decrease with this medication. Because of these potential side effects, my patients who are taking a resin in the morning and at night also take one multivitamin and mineral preparation a day that contains iron and folic acid, usually at lunchtime.

If you are taking a bile acid resin, your blood triglyceride level may increase. This increase is often transient, but it persists in some patients and may require the addition of a second lipid-lowering drug (such as nicotinic acid or gemfibrozil) to lower the triglyceride level. One such patient was Don Whisner, a 59-year-old-man who was originally in the Coronary Primary Prevention Trial. After the study, he was taking Colestid, two scoops in the morning and two scoops in the evening. His blood cholesterol and LDL cholesterol were lower, his HDL was about the same, but his triglyceride level was above

300 mg/dl. I added Lopid, two capsules twice daily, and he had the following remarkable response:

Lipid profile	Before treatment	Diet and Colestid	Diet, Colestid, and Lopid
Cholesterol	363	255	150
LDL cholesterol	274	150	86
HDL cholesterol	45	42	54
LDL/HDL Ratio	6.1	3.6	1.6
Triglyceride	251	315	48

This is a dramatic example—one of the most dramatic known to me—of how combined treatment with a bile acid sequestrant and a triglyceride-lowering drug can alter *all* the numbers for the better.

Effect on coronary heart disease. Cholestyramine was shown in the Lipid Research Clinics Coronary Primary Prevention Trial (see Chapter 3) to reduce the incidence of coronary heart disease in healthy middle-aged male volunteers with high blood cholesterol and LDL cholesterol levels. The general rule of thumb is that for each 1 percent lowering in blood cholesterol, there is a 2 percent reduction in the risk of coronary heart disease. For example, if you are able to lower your total cholesterol 25 percent, as cholestyramine has helped many patients to do, you have reduced your risk of coronary heart disease by 50 percent.

Nicotinic Acid

In chemical terms, the word *niacin* is synonymous with nicotinic acid; however, nutritionists often use niacin as a generic descriptor for both nicotinic acid and one of its derivatives, nicotinamide, which is important as a co-factor for hundreds of enzymatic reactions in the body. The distinction between nicotinic acid and nicotinamide is particularly important when the goal is to improve the blood lipid profile. Nicotinic acid does; nicotinamide doesn't. Therefore, here and elsewhere in this book I always use the phrase nicotinic acid when referring to it as a drug. Your diet generally contains about 15–35 mg of niacin (Vitamin B_3). At least 60 times that much is required as nicotinic acid when the treatment of a lipid problem is undertaken. Information about nicotinic acid is summarized in Table 16-5.

Usual dose. The average adult dose of nicotinic acid is one and one-half to three grams a day, although as much as six grams a day

Table 16-5. Facts about Nicotinic Acid

Name of drug:	Nicotinic acid
Supplied as:	Regular tablets: 250 mg; 500 mg Sustained release capsules (Slo-Niacin): 250 mg, 500 mg, 750 mg Timed release tempules: 125 mg, 250 mg, 500 mg
Usual dose:	500 to 1,000 mg three times a day
Major effect:	Lowers total and LDL cholesterol and triglyceride levels; raises HDL cholesterol
Mechanism of action:	Decreases production of VLDL in liver
Side effects:	Flushing; itching; feeling of warmth; irritates stomach
Precautions:	Can increase blood sugar and uric acid; can affect liver function; can activate peptic ulcer

Costs:[a]	Generic (regular and sustained release)
	   $6.00 to $12.00 per 100 tablets
	   $12.00 to $24.00 per 100 capsules
	Nicolar (regular)
	   $34.50 per 100 500 mg tablets
	Nicobid (timed release)
	   $43.06 per 100 125 mg tempules
	   $49.10 per 100 250 mg tempules
	   $51.32 per 100 500 mg tempules
	   $245.76 per 500 500 mg tempules

[a]See note to Table 16-4.

has been prescribed. It is usually taken three times a day with meals. I usually start my patients on a very low or "homeopathic" dose of 250 mg three times a day, which does not affect the blood cholesterol or triglyceride levels but helps them get used to the drug's annoying side effects. If you work, it is best to start treatment on a weekend for this reason.

Nicotinic acid may be obtained at your pharmacy without a doctor's prescription. When doses of nicotinic acid high enough to lower your blood lipids are used, however, a number of serious side effects can occur. Consequently, treatment with nicotinic acid for a blood lipid problem should be undertaken only under the care of your physician. Generic preparations are much more economical.

Only the kinds of nicotinic acid listed in Table 16-5 are effective in lowering your blood lipid levels; as pointed out above, at least one cousin of niacin, called nicotinamide, is *not*. Two preparations of nicotinic acid are available: regular tablets and sustained release capsules. The nicotinic acid in sustained release capsules is more gradually released from the stomach into the blood, and the annoying minor side effects are therefore less marked; but its users have a higher incidence of serious side effects. In contrast, regular nicotinic acid has a greater incidence of annoying side effects but a lower incidence of serious side effects. Since regular nicotinic acid is also more effective than sustained release nicotinic acid in lowering cholesterol and triglyceride and increasing HDL cholesterol, it is the form I recommend.

Major effect. Many of my patients have a 10 to 20 percent decrease in both their blood cholesterol and triglyceride levels when they are treated with nicotinic acid. The LDL cholesterol level usually falls, and the HDL cholesterol level usually increases. In regard to the risk of coronary heart disease, the entire blood lipoprotein profile improves.

In Chapter 9 you read about Howard Needle, whose diet by itself led to insufficient improvements in his lipid profile. Adding nicotinic acid lowered his blood cholesterol further from 241 mg/dl to 188 mg/dl, his LDL cholesterol from 161 to 109 mg/dl, and his triglyceride from 242 to 156 mg/dl, and raised his HDL cholesterol from 33 to 48 mg/dl.

Mechanism of action. Nicotinic acid has its primary action in the liver, where it decreases production of the triglyceride-rich VLDL particles. A fall in the blood triglyceride level often occurs on nicotinic acid. Since VLDL is eventually converted in the blood into cholesterol-rich LDL, nicotinic acid often produces a decrease in the LDL cholesterol as well. A significant increase in the "protective" HDL cholesterol also occurs, and the LDL/HDL ratio can improve dramatically.

Side effects. People tend to feel a warmth or flushing of the face and a general itchiness about half an hour after taking nicotinic acid. If you don't experience any flushing, you should check to make sure you are not taking nicotinamide, which does not produce these effects. These side effects last only 15 to 30 minutes, but in some patients they are severe enough to be intolerable. These annoying side effects can be prevented by taking one adult aspirin 30 minutes before the nicotinic acid is taken. Alternatively, taking nicotinic acid with food helps to decrease both the amount of flushing and the irritation of the stomach that nicotinic acid sometimes causes.

Precautions. Unlike the bile acid binding resins, nicotinic acid enters the bloodstream and can have an effect on certain organs in your body. In particular, it can irritate the liver cells, producing an increased release of certain enzymes into the blood that can be detected by special blood tests called "liver function tests." These changes usually last only a few weeks and are moderate in degree; but occasionally the adverse effect on the liver is more marked and treatment with nicotinic acid must be stopped. Such an effect of nicotinic acid on the liver cells is usually reversible, and the cells return to their normal state in two or three months. Nicotinic acid should be used with caution in patients with a history of peptic or duodenal ulcers, and not be given at all to those with an active ulcer under treatment.

You may have read about or experienced attacks of gout in the big toe or other joints. Gout is caused by very high levels of uric acid in the blood. Those who have a high uric acid level must take nicotinic acid with caution, since it can actually increase the uric acid level enough to bring on an attack of gout. Nicotinic acid can also increase the blood sugar level, and its use in patients with diabetes or a high blood sugar level is accordingly not recommended.

One of my patients being treated with nicotinic acid developed blurring of vision. Careful examination by an eye doctor disclosed swelling in an important part of the eye called the retina. Treatment with nicotinic acid was discontinued and his vision returned to normal. This adverse effect of nicotinic acid on the eye is fortunately rare and reversible.

Another unusual side effect of nicotinic acid is the development of a dark brown discoloration of the skin in the armpits or in the groin (called "acanthosis nigracans").

Effect on coronary heart disease. In the Coronary Drug Project, nicotinic acid was one of the drugs given to men with coronary heart disease. After five years, those taking two grams a day of nicotinic acid had significantly less coronary heart disease than a corresponding group treated with a placebo. Both groups were reexamined ten years after the end of the study; those previously treated with nicotinic acid had 20 percent fewer events from coronary heart disease than those previously treated with a placebo. This is remarkable when you consider that most of these men had not been treated with nicotinic acid for ten years.

HMG CoA Reductase Inhibitors

Everyone knows about penicillin, an antibiotic derived from the mold *Penicillium* that was discovered in the 1930s by Alexander Fleming. This same mold also produced a compound called "compactin," which was discovered in the 1970s by Japanese researchers.

Table 16-6. Facts about HMG CoA Reductase Inhibitors

Name of drug:	Lovastatin (Mevacor®)
Supplied as:	Tablet: 20 mg or 40 mg
Usual dose:	20 to 40 mg two times a day
Major effect:	Lowers total and LDL cholesterol; may also lower triglycerides and raise HDL cholesterol in high doses
Mechanism of action:	Inhibits cholesterol synthesis; induces LDL receptors in liver
Side effects:	Headache, rash, and muscle aches
Precautions:	Persistent abnormal tests of liver function (2% of patients); marked irritation of muscle cells (myositis); not to be used in heart, liver, or kidney transplant patients; huge doses cause cataracts in dogs
Costs:[a]	$93.75 per bottle of 60 20 mg tablets $168.75 per bottle of 60 40 mg tablets

[a]See note to Table 16-4.

Compactin has a special characteristic that enables it to interfere with the liver's production of cholesterol by inhibiting the enzyme (called HMG CoA reductase) that regulates the entire pathway of cholesterol production.

Compactin is no longer used because it was rumored to produce lymphatic tumors in dogs. A similar compound, previously called mevinolin but now called lovastatin, is marketed as Mevacor®. Lovastatin and another HMG CoA reductase inhibitor, simvastatin, are effective in lowering the blood cholesterol and LDL cholesterol levels, even in patients with the inherited blood cholesterol problem known as familial hypercholesterolemia (see Chapter 7). The basic information on these drugs is given in Table 16-6.

Usual dose. Lovastatin is given in a dose of 20 to 80 milligrams (mg) per day. It comes in a small pill (containing either 20 or 40 mg) that is easy to take. On the lowest dose, 20 mg a day, the medicine is taken with the evening meal; if two pills are required, they are taken in the morning and evening. Some patients with very high LDL cholesterol levels, such as those found in familial hypercholesterolemia, will require the maximum dose of 80 mg a day.

Major effect. Lovastatin produced a fall in LDL cholesterol of 30 to 40 percent in patients with familial hypercholesterolemia. The HDL cholesterol level of these patients increased by about 10 percent, and their triglyceride level fell about 30 percent. Many of my patients do not have the extreme cholesterol levels found in familial hypercholesterolemia, but they do often have premature coronary heart disease and an LDL cholesterol level between 160 mg/dl and 200 mg/dl after diet treatment. These patients respond very well to one or two doses of lovastatin per day. Their total cholesterol and LDL cholesterol levels often fall 50 to 100 mg/dl. If you already have coronary heart disease and a blood cholesterol problem that has not responded to a low-fat diet, discuss with your doctor the possible addition of lovastatin to your treatment.

Beverly Grand, a 69-year-old woman, was unable to tolerate cholestyramine or nicotinic acid. Despite a good low-fat diet, her blood cholesterol and LDL cholesterol levels were 297 mg/dl and 199 mg/dl, respectively. On one pill (20 mg) of lovastatin with dinner, these levels fell to 207 mg/dl and 139 mg/dl, respectively, in just four weeks.

Mechanism of action. The inhibitors of HMG CoA reductase decrease the production of cholesterol by the liver. This sends a signal to the liver cell to make more LDL receptors. The LDL receptors are then transported to the surface of liver cells, where they bind the LDL in the blood and take the bound LDL into the liver for disposal (see Figure 7-3, right).

Side effects. Most of my patients report no side effects at all from lovastatin. Some experience headaches, mild rashes, muscle aches, or increased gas. Occasionally a patient will complain of difficulty with sleeping (insomnia) or nightmares.

Precautions. The HMG CoA reductase inhibitors are the newest group of cholesterol-lowering drugs. Lovastatin has just recently (1987) been approved by the Food and Drug Administration for prescription use. In about two out of 100 patients, lovastatin produces an irritation of the liver cells, causing them to release abnormal amounts of enzymes into the blood. This abnormality, also a side effect of nicotinic acid, can be detected by a liver function test.

In one of my patients, lovastatin produced such an adverse effect on her liver that she developed hepatitis. Lovastatin was discontinued, and over several months her liver function tests gradually returned to normal. This patient had a blood cholesterol level of over 450 mg/dl, could not tolerate the bile acid resins, and wished to resume treatment with lovastatin. She did, her cholesterol level promptly fell again to 200 mg/dl, and the abnormalities in her liver function tests did not return. The adverse effect of lovastatin on the liver cells appears reversible.

Another precaution for those taking lovastatin involves a type of cataract in the eyes called a subscapular cataract. These cataracts occurred in dogs receiving 50 times the dose of lovastatin given humans. However, many people develop subscapular cataracts after age 40 as a normal part of the aging process. The frequency of these cataracts in patients on lovastatin does not appear to be any greater than in the population generally.

As we have seen, small tumors called lymphomas were reportedly discovered in the intestines of dogs treated with a cousin of lovastatin, compactin. However, since this report has not been published in the medical literature, no reliable assessment of it can be made. Subsequent experiments with mice and rabbits have not found any evidence that lovastatin causes lymphomas.

Lovastatin can cause an irritation of the muscle cells (myositis), especially in patients who have had a heart, kidney, or liver transplant and are on special drugs to prevent the rejection of the transplanted organ. Lovastatin can cause such patients' muscle cells to release toxic materials that adversely affect the cells in the kidney and can lead to kidney failure. Severe reactions of the muscle cells have also been reported in patients treated with the combination of lovastatin and gemfibrozil (Lopid®). It seems clear that lovastatin should not be used by patients with heart, kidney, or liver transplants, and should be used with caution in combination with Lopid.

We have less experience with lovastatin and the other HMG CoA reductase inhibitors than with other cholesterol-lowering agents such as the bile acid resins or nicotinic acid. We do not yet know their long-term safety record. We do know that lovastatin is easier to take than bile acid resins or nicotinic acid, and at least as effective in improving lipid levels. My patients have experienced few if any annoying side effects when taking lovastatin, and many prefer it to the other medications for that reason.

Effect on coronary heart disease. Lovastatin has not yet been shown to decrease coronary heart disease, but such an effect can be predicted with some confidence from its excellent performance in reducing total and LDL cholesterol levels.

Combining lovastatin and a bile acid sequestrant. Lovastatin can also be used in combination with a bile acid sequestrant. This is a potentially powerful combination because each drug induces LDL receptors by a different mechanism (see Figure 7-3).

Sylvia Bondroff had quadruple bypass surgery at 63 after two years of angina pectoris. She had a repeat heart catheterization three years later, by which time one of her bypasses was completely blocked. Despite a diet low in total fat, saturated fat, and cholesterol, her cholesterol level when I first saw her was 386 mg/dl and her LDL cholesterol was 246 mg/dl; her HDL was 60 mg/dl and her triglyceride 229 mg/dl.

Questran, two packets twice a day, lowered her cholesterol to 277 mg/dl and her LDL cholesterol to 184 mg/dl—not low enough. Her HDL cholesterol was 55 mg/dl at this point, and her triglyceride 188 mg/dl. Unable to tolerate this much Questran, she was reduced to one packet twice a day. Mevacor was added, one pill (20 mg) twice a day, to excellent effect. Her latest cholesterol level was 217 mg/dl and her LDL cholesterol only 119 mg/dl; her HDL remained at 55 mg/dl, and her triglyceride remained borderline high at 213 mg/dl.

Fibric Acid Derivatives

Two fibric acid derivatives, gemfibrozil (Lopid®) and clofibrate (Atromid-S®), are primarily used to treat patients with an elevated triglyceride level rather than as first-line drugs to treat elevated LDL cholesterol levels. The basic information on these drugs is given in Table 16-7.

Usual dose. Gemfibrozil is available as 300 mg and 600 mg capsules and clofibrate as 500 mg capsules. The dose of gemfibrozil is 1.2 grams (two 300 mg capsules or one 600 mg capsule twice a day) and of clofibrate two grams (two capsules twice a day).

Major effect. The major effect of the fibric acid derivatives is to lower the blood levels of triglyceride and VLDL, the major carrier of triglyceride in the blood. The level of HDL cholesterol often increases to a significant degree, especially with gemfibrozil. The total cholesterol and LDL cholesterol levels may fall modestly (about 10 percent), although in some patients the LDL cholesterol level may actually increase.

Mechanism of action. Both drugs increase the removal of the triglyceride-rich VLDL from the blood by increasing the activity of lipoprotein lipase (see Chapter 8), the enzyme that breaks down triglyceride. Both also increase the amount of cholesterol put out from the liver into the bile, and gemfibrozil slows down the production of triglyceride inside the liver cell.

Side effects. Side effects of the fibric acid derivatives include abdominal discomfort, a feeling of nausea or fullness in the stomach, and diarrhea. Some patients experience a decreased libido, and others report increased appetite and weight gain. Some patients also develop muscle aches, which can become so severe that the drug needs to be discontinued.

Precautions. Like nicotinic acid and lovastatin, these drugs may

Table 16-7. Facts about Fibric Acid Derivatives

Names of drugs:	Gemfibrozil (Lopid®) Clofibrate (Atromid-S®)

Supplied as:	Capsules
	  Gemfibrozil: 300 mg or 600 mg
	  Clofibrate: 500 mg

Usual dose:	Gemfibrozil: one 600 mg or two 300 mg capsules twice daily Clofibrate: two capsules twice daily
Major effect:	Lowers triglyceride levels and raises HDL cholesterol; modest lowering of total and LDL cholesterol
Mechanism of action:	Increases the breakdown of VLDL and triglyceride in blood; may also decrease VLDL production in liver
Side effects:	Discomfort in stomach and intestine; muscle aches; diar- rhea; decreased libido; increased appetite
Precautions:	Increased chance of developing gallstones; abnormal liver function tests; patients on blood thinners need less anticoagulant; clofibrate caused increased mortality in WHO study; can cause irregular heartbeats

Costs:[a]	Lopid
	  $37.13 per bottle of 100 300 mg capsules
	  $176.35 per bottle of 500 300 mg capsules
	  $44.54 per bottle of 60 600 mg capsules
	Atromid-S
	  $41.25 per bottle of 100

[a]See note to Table 16-4.

irritate the cells in the liver; the irritation is usually mild, but can be severe enough to require that the drug be discontinued. There is an increased risk of developing gallstones with prolonged treatment (for example, five years). Rarely, a patient may develop a serious cardiac arrhythmia from taking one of these medications. Patients on a blood thinner such as one of the coumarin derivatives need to decrease their dose by one-third to one-half when taking a fibric acid derivative.

In some patients with familial combined hyperlipidemia (see Chapter 8), who have increased levels of both cholesterol and triglyceride, treatment with fibric acid derivatives lowers the triglyceride level but actually increases the LDL cholesterol level. If this happens to you, it is important for your doctor to check your LDL/HDL ratio. If that ratio has in fact increased, either treatment with the fibric acid derivative should be discontinued or a bile acid sequestrant should be added to the regimen.

In the World Health Organization (WHO) study, the group treated with clofibrate had a higher incidence of total deaths from all causes than those on placebo. The use of clofibrate has been curtailed significantly since these results were reported, and is today chiefly confined to patients with an unusual blood lipid problem called type 3 disease, which was reviewed for you in Chapter 8. No such excess of mortality was found for gemfibrozil in the Helsinki Heart Study (see Chapter 3), which evaluated the effect and long-term safety of that drug.

Effect on coronary heart disease. In the Helsinki Heart Study, gemfibrozil produced a significant decrease in heart attacks and death from coronary heart disease. This effect was mediated by two changes in the blood; the average LDL level fell about 10 percent, and the HDL cholesterol level increased to a similar extent. Clofibrate produced a significant decrease in coronary heart disease in the World Health Organization study, but this effect was more than offset by a significant increase in death from other causes.

Probucol

Probucol (Lorelco®) is another drug used for elevated blood cholesterol and LDL cholesterol levels. It is not indicated where a high blood triglyceride level is the primary problem of concern. Probucol is derived from a chemical called butylphenol and does not resemble any other cholesterol-lowering drug. Information about probucol is summarized in Table 16-8.

Usual dose. Probucol is available as a 250 mg tablet or a 500 mg tablet. The usual daily dose is one gram: two 250 mg tablets or one 500 mg tablet taken twice daily with morning and evening meals.

Major effect. Probucol decreases LDL cholesterol 10 to 20 percent; it also decreases HDL cholesterol by 10 to 30 percent. The total cholesterol level may not change appreciably. Most of the effect of probucol on HDL is on the subfamily of HDL called HDL_3; it has only a minor effect on the subfamily HDL_2, which may be responsible for HDL's protective effect against the development of coronary heart disease. The triglyceride level is not affected by probucol.

Mechanism of action. Probucol is not absorbed completely into the intestine, and on average only about 10 percent of the administered dose gets into the blood. Probucol is stored in the fat tissue and is fully excreted from the body in the bile. It takes a while to build up a constant level of probucol in the blood, and after this is achieved

Table 16-8. Facts about Probucol

Name of drug:	Probucol (Lorelco®)
Supplied as:	Tablets: 250 mg or 500 mg
Usual dose:	One 500 mg or two 250 mg tablets twice daily
Major effect:	Lowers total and LDL cholesterol; also lowers HDL cholesterol
Mechanism of action:	Increases the removal of LDL from blood
Side effects:	EKG abnormality; diarrhea; flatulence; headache; rash; insomnia
Precautions:	Causes irregular heartbeats (arrhythmias) in beagle dogs and rhesus monkeys
Cost:[a]	$52.02 per bottle of 120 250 mg tablets $80.10 per bottle of 100 500 mg tablets

[a]See note to Table 16-4.

it takes a while for it to be cleared from the body if treatment is stopped. Probucol is lipophilic, meaning that it mixes very well with fat and is readily incorporated into your body's fat cells. Thus if you begin treatment with probucol and then discontinue it later, *it may take up to three months until all the probucol is removed from your body.*

Because probucol is lipophilic, it is incorporated into the cholesterol-rich core of LDL itself. The incorporation of probucol into LDL produces an increased removal of LDL from the blood. This occurs by a mechanism other than the LDL receptor. A different mechanism apparently reduces HDL, one that decreases the production of HDL and its major apolipoprotein, apoA1, in the liver.

Side effects. Side effects of probucol include diarrhea, nausea, increased gas (flatulence), headache, insomnia, and rash.

Precautions. Probucol has been shown to cause irregular heartbeats (arrhythmias) in beagle dogs and rhesus monkeys. In humans, abnormalities may show up on an EKG. The drug should be used with considerable caution or not at all if you have an arrhythmia.

Effect on coronary heart disease. The precise effect of probucol on coronary heart disease is not known, although there are isolated reports that treatment with probucol reduced the size of cholesterol deposits (xanthomas) in patients with familial hypercholesterolemia and slowed the development of atherosclerosis in Watanabe rabbits with familial hypercholesterolemia.

Do Children and Adolescents Require Drug Treatment for Blood Lipid Problems?

Generally speaking, I am more conservative in recommending drug treatment for children with blood lipid problems. Clearly, children with astronomically high blood cholesterol levels (between 600 and 1,000 mg/dl) are candidates not only for drug treatment, but for other, more dramatic measures such as liver transplants. (These children are invariably homozygotes for familial hypercholesterolemia: see Chapter 7.)

The child or adolescent who has a cholesterol level of about 300 mg/dl, an LDL cholesterol level of about 240 mg/dl, and a normal triglyceride level usually carries one faulty gene for familial hypercholesterolemia. These FH heterozygotes, who are far more numerous than FH homozygotes, constitute the largest class of very young people for whom drug treatment may be necessary.

My practice is to initiate drug treatment for a child or adolescent under the following conditions:

1. After a good low-cholesterol, low-saturated-fat diet, the blood cholesterol level is still above 230 mg/dl and the LDL cholesterol level above 160 mg/dl.

2. There is a family history of premature coronary heart disease.

3. The child is otherwise healthy and shows every evidence of normal growth and development.

4. The child is of school age.

If these four conditions apply to your child, treatment with a bile·acid sequestrant should be discussed with the child's doctor. None of the other drugs, including nicotinic acid and lovastatin, has been systemically studied in children or adolescents.

As an example, Laurie Beczkowski, a 15-year-old girl, was first seen with a cholesterol level of 377 mg/dl, LDL cholesterol of 285 mg/dl, HDL cholesterol of 45 mg/dl, and triglyceride of 149 mg/dl. After almost five months on a good diet, her blood cholesterol fell to 294 mg/dl, her LDL cholesterol to 241 mg/dl, her triglyceride to 71 mg/dl, but her HDL cholesterol remained borderline low at 39 mg/dl. Her mother had a cholesterol level over 400 mg/dl and tendon xanthomas, indicating that familial hypercholesterolemia was present in this family. Also the patient's mother's brother had died of a heart attack at age 38 and had actually developed angina pectoris in his twenties.

Because of the striking family history of premature coronary heart disease, the presence of a genetic cholesterol problem, and the inadequate results from the diet, I prescribed Questran, starting with a low dose of one scoop twice a day. After four weeks, Laurie's cholesterol fell to 248 mg/dl and her LDL cholesterol to 184 mg/dl; her HDL cholesterol increased to 42 mg/dl, and her triglyceride remained normal at 110 mg/dl. She will require two scoops twice a day to lower her cholesterol further.

What about children with high blood triglyceride levels? Children with triglyceride levels above 500 mg/dl are rare indeed. Over the past fifteen years I have had only two preadolescent patients with a type 5 problem (see Chapter 8), one girl and one boy. Although both had sky-high blood triglyceride levels (above 3,000 mg/dl), both responded very well to a special diet restricted in total fat (about 20 to 25 percent of calories) and an accompanying program of weight reduction or weight control. Even in children with such extreme triglyceride elevations, diet alone can be adequate.

There are reports of children with even higher triglyceride levels, as high as 10,000 mg/dl. Diet treatment can reportedly reduce these levels to between 1,000 and 2,000 mg/dl. Even with these children drugs are not used because they are not specific for the underlying genetic problem, the body's inability to make lipoprotein lipase.

Summary

1. A diet modified in total fat, saturated fat, and cholesterol remains the cornerstone of treatment for those with blood cholesterol or triglyceride problems. Weight reduction and maintenance of ideal body weight are also important factors in the management of blood lipid problems, particularly where an increased blood triglyceride level is part of the problem.

2. However, in many patients with a significant blood lipid problem or with coronary heart disease, it is necessary to add a lipid-lowering drug to the treatment program. The criteria for adding a lipid-lowering drug are outlined in this chapter.

3. The presence of coronary heart disease, or of two or more risk factors for coronary heart disease, must be considered when deciding whether or not to add a lipid-lowering drug to diet treatment.

4. Treatment of blood lipid problems, even by a nonprescription drug such as nicotinic acid, should always be undertaken *under the supervision of a physician.*

5. Three lipid-lowering drugs, cholestyramine, nicotinic acid, and gemfibrozil, have been found to decrease the incidence of coronary

heart disease. Others are promising, but have not been in use long enough to make so broad a claim.

6. Treatment with lipid-lowering drugs is much less frequently advisable for children or adolescents than for adults. Treatment of a high triglyceride level in children with drugs is not necessary.

Appendixes

Cholesterol and Triglyceride Levels of Children and Adults

The information in this Appendix comes from Lipid Research Clinics Population Studies Data Book, Vol. I, The Prevalence Study (NIH Publication No. 80-1527, July 1980)

Table A-1. Percentile Values of Blood Cholesterol in the First Two Decades of Life (mg/dl)

Age	Number	Percentile				
		5th	25th	50th	75th	95th
0–4						
Males	238	114	137	151	171	203
Females	186	112	139	156	172	200
5–9						
Males	1,253	121	143	159	175	203
Females	1,118	126	146	163	179	205
10–14						
Males	2,278	119	140	155	173	202
Females	2,087	124	144	158	174	201
15–19						
Males	1,980	113	132	146	165	197
Females	2,079	120	140	155	172	203

Table A-2. Percentile Values of LDL Cholesterol in the First Two
Decades of Life (mg/dl)

Age	Number	Percentile				
		5th	25th	50th	75th	95th
5–9						
Males	131	63	80	90	103	129
Females	114	68	88	98	115	140
10–14						
Males	284	64	81	94	109	132
Females	244	68	81	94	110	136
15–19						
Males	298	62	80	93	109	130
Females	294	59	78	93	111	137

Table A-3. Percentile Values of HDL Cholesterol in the First Two
Decades of Life (mg/dl)

Age	Number	Percentile				
		5th	25th	50th	75th	95th
5–9						
Males	142	38	49	54	63	74
Females	124	36	47	52	61	73
10–14						
Males	296	37	46	55	61	74
Females	247	37	45	52	58	70
15–19						
Males	299	30	39	46	52	63
Females	295	35	43	51	61	74

Table A-4. Percentile Values of Blood Triglycerides in the First Two Decades of Life (mg/dl)

Age	Number	Percentile				
		5th	25th	50th	75th	95th
0–4						
Males	238	29	40	51	67	99
Females	186	34	45	59	77	112
5–9						
Males	1,253	30	40	51	65	101
Females	1,118	32	44	55	71	105
10–14						
Males	2,278	32	45	59	78	125
Females	2,087	37	54	70	90	131
15–19						
Males	1,980	37	54	69	91	148
Females	2,079	39	53	68	87	132

Table A-5. Percentile Values of Blood Cholesterol for Men and Women Aged 20 to 70+ Years

Age	Blood cholesterol level (mg/dl)									
	Percentile, men					Percentile, women				
	5th	25th	50th	75th	95th	5th	25th	50th	75th	95th
20–24	124	146	165	186	218	125	149	170	190	228
25–29	133	159	178	202	244	130	155	173	193	229
30–34	138	167	190	213	254	131	158	176	196	238
35–39	146	176	197	223	270	141	164	183	205	245
40–44	151	182	203	228	268	147	171	192	215	253
45–49	158	188	210	234	276	152	178	201	226	268
50–54	158	187	210	235	277	163	192	215	240	285
55–59	156	189	212	235	276	169	200	223	248	294
60–64	159	188	210	235	276	173	202	226	252	296
65–69	158	190	210	233	274	171	205	226	252	297
70+	151	182	205	229	270	167	199	224	251	288

Table A-6. Percentile Values of LDL Cholesterol for Men and Women
Aged 20 to 70 + Years

	Blood LDL cholesterol level (mg/dl)									
	Percentile, men					Percentile, women				
Age	5th	25th	50th	75th	95th	5th	25th	50th	75th	95th
20–24	66	85	101	118	147	57	82	102	118	159
25–29	70	96	116	138	165	71	90	108	126	164
30–34	78	107	124	144	185	70	91	109	128	156
35–39	81	110	131	154	189	75	96	116	139	172
40–44	87	115	135	157	186	74	104	122	146	174
45–49	98	120	141	163	202	79	105	127	150	186
50–54	89	118	143	162	197	88	111	134	160	201
55–59	88	123	145	168	203	89	120	145	168	210
60–64	83	121	143	165	210	100	126	149	168	224
65–69	98	125	146	170	210	92	125	151	184	221
70 +	88	119	142	164	186	96	127	147	170	206

Table A-7. Percentile Values of HDL Cholesterol for Men and Women
Aged 20 to 70 + Years

	Blood HDL cholesterol level (mg/dl)									
	Percentile, men					Percentile, women				
Age	5th	25th	50th	75th	95th	5th	25th	50th	75th	95th
20–24	30	38	45	51	63	33	44	51	62	79
25–29	31	37	44	50	63	37	47	55	63	83
30–34	28	38	45	52	63	36	46	55	64	77
35–39	29	36	43	49	62	34	44	53	64	82
40–44	27	36	43	51	67	34	48	56	65	88
45–49	30	38	45	52	64	34	47	58	68	87
50–54	28	36	44	51	63	37	50	62	71	92
55–59	28	38	46	55	71	37	50	60	73	91
60–64	30	41	49	61	74	38	51	61	75	92
65–69	30	39	49	62	78	35	49	62	73	98
70 +	31	40	48	56	75	33	48	60	71	92

Table A-8. Percentile Values of Blood Triglyceride for Men and Women
Aged 20 to 70+ Years

Age	Blood triglyceride level (mg/dl)									
	Percentile, men					Percentile, women				
	5th	25th	50th	75th	95th	5th	25th	50th	75th	95th
20–24	44	63	86	119	201	40	60	81	108	165
25–29	46	70	95	136	249	40	58	78	107	172
30–34	50	75	104	149	266	41	58	77	106	176
35–39	54	81	113	170	321	41	60	80	113	194
40–44	55	86	122	174	320	47	65	88	122	209
45–49	58	89	124	174	327	47	69	94	132	228
50–54	58	87	124	180	320	54	77	101	141	238
55–59	58	87	119	170	286	56	81	108	148	257
60–64	58	87	119	169	291	57	81	108	148	240
65–69	57	83	112	149	267	60	83	112	157	241
70+	58	83	111	149	258	60	85	111	150	235

Calorie, Fat, and Cholesterol Content of Commonly Eaten Foods

The tables that follow were prepared for this book by Ginny Hartmuller, M.S., R.D, and Judith Chiostri, M.S., R.D. Their sources were the USDA *Handbook 8* series; *Pennington and Church's Food Values*, 1985; *The Fast Food Guide* (Center for Science in the Public Interest), 1986; and manufacturers' data.

There are a number of foods for which reliable figures could not be obtained. It is also not possible to include every food and brand. Nevertheless, there is a lot of information here that I hope you will find useful. Finally, note that some variation between brands and homemade recipes should be expected.

The figures are of course in many cases approximations or averages. As an example, 1 homemade biscuit is listed as having 103 calories, 4.8 grams of fat, etc., but these figures would obviously vary depending on the size of the biscuit and the ingredients used. And indeed, one person's idea of a medium-sized apple or a pat of butter will differ from another's.

The sequence of the tables is alphabetical by food category, with cross-references as necessary:

Beverages
Candy and Candy Bars
Cereals and Grains
Chips and Snacks
Combination Foods (Entrées and
    Frozen Meals)
Dairy Products and Eggs
Desserts and Cookies
Fast Foods
Fats and Oils
Fruits
Grain Products (Bread, Crackers,
    etc.)

Juices, Fruit and Vegetable
Legumes
Meat, Fish, and Poultry
Miscellaneous
Nuts and Seeds
Sausages and Luncheon Meats
Soups, Sauces, and Gravies
Soy Protein Products
Sugar and Sweet Foods
    (see Miscellaneous)
Vegetables

The following abbreviations are used:

avg	average	ord	order	sl	slice(s)
cnd	canned	oz.	ounce	sm	small
fl.oz.	fluidounce	pc(s)	piece(s)	sv	serving
frz	frozen	pkg	package	Tb	tablespoon
lg	large	pkt	packet	tr	trace (<0.1)
med	medium-sized	rec	recipe	tsp	teaspoon
n/a	not available				

Food	Portion	Total cal.	Total fat (gm)	Sat. fat (gm)	Chol. (mg)
BEVERAGES					
See also Dairy Products; Juices, Fruit and Vegetable					
ALCOHOLIC BEVERAGES					
Beer, regular	12 fl.oz.	148	0.0	0.0	0
Beer, light (brands vary)	12 fl.oz	100	0.0	0.0	0
Cordials and liqueurs	1 fl.oz.	97	0.0	0.0	0
Gin/rum/vodka/whiskey, 80 proof	1 fl.oz.	65	0.0	0.0	0
Gin/rum/vodka/whiskey, 86 proof	1 fl.oz.	70	0.0	0.0	0
Wine:					
Champagne	4 fl.oz.	84	0.0	0.0	0
Dessert-type, dry	3.5 fl.oz.	126	0.0	0.0	0
Dessert-type, sweet	3.5 fl.oz.	153	0.0	0.0	0
Sherry	2 fl.oz.	84	0.0	0.0	0
Table, red	3.5 fl.oz.	76	0.0	0.0	0
Table, white	3.5 fl.oz.	80	0.0	0.0	0
COFFEE AND TEA					
Coffee, regular, brewed	6 fl.oz.	3	0.0	0.0	0
Coffee, regular, instant	6 fl.oz.	3	0.0	0.0	0
Coffee, flavored, instant:					
Almond Mocha	8 fl.oz.	85	1.4	1.0	tr
Bavarian Mint	8 fl.oz.	82	1.4	1.0	tr
Café Amaretto	6 fl.oz.	51	2.4	2.1	tr
Café Français	6 fl.oz.	58	3.4	2.9	tr
Café Vienna	6 fl.oz.	64	2.4	2.1	tr
Irish Mocha Mint	6 fl.oz.	54	2.6	2.2	tr
Orange Cappuccino	6 fl.oz.	64	2.4	2.0	tr
Suisse Mocha	6 fl.oz.	56	2.8	2.4	tr
Tea, brewed or instant, plain	8 fl.oz.	0	0.0	0.0	0

Food	Portion	Total cal.	Total fat (gm)	Sat. fat (gm)	Chol. (mg)
CARBONATED DRINKS					
Coca-Cola, regular	12 fl.oz.	144	0.0	0.0	0
Pepsi-Cola, regular	12 fl.oz.	156	0.0	0.0	0
Ginger ale, regular	12 fl.oz.	113	0.0	0.0	0
Grape or orange, regular	12 fl.oz.	179	0.0	0.0	0
Diet sodas	12 fl.oz.	1	0.0	0.0	0
Seltzer water, plain	12 fl.oz.	0	0.0	0.0	0
Seltzer water, flavored	12 fl.oz.	0	0.0	0.0	0

BREAD
See Grain Products

CANDY AND CANDY BARS

CANDY					
Butterscotch chips	1 oz.	150	7.0	6.0	tr
Butterscotch hard candy	6 pcs	116	2.5	tr	0
Caramels, plain or choco-late	3	112	2.9	1.3	8
Chocolate chips, semi-sweet	¼ cup	220	12.2	6.3	tr
Choc.-covered almonds	1 oz.	159	12.2	4.1	3
Choc.-covered peanuts	1 oz.	153	9.0	2.6	tr
Choc.-covered raisins	1 oz.	115	3.7	1.9	3
Chocolate kisses	6	154	9.0	5.2	6
Gumdrops	28	97	0.2	tr	0
Hard candy	8 pcs	108	0.3	tr	0
Jelly beans	10	66	0.0	0.0	0
Life Savers	5	39	0.1	0.0	0
M & M's, plain	1.6 oz. pkg	220	10.0	3.5	5
M & M's, peanut	1.7 oz. pkg	240	12.0	3.8	5
Marshmallow	1 lg	25	0.0	0.0	0
Peanut Butter Cup, Reese's	2	184	10.7	6.0	5
Sugar-coated almonds	7	128	5.2	0.4	0

CANDY BARS					
Almond Joy	1 oz.	151	7.8	3.6	1
Bit-O-Honey	1 oz.	121	3.6	0.8	0
Chunky, original	1 oz.	143	7.1	3.5	2
Nestlé Crunch	1.1 oz.	160	8.0	5.0	6
Hershey Golden Almond	1 oz.	161	11.0	4.7	5
Hershey Krackel	1.0 oz.	179	9.7	5.6	7
Hershey Milk Choc., plain	1.0 oz.	160	9.4	7.0	10

Food	Portion	Total cal.	Total fat (gm)	Sat. fat (gm)	Chol. (mg)
Hershey Milk Choc., w/almonds	1.1 oz.	160	9.5	6.0	5
Kit Kat	1.5 oz.	210	11.0	6.5	8
Milky Way	2.1 oz.	260	9.0	4.7	6
Mounds Bar	1 oz.	147	6.9	3.5	1
Mr. Goodbar	1.6 oz.	250	15.0	7.8	7
Oh Henry	1 oz.	139	7.1	2.2	1
Peppermint Patty	1 oz.	124	2.3	1.4	1
Snickers	2 oz.	270	13.0	4.4	3
Three Musketeers	2.3 oz.	280	8.0	4.8	6
Twix	1.7 oz.	173	6.0	3.8	4

CEREALS AND GRAINS

COOKED

Barley, pearled, quick-cook, dry	¼ cup	172	0.5	tr	0
Bulgur wheat, cooked	1 cup	227	0.9	0.1	0
Cream of rice, cooked	¾ cup	95	0.1	0.0	0
Cream of wheat, cooked	¾ cup	100	0.4	0.1	0
Farina, cooked	¾ cup	87	0.1	0.0	0
Grits, corn, cooked	1 cup	146	0.5	tr	0
Oats, reg/quick, cooked	¾ cup	108	1.8	0.3	0
Oats, instant, prepared	1 pkt	104	1.7	0.3	0
Ralston, cooked	¾ cup	100	0.6	0.1	0
Rice, white, cooked	1 cup	170	0.2	0.0	0
Wheatena, cooked	¾ cup	101	0.8	0.1	0

READY-TO-EAT

All-Bran	1 oz.	71	0.5	tr	0
Alpha Bits	1 oz.	111	0.6	0.1	0
100% Bran	1 oz.	76	1.4	0.3	0
Bran Chex	1 oz.	91	0.8	0.1	0
Bran flakes (40% bran)	1 oz.	92	0.5	0.1	0
Cap'n Crunch	1 oz.	119	2.6	1.7	0
Cheerios	1 oz.	111	1.8	0.3	0
Corn flakes	1 oz.	110	0.1	tr	0
Cracklin' Oat Bran	1 oz.	108	4.1	1.1	0
Frosted Mini-Wheats	1 oz.	102	0.3	tr	0
Fruit & Fiber	1 oz.	87	0.3	tr	0
Granola, Nature Valley	1 oz.	126	4.9	3.3	0
Grape-Nuts	1 oz.	101	0.1	tr	0
Heartland Natural	1 oz.	123	4.4	4.0	0
Honeynut Cheerios	1 oz.	107	0.7	0.1	0
Kix	1 oz.	110	0.7	0.2	0

Food	Portion	Total cal.	Total fat (gm)	Sat. fat (gm)	Chol. (mg)
Life	1 oz.	104	0.5	0.1	0
Product 19	1 oz.	108	0.2	tr	0
Puffed Rice	½ oz.	57	0.1	tr	0
Puffed Wheat	½ oz.	52	0.2	tr	0
Quaker 100% Natural	1 oz.	133	6.1	4.1	0
Raisin Bran	1 oz.	87	0.5	0.1	0
Rice Krispies	1 oz.	112	0.2	tr	0
Shredded Wheat	1 oz.	102	0.6	0.1	0
Shredded Wheat	1 bisc	83	0.3	tr	0
Special K	1 oz.	111	0.1	tr	0
Total	1 oz.	100	0.6	0.1	0
Wheat Chex	1 oz.	104	0.7	0.1	0
Wheat germ, toasted	1 oz.	108	3.0	0.5	0
Wheaties	1 oz.	99	0.5	0.1	2

CHICKEN
See Meat, Fish, and Poultry; Combination Foods

CHIPS AND SNACKS
See also Desserts and Cookies; Fast Foods; Grain Products

Food	Portion	Total cal.	Total fat (gm)	Sat. fat (gm)	Chol. (mg)
Cheese Puffed Balls, Cheetos	1 oz.	161	10.6	2.6	1
Cheese Puffs, Cheetos	1 oz.	159	10.0	2.4	1
Corn chips, Fritos	1 oz.	155	9.7	1.6	tr
Cracker Jacks	1 oz.	114	1.0	0.1	0
Fruit Roll-ups	1 roll	50	0.0	0.0	0
Funyums	1 oz.	140	6.4	1.2	tr
Granola Bar, Nature Valley	1 bar	110	5.0	4.3	0
Granola Bar, Quaker, chewy	1 bar	130	5.0	4.3	0
Granola Snack, Nature Valley	1 pouch	140	7.0	5.6	0
Popcorn, commercial popped	1 cup	54	0.7	0.3	0
Pork rinds, fried	1 oz.	151	9.3	3.7	24
Potato chips	1 oz.	151	9.8	2.6	0
Potato chips, BBQ	1 oz.	149	9.5	2.4	tr
Potato chips, sour cream and onion	1 oz.	153	9.5	2.4	1
Potato sticks	1 oz.	152	10.2	3.0	0
Pretzels	1 oz.	111	1.0	0.5	0
Tortilla chips, Doritos	1 oz.	139	6.6	1.0	0
Tortilla chips, Tostitos	1 oz.	145	7.7	1.4	tr

Food	Portion	Total cal.	Total fat (gm)	Sat. fat (gm)	Chol. (mg)
Tortilla chips, cheese-fla-vored	1 oz.	144	6.9	1.2	tr

COMBINATION FOODS (ENTREES AND FROZEN MEALS)

Food	Portion	Total cal.	Total fat (gm)	Sat. fat (gm)	Chol. (mg)
Beans and franks, cnd	8 oz.	355	14.0	4.8	8
Beans, refried, and sausage	½ cup	194	13.0	4.2	2
Beef and macaroni, Franco-American, cnd	7.5 oz.	220	8.0	3.5	40
Beef Oriental, Stouffer	9.1 oz.	280	9.0	3.7	45
Beef Pie, Banquet, frz	8 oz.	409	20.0	8.5	65
Beef Pie, Swanson	8 oz.	430	23.0	9.6	65
Beef Stew, Bounty, cnd	7.5 oz.	145	4.0	1.7	47
Beef Stew, Heinz, cnd	7.5 oz.	166	3.6	0.8	42
Beef Stew, Stouffer, frz	10 oz.	310	17.0	7.3	70
Burrito and guacamole, frz	6 oz.	354	16.0	7.0	30
Chicken a la King, Swanson, cnd	5.2 oz.	180	12.0	3.0	41
Chicken a la King, Banquet, frz	5 oz.	138	4.7	1.6	39
Chicken Dinner, Swanson, frz	14 oz.	870	43.0	10.0	80
Chicken Pie, Banquet, frz	8 oz.	427	23.2	9.8	45
Chicken Pie, Swanson, Hungryman, frz	16 oz.	780	44.0	15.0	80
Chicken Stew, Bounty, cnd	7.5 oz.	160	7.0	2.0	45
Chili with Beans, Heinz, cnd	7.7 oz.	326	17.2	6.5	43
Chili with Beans, Stokely, cnd	1 cup	390	26.0	9.6	52
Chili w/o Beans, Stokely, cnd	1 cup	430	35.0	14.0	120
Chow Mein, Beef, La Choy, cnd	1 cup	72	2.3	1.0	23
Chow Mein, Chicken, La Choy, cnd	1 cup	68	2.3	0.7	29
Corn fritter	3.5 oz.	377	21.5	6.0	150
Egg Rolls, Chicken, La Choy, frz	4	120	5.2	0.9	45
Enchiladas, Beef, Van de Kamps, cnd	6 oz.	214	10.0	6.1	29
Hash, corned beef, cnd	3.5 oz.	184	12.5	3.6	35
Lasagna, Stouffer, frz	10.5 oz.	385	14.0	8.6	90
Lasagna, Green Giant, frz	7 oz.	290	11.2	6.0	51

Food	Portion	Total cal.	Total fat (gm)	Sat. fat (gm)	Chol. (mg)
Macaroni and Cheese, Stouffer, frz	6 oz.	260	12.0	4.0	12
Pizza, Cheese, Celeste, frz	¼ pizza	320	12.8	6.6	32
Pizza, Deluxe, Celeste, frz	¼ pizza	367	18.6	9.5	52
Pizza, Pepperoni, Celeste, frz	¼ pizza	356	18.2	9.2	43
Pizza, Sausage, Celeste, frz	¼ pizza	375	19.5	10.1	52
Pizza, French bread, frz:					
Cheese	5.1 oz.	330	13.0	6.9	33
Pepperoni	5.4 oz.	410	20.0	10.1	45
Sausage	6 oz.	420	20.0	9.3	50
Ravioli, Beef, Franco-American, cnd	7.5 oz.	230	6.0	3.4	19

COOKIES
See Desserts and Cookies

DAIRY PRODUCTS AND EGGS

Food	Portion	Total cal.	Total fat (gm)	Sat. fat (gm)	Chol. (mg)
BUTTER	1 pat	36	4.0	2.5	11
CHEESE					
American, processed	1 oz.	106	8.9	5.6	27
American, low-fat, Lite-Line	1 oz.	50	2.0	1.3	10
American, part-skim, Light 'n Lively	1 oz.	70	4.0	2.5	15
Cheddar	1 oz.	114	9.4	6.0	30
Cheddar, Golden Image, Kraft	1 oz.	110	9.0	2.0	5
Colby, part-skim, Kraft Natural Lights	1 oz.	80	5.0	3.0	20
Cottage, creamed	½ cup	117	5.1	3.2	17
Cottage, low-fat (1%)	½ cup	82	1.2	0.7	5
Cream	1 oz.	99	9.9	6.2	31
Lo-Chol Light (muenster-type), Dorman's	1 oz.	70	5.0	0.3	3
Mozzarella, whole milk	1 oz.	90	7.0	4.4	25
Mozzarella, part-skim	1 oz.	79	4.9	3.1	15
Parmesan, grated	1 Tb	23	1.5	1.0	4
Swiss	1 oz.	107	7.8	5.0	26

Food	Portion	Total cal.	Total fat (gm)	Sat. fat (gm)	Chol. (mg)
CREAM					
Half and half	1 Tb	20	1.7	1.1	6
Heavy whipping cream	1 Tb	52	5.6	3.5	21
Light table cream	1 Tb	29	2.9	1.8	10
Sour cream	1 Tb	26	2.5	1.6	5
Whipped cream topping, canned	1 Tb	8	0.7	0.4	2
FROZEN DESSERTS					
Ice cream, vanilla (10% fat)	1 cup	269	14.0	8.9	59
Ice cream, vanilla (16% fat)	1 cup	349	23.7	14.7	88
Ice milk, vanilla	1 cup	184	5.6	3.5	18
Sherbet	1 cup	270	3.8	2.4	14
Sorbet	1 cup	200	0.0	0.0	0
MILK					
Whole	1 cup	150	8.2	5.1	33
2%, low-fat	1 cup	121	4.7	2.9	18
1%, low-fat	1 cup	102	2.6	1.6	10
Skim, nonfat	1 cup	86	0.4	0.3	4
Chocolate milk, low-fat	1 cup	179	5.0	3.1	17
Buttermilk	1 cup	99	2.2	1.3	9
NONDAIRY PRODUCTS					
Coffee whitener, liquid	½ oz.	20	1.5	0.3	0
Coffee whitener, powdered	1 tsp	11	0.7	0.7	0
Whipped topping, cnd	1 Tb	11	0.9	0.8	0
Whipped topping, frz	1 Tb	13	1.0	0.9	0
YOGURT					
Whole milk, plain	1 cup	139	7.4	4.8	29
Low-fat, plain	1 cup	144	3.5	2.3	14
Skim, plain	1 cup	127	0.4	0.3	4
Low-fat, vanilla, coffee	1 cup	194	2.8	1.8	11
Low-fat, fruit-flavored	1 cup	225	2.6	1.7	10
Nonfat, fruit-flavored	1 cup	200	0.3	0.2	3
EGGS, CHICKEN					
Whole	1 egg	79	5.6	1.7	210
Egg white	1 white	16	tr	0.0	0
Egg yolk	1 yolk	63	5.6	1.7	210
EGG SUBSTITUTE					
Egg Beaters, Fleischmann's	¼ cup	40	0.0	0.0	tr

Food	Portion	Total cal.	Total fat (gm)	Sat. fat (gm)	Chol. (mg)
DESSERTS AND COOKIES					
DESSERTS					
Brownies, from mix	1	130	5.0	2.3	27
Brownies, Sara Lee	1	192	9.7	4.6	54
Cake:					
Angelfood, from mix	1/12 cake	126	0.0	0.0	0
Cheesecake, from mix	1/8 cake	300	14.3	8.9	30
Choc. w/choc. icing	1 pc	233	10.8	5.5	26
German Choc. Cake, Pepperidge Farm	1 pc	297	16.0	9.9	46
Pound	1 pc	142	8.8	3.4	51
Strawberry shortcake	1 pc	344	8.9	3.7	15
Yellow w/choc. icing	1 pc	292	12.3	6.3	39
Custard, baked	1/2 cup	153	7.3	3.5	154
Danish pastry, apple	1 sm	121	4.9	1.8	9
Danish pastry, cheese	1 sm	131	7.2	4.1	23
Doughnuts:					
Cake	1 sm	105	5.8	2.5	23
Sugar-coated	1 sm	153	9.5	4.3	15
Raised/yeast	1 sm	124	8.0	4.0	12
Jelly center	1	226	8.8	4.5	16
Eclairs, choc. icing/custard fill	1	316	15.4	7.3	195
Gelatin (Jello) all flavors	1/2 cup	81	tr	tr	0
Pie:					
Apple, homemade	1/8 pie	282	11.9	4.2	4
Apple, Mrs. Smith's, frz	1/8 pie	390	17.0	6.5	7
Banana custard, homemade	1/8 pie	353	14.8	6.0	92
Blueberry, homemade	1/8 pie	387	17.3	6.3	4
Lemon Meringue, Mrs. Smith's, frz	1/8 pie	310	10.0	4.2	35
Pecan, Mrs. Smith's, frz	1/8 pie	510	23.0	5.6	30
COOKIES					
Animal Crackers	15	120	2.9	0.8	8
Chocolate chip cookie	1	50	2.3	0.9	4
Chocolate sandwich cookie	1	49	2.1	0.9	4
Fig bar	1	53	1.0	0.4	6
Gingersnap	3 sm	50	1.1	0.5	5
Golden Fruit cookie	1	63	0.6	0.3	5
Oatmeal cookie	1	80	3.2	1.1	13
Sugar cookie	1	89	3.4	1.4	6

Food	Portion	Total cal.	Total fat (gm)	Sat. fat (gm)	Chol. (mg)
Sugar wafer	2	53	2.1	0.9	4
Vanilla wafer	3	51	1.8	0.6	7

EGGS
See Dairy Products and Eggs

FAST FOODS

ARBY'S
Roast beef sandwich	1	353	15.0	n/a	39
Junior roast beef sandwich	1	218	8.0	n/a	20
Chicken breast sandwich	1	592	27.0	n/a	57
French fries	1 sm ord	211	8.0	n/a	6
Sausage and egg croissant	1	499	33.0	n/a	645

ARTHUR TREACHER'S
Chicken sandwich	1	341	19.2	2.8	32
Fish sandwich	1	440	24.0	4.2	42
Chowder	6 oz.	112	5.4	1.7	9
Cole slaw	3 oz.	123	8.2	1.1	7
Krunch Pups	2 oz.	203	14.8	3.7	25
Chips	4 oz.	276	13.2	2.3	1
Fried fish	5.2 oz.	355	19.8	2.8	56
Broiled fish	5 oz.	245	14.2	n/a	n/a

BURGER KING
Whopper	1	628	36.0	12.0	90
Hamburger	1	275	12.0	5.0	37
Whopper Junior	1	322	17.0	6.0	41
Whaler Fish Sandwich	1	488	27.0	6.0	77
Chicken Tenders	6	204	10.0	2.0	47
Onion rings	1 ord	274	16.0	3.0	0
French fries	1 sm ord	227	13.0	7.0	14
Great Danish	1	500	36.0	23.0	6

CHURCH'S
Chicken breast, fried	1	278	17.3	n/a	n/a
Chicken thigh, fried	1	306	21.6	n/a	n/a
Chicken leg, fried	1	147	8.6	n/a	n/a
Corn on the cob	1 ear	236	9.3	n/a	n/a
French fries	1 sm ord	256	13.0	n/a	n/a
Catfish, fried	3 pcs	201	12.0	n/a	n/a
Pecan pie	1 ord	367	20.0	n/a	n/a

Food	Portion	Total cal.	Total fat (gm)	Sat. fat (gm)	Chol. (mg)
HARDEE'S					
Biscuit, plain	1	257	12.4	n/a	0
Hamburger	1	244	9.2	n/a	20
Big Deluxe Burger	1	503	28.9	n/a	54
Roast beef sandwich	1	312	12.4	n/a	68
Large roast beef sandwich	1	440	21.5	n/a	86
Hot ham and cheese sandwich	1	316	9.6	n/a	57
Side salad	1	90	0.4	n/a	0
Chef salad	1	309	13.0	n/a	172
French fries	1 sm ord	252	12.4	n/a	0
KENTUCKY FRIED CHICKEN					
Original Recipe:					
Chicken breast, fried	1	276	17.3	4.6	96
Chicken drumstick, fried	1	147	8.8	2.3	81
Chicken thigh, fried	1	278	19.2	5.3	122
Extra Crispy:					
Chicken breast, fried	1	354	23.7	6.0	66
Chicken drumstick, fried	1	173	10.9	2.8	65
Chicken thigh, fried	1	371	26.3	6.9	121
Biscuit	1	269	13.6	3.5	tr
Mashed potato with gravy	1	62	1.4	0.4	tr
Kentucky Fries	1	268	12.8	3.1	2
Corn on the cob	1 ear	176	3.1	0.5	tr
Cole slaw	1 ord	103	5.7	0.8	4
Baked beans	1 ord	105	1.2	0.4	tr
LONG JOHN SILVER'S					
Baked Fish with Sauce	1 ord	151	2.0	n/a	n/a
Batter Fried Fish	1 pc	202	12.0	n/a	31
Kitchen Breaded Fish	1 pc	122	6.0	n/a	25
Ocean Chef Salad	1 ord	229	8.0	n/a	64
MCDONALD'S					
Big Mac	1	570	35.0	11.5	83
Biscuit	1	330	18.0	7.6	9
English muffin, buttered	1	186	5.0	2.3	15
Egg McMuffin	1	340	16.0	5.9	259
Sausage McMuffin with Egg	1	517	33.0	12.7	287
Quarter Pounder	1	427	24.0	9.0	81
McD.L.T.	1	680	44.0	14.8	101
Hamburger	1	263	11.0	4.4	29
French fries	1 sm ord	220	11.5	4.6	9
Fillet-O-Fish	1	435	26.0	5.6	47

Food	Portion	Total cal.	Total fat (gm)	Sat. fat (gm)	Chol. (mg)
Chicken McNuggets	6	323	20.0	5.0	62
Hot cakes with butter and syrup	1 ord	500	10.0	3.8	47
Soft-serve cone	1	189	5.0	2.0	24
Chocolate shake	1	383	9.0	4.0	30
PIZZA HUT					
Thin and Crispy (serving is ½ of 10"):					
Cheese	1 sv	450	15.0	n/a	n/a
Pepperoni	1 sv	430	17.0	n/a	n/a
Supreme	1 sv	510	21.0	n/a	n/a
Thick and Chewy (serving is ½ of 10"):					
Cheese	1 sv	560	14.0	n/a	n/a
Pepperoni	1 sv	560	18.0	n/a	n/a
Supreme	1 sv	640	22.0	n/a	n/a
ROY ROGERS					
Chicken breast, fried	1	412	23.7	n/a	118
Chicken wing, fried	1	192	12.8	n/a	47
Chicken thigh, fried	1	296	19.5	n/a	85
Chicken drumstick, fried	1	140	8.0	n/a	40
Roast beef sandwich	1	317	10.0	n/a	55
Large roast beef sandwich	1	360	12.0	n/a	73
Hamburger (¼ lb)	1	456	28.0	n/a	73
Biscuit	1	231	12.0	n/a	0
French fries	1 sm ord	268	14.0	n/a	42
Breakfast Crescent Sandwich	1	401	27.0	n/a	148
TACO BELL					
Beef Burrito	1	466	21.0	n/a	n/a
Enchirito	1	454	21.0	n/a	n/a
Taco	1	186	34.0	n/a	n/a
WENDY'S					
Big Classic	1	470	25.0	n/a	80
Small Hamburger (Kid's Meal)	1	200	9.0	n/a	35
Single Burger on Roll	1	350	16.0	n/a	75
Chicken Breast Filet Sandwich	1	340	13.0	n/a	60
Plain Baked Potato	1	250	2.0	n/a	tr
Broccoli and Cheese Potato	1	500	25.0	n/a	22
Sour Cream and Chive Potato	1	460	24.0	n/a	15

Food	Portion	Total cal.	Total fat (gm)	Sat. fat (gm)	Chol. (mg)
Chili	8 oz.	240	8.0	n/a	25
Frosty Dairy Dessert	1 ord	400	14.0	n/a	50
Taco Salad	1 ord	430	19.0	n/a	45
Chocolate chip cookie	1	320	17.0	n/a	5
Breakfast Sandwich	1	370	19.0	n/a	200
French toast	1 ord	400	19.0	n/a	115
Wheat toast with margarine	1 ord	190	8.0	n/a	5

FATS AND OILS

ANIMAL FATS

Food	Portion	Total cal.	Total fat (gm)	Sat. fat (gm)	Chol. (mg)
Beef tallow	1 Tb	116	12.8	6.4	14
Butter	1 Tb	108	12.2	7.6	33
Chicken fat	1 Tb	115	12.8	3.8	11
Lard (pork fat)	1 Tb	116	12.8	5.0	12
Turkey fat	1 Tb	115	12.8	3.8	13

VEGETABLE OILS

Food	Portion	Total cal.	Total fat (gm)	Sat. fat (gm)	Chol. (mg)
Canola (rapeseed)	1 Tb	120	13.6	0.9	0
Cocoa butter	1 Tb	120	13.6	8.1	0
Coconut	1 Tb	120	13.6	11.8	0
Corn	1 Tb	120	13.6	1.7	0
Cottonseed	1 Tb	120	13.6	3.5	0
Olive	1 Tb	119	13.5	1.8	0
Palm	1 Tb	120	13.6	6.7	0
Palm kernel	1 Tb	120	13.6	11.1	0
Peanut	1 Tb	119	13.5	2.3	0
Safflower	1 Tb	120	13.6	1.2	0
Sesame	1 Tb	120	13.6	1.9	0
Soybean	1 Tb	120	13.6	2.0	0
Sunflower	1 Tb	120	13.6	1.4	0

MARGARINE

Food	Portion	Total cal.	Total fat (gm)	Sat. fat (gm)	Chol. (mg)
Regular, hard stick	1 tsp	34	3.8	0.7	0
Corn oil, stick	1 tsp	34	3.8	0.7	0
Corn oil, soft, tub	1 tsp	34	3.8	0.6	0
Sunflower/soy, stick	1 tsp	34	3.8	0.6	0
Sunflower/soy, soft	1 tsp	34	3.8	0.6	0
Soybean liquid	1 tsp	34	3.8	0.6	0

COMMERCIAL SALAD DRESSINGS

Food	Portion	Total cal.	Total fat (gm)	Sat. fat (gm)	Chol. (mg)
Blue cheese	1 Tb	77	8.0	1.5	3
French, low-calorie	1 Tb	22	0.9	0.1	1

Food	Portion	Total cal.	Total fat (gm)	Sat. fat (gm)	Chol. (mg)
French, regular	1 Tb	67	6.4	1.5	9
Italian, low-calorie	1 Tb	16	1.5	0.2	1
Italian, regular	1 Tb	69	7.1	1.0	10
Mayonnaise, regular	1 Tb	100	11.0	1.6	8
Mayonnaise, "Light"	1 Tb	50	5.0	1.0	5
Mayonnaise, imitation	1 Tb	35	2.9	0.5	4
Mayonnaise-type salad dressing	1 Tb	57	4.9	0.7	4
Russian, low-calorie	1 Tb	23	0.7	0.1	1
Russian, regular	1 Tb	76	7.8	1.1	3
Thousand Island, low-calorie	1 Tb	24	1.6	0.2	2
Thousand Island, regular	1 Tb	59	5.6	0.9	4
SHORTENING					
Crisco (hydrogenated soy/ cottonseed)	1 Tb	113	12.8	3.2	0

FISH
See Meat, Fish, and Poultry

FROZEN MEALS
See Combination Foods

FRUITS
See also Juices, Fruit and Vegetable

Food	Portion	Total cal.	Total fat (gm)	Sat. fat (gm)	Chol. (mg)
Apple, with skin	1 med	81	0.5	0.1	0
Applesauce, sweetened	½ cup	97	0.2	tr	0
Apricot halves, cnd, heavy syrup	4	75	0.1	tr	0
Banana	1 med	105	0.6	0.2	0
Cantaloupe	1 cup pcs	57	0.4	tr	0
Carambola (star fruit)	1 med	42	0.4	tr	0
Cherries, raw	10	49	0.7	0.1	0
Cranberry sauce, jellied	½ cup	209	0.2	0.0	0
Dates, dried	10	228	0.4	tr	0
Figs, raw	1 med	37	0.2	tr	0
Fruit cocktail, cnd, juice pack	½ cup	56	tr	tr	0
Grapefruit, raw	½ med	38	0.1	tr	0
Honeydew melon, raw	¼ sm	33	0.3	tr	0
Kiwi fruit	1 med	46	0.3	tr	0

Food	Portion	Total cal.	Total fat (gm)	Sat fat (gm)	Chol. (mg)
Mango	1 med	135	0.6	0.1	0
Nectarine	1 med	67	0.6	tr	0
Orange, navel	1 med	65	0.1	tr	0
Peach, raw	1 med	37	0.1	tr	0
Pear, raw	1 med	98	0.7	tr	0
Pineapple, raw	1 cup pcs	77	0.7	tr	0
Plum, raw	1 med	36	0.4	tr	0
Pomegranate, raw	1 med	104	0.5	tr	0
Prunes, dried	10	201	0.4	tr	0
Raisins, seedless	⅔ cup	300	0.5	0.2	0
Strawberries, raw	1 cup	45	0.6	tr	0
Tangelo, raw	1 med	39	0.1	0.0	0
Tangerine, raw	1 med	37	0.2	tr	0

GRAIN PRODUCTS (BREAD, CRACKERS, ETC.)

See also Cereals and grains

BREAD

Food	Portion	Total cal.	Total fat (gm)	Sat fat (gm)	Chol. (mg)
Brown w/raisins	½" sl	80	tr	0.0	2
Cornbread from mix	⅛ rec	160	4.0	1.5	34
Cracked wheat	1 sl	66	0.9	0.2	tr
French	1 sl	70	1.0	0.2	0
Matzo	1 pc	117	0.3	0.0	0
Mixed grain	1 sl	64	0.9	0.2	tr
Pumpernickel	1 sl	82	0.8	0.1	0
Raisin	1 sl	70	1.0	0.3	1
Rye	1 sl	66	0.9	0.1	0
White	1 sl	64	0.9	0.2	tr
Whole wheat	1 sl	61	1.1	0.3	tr

CRACKERS

Food	Portion	Total cal.	Total fat (gm)	Sat fat (gm)	Chol. (mg)
Cheese	5	81	4.9	1.2	6
Cheese cracker w/peanut butter	2 oz.	205	13.5	3.5	18
Goldfish, asst. flavors	12	30	2.0	0.5	4
Goldfish, pretzel	12	30	1.0	0.3	2
Graham	2	60	1.5	0.6	3
Hi Ho, Sunshine	4	82	4.4	1.0	6
Melba toast	1 pc	15	0.2	0.1	1
Oyster	33	120	3.3	1.2	8
Ritz	3	54	2.9	0.8	5
Ry-Krisp	2 triples	50	0.2	0.1	1
Saltines	2	26	0.6	0.2	1
Triscuits	2	42	1.5	0.4	2
Wheat Thins	4	36	1.4	0.4	2
Zwieback	1 pc	31	0.7	0.3	2

Food	Portion	Total cal.	Total fat (gm)	Sat. fat (gm)	Chol. (mg)
ROLLS					
Brown & Serve	1	92	2.2	0.6	2
Crescent, from refrigerator dough	1	100	5.0	2.7	6
Dinner/pan	1	85	2.1	0.6	2
French	1	137	0.4	0.1	0
Hamburger	1	114	2.1	0.5	1
Hot dog/frankfurter	1	116	2.1	0.5	1
Kaiser/Hoagie	1 lg	470	8.4	2.1	4
Sandwich	1	162	3.1	0.8	1
OTHER GRAIN PRODUCTS					
Bagel, plain	1 med	163	1.4	0.2	0
Biscuit, from mix	1	93	3.3	1.2	2
Biscuit, from refrigerator dough	1	91	3.1	1.2	2
Biscuit, homemade	1	103	4.8	1.5	2
Bread crumbs	1 cup	345	4.0	1.0	2
Chow mein noodles	½ cup	153	8.8	2.5	4
Croutons	.7 oz.	70	0.0	0.0	0
English muffin	1	135	1.1	0.2	tr
Flour, all-purpose	1 Tb	25	0.1	0.0	0
Macaroni, cooked (1 oz. uncooked)	⅗ cup	102	0.4	0.0	0
Muffin, blueberry	1 sm	126	4.3	1.5	25
Muffin, bran	1 sm	112	5.1	1.8	26
Muffin, corn	1 sm	130	4.2	1.4	25
Noodles, egg	1 cup	160	2.4	0.8	50
Noodles, ramen	1 cup	202	6.8	1.5	0
Pancake, homemade	1 med	104	3.2	1.1	27
Spaghetti, cooked	1 cup	216	0.7	0.1	0
Stuffing, from mix	½ cup	198	12.2	3.0	1
Stuffing, Stove Top	½ cup	176	8.9	2.2	1
Taco shell	1	50	2.2	1.0	0
Tortilla, corn	1	67	1.1	0.1	0
Tortilla, flour	1	95	1.8	0.6	2
Waffle, homemade	1 lg	245	12.6	4.2	39
Waffle, frz	1 avg	95	3.2	1.0	24
JUICES, FRUIT AND VEGETABLE					
Apple juice	8 fl.oz.	116	0.3	tr	0
Apricot nectar	8 fl.oz.	141	0.2	tr	0
Cranberry Juice Cocktail	8 fl.oz.	147	0.1	0.0	0
Grape juice	8 fl.oz.	155	0.2	0.1	0
Grapefruit juice	8 fl.oz.	93	0.2	tr	0

Food	Portion	Total cal.	Total fat (gm)	Sat. fat (gm)	Chol. (mg)
Orange juice	8 fl.oz.	112	0.1	tr	0
Pineapple juice	8 fl.oz.	139	0.2	tr	0
Prune juice	8 fl.oz.	181	0.1	tr	0
Tomato juice	8 fl.oz.	41	0.2	0.0	0
V-8 juice	8 fl.oz.	53	0.1	0.0	0

LEGUMES

Food	Portion	Total cal.	Total fat (gm)	Sat. fat (gm)	Chol. (mg)
Beans with BBQ Sauce (Campbell)	7¾ oz.	270	4.0	1.5	0
Beans with Molasses Sauce (Heinz)	7¾ oz.	251	0.9	0.2	0
Beans with Tomato Sauce (Heinz)	8 oz.	232	1.9	0.4	0
Black-eyed peas, frz	⅔ cup	130	0.4	0.2	0
Butter beans, frz	½ cup	138	0.6	0.1	0
Cowpeas, cooked	3.5 oz.	76	0.3	0.1	0
Garbanzo beans (chick-peas), cooked	3.5 oz.	179	2.4	0.5	0
Kidney beans, cnd	½ cup	100	0.4	0.1	0
Lentils, cooked	⅔ cup	106	tr	tr	0
Lima beans, cooked	⅝ cup	159	0.7	0.2	0
Pork and beans, with tomato sauce	1 cup	250	4.0	2.0	4
Soybeans, cooked	½ cup	130	5.7	0.8	0
Split peas, cooked	½ cup	104	0.3	0.1	0
White beans, cooked	½ cup	118	0.6	0.2	0

LUNCHEON MEATS
See Sausages and Luncheon Meats

MEAT, FISH, AND POULTRY
See also Sausages, and Luncheon Meats; Combination Foods

MEAT

Beef

Food	Portion	Total cal.	Total fat (gm)	Sat. fat (gm)	Chol. (mg)
Liver, braised	3 oz.	137	4.2	1.6	331
Brisket:					
Lean and fat, braised	3 oz.	347	29.6	12.3	78
Lean only, braised	3 oz.	223	13.5	5.3	77
Chuck roast:					
Lean and fat, braised	3 oz.	325	25.9	10.8	87
Lean only, braised	3 oz.	230	13.0	5.3	90

Food	Portion	Total cal.	Total fat (gm)	Sat. fat (gm)	Chol. (mg)
Flank steak:					
Lean and fat, braised	3 oz.	218	13.2	5.6	61
Lean only, braised	3 oz.	208	11.8	5.0	60
Rib roast:					
Lean and fat, roasted	3 oz.	324	27.1	11.4	72
Lean only, roasted	3 oz.	204	11.7	4.9	68
Shortribs:					
Lean and fat, braised	3 oz.	400	36.7	15.1	80
Lean only, braised	3 oz.	251	15.4	6.6	79
Bottom round:					
Lean and fat, braised	3 oz.	222	12.6	4.8	81
Lean only, braised	3 oz.	189	8.2	2.9	81
Eye of round:					
Lean and fat, roasted	3 oz.	206	12.1	4.9	62
Lean only, roasted	3 oz.	155	5.5	2.1	59
Porterhouse steak:					
Lean and fat, broiled	3 oz.	254	18.0	7.5	70
Lean only, broiled	3 oz.	185	9.2	3.7	68
Ground:					
Extra-lean, broiled	3 oz.	217	13.9	5.5	71
Lean, broiled	3 oz.	231	15.7	6.2	74
Regular, broiled	3 oz.	246	17.6	6.9	76
Pork (Fresh)					
Liver, braised	3 oz.	141	3.7	1.2	302
Leg or ham:					
Lean and fat, roasted	3 oz.	250	17.6	6.4	79
Lean only, roasted	3 oz.	187	9.4	3.2	80
Loin:					
Lean and fat, roasted	3 oz.	271	20.7	7.5	77
Lean only, roasted	3 oz.	204	11.8	4.1	77
Shoulder:					
Lean and fat, roasted	3 oz.	277	21.8	7.9	81
Lean only, roasted	3 oz.	207	12.7	4.4	82
Pork (Cured)					
Bacon, regular, broiled	3 sl	109	9.4	3.3	16
Bacon, Canadian, grilled	2 sl	86	3.9	1.3	27
Ham, extra-lean (5% fat)	3 oz.	111	4.2	1.5	39
Ham, regular (11% fat)	3 oz.	156	9.0	3.0	45
Ham roast	3 oz.	192	12.9	4.3	52

Food	Portion	Total cal.	Total fat (gm)	Sat. fat (gm)	Chol. (mg)
Veal					
Cutlet, lean only, broiled	3 oz.	176	5.7	2.5	84
Loin chop, lean only, broiled	3 oz.	184	9.4	4.0	84
Lamb					
Leg chop, lean only, broiled	3 oz.	150	6.5	2.1	71
Loin chop, lean only, broiled	3 oz.	153	6.9	2.3	71
Leg roast, lean only, roasted	3 oz.	150	6.5	2.1	71
Shoulder, lean only, roasted	3 oz.	188	10.9	3.3	82
FISH AND SHELLFISH					
Fish					
Anchovies, cnd in oil, drained	5	142	1.9	0.4	20
Catfish, raw	3 oz.	99	3.6	0.8	49
Caviar	1 Tb	40	2.9	0.7	94
Cod, baked, no added fat	3 oz.	89	0.7	0.1	47
Fishsticks, commercial	3.5 oz.	272	12.2	3.1	112
Haddock, baked, no added fat	3 oz.	95	0.8	0.1	63
Halibut, baked, no added fat	3 oz.	119	2.5	0.4	35
Herring, cooked, no added fat	3 oz.	172	9.9	2.2	65
Mackerel, cnd, drained	3.5 oz.	156	6.3	1.8	79
Orange roughy, raw	3.5 oz.	126	7.0	0.1	20
Salmon, Atlantic, raw	3.5 oz.	142	6.3	1.0	55
Salmon, pink, cnd	3 oz.	118	5.1	1.3	43
Salmon, Sockeye, cnd	3 oz.	130	6.2	1.4	37
Sardine, cnd in oil, drained	3.5 oz.	208	11.5	1.5	142
Snapper, cooked, no added fat	3 oz.	109	1.5	0.3	40
Swordfish, cooked, no added fat	3 oz.	132	4.4	1.2	43
Trout, rainbow, cooked, no added fat	3 oz.	129	3.7	0.7	62
Tuna, light, oil-packed, drained	3 oz.	169	7.0	1.3	15
Tuna, light, water-packed, drained	3 oz.	111	0.4	0.1	15

Food	Portion	Total cal.	Total fat (gm)	Sat. fat (gm)	Chol. (mg)
Tuna, white, oil-packed, drained	3 oz.	158	6.9	1.2	26
Tuna, white, water-packed, drained	3 oz.	116	2.1	0.6	35
Whitefish, smoked	3 oz.	92	0.8	0.2	28
Shellfish					
Crustaceans:					
Crab, Alaska king, cooked	3 oz.	82	1.3	0.1	45
Crab, blue, cooked	3 oz.	87	1.5	0.2	85
Crayfish, cooked	3 oz.	97	1.2	0.2	151
Lobster, cooked	3 oz.	83	0.5	0.1	61
Shrimp, steamed	3 oz.	84	0.9	0.2	166
Shrimp, fried	3 oz.	206	10.4	1.8	150
Mollusks:					
Clams, raw	3 oz.	63	0.8	0.1	29
Clams, cnd, drained	3 oz.	126	1.7	0.2	57
Clams, fried	3 oz.	171	9.5	2.3	52
Mussels, steamed	3 oz.	147	3.8	0.7	48
Octopus, raw	3 oz.	70	0.9	0.2	41
Oyster, raw	3 oz.	59	2.1	0.5	47
Oyster, cnd, drained	3 oz.	58	2.1	0.5	46
Oyster, fried	3 oz.	167	10.7	2.7	69
Scallops, raw	3 oz.	75	0.6	0.1	28
Squid, raw	3 oz.	78	1.2	0.3	198
POULTRY					
Chicken					
Liver, simmered	½ cup	109	3.8	1.3	442
Breast:					
With skin, roasted	½	193	7.6	2.2	83
Skin removed, roasted	½	142	3.1	0.9	73
With skin, fried	½	218	8.7	2.4	88
Skin removed, fried	½	161	4.1	1.1	78
Drumstick:					
With skin, roasted	1	112	5.8	1.6	48
Skin removed, roasted	1	76	2.5	0.7	41
With skin, fried	1	120	6.7	1.8	44
Skin removed, fried	1	82	3.4	0.9	40
Leg:					
With skin, roasted	1	265	15.0	4.2	105
Skin removed, roasted	1	182	8.0	2.2	89
With skin, fried	1	285	16.0	4.4	105
Skin removed, fried	1	195	8.8	2.3	93

Food	Portion	Total cal.	Total fat (gm)	Sat. fat (gm)	Chol. (mg)
Thigh:					
With skin, roasted	1	153	9.3	2.5	58
Skin removed, roasted	1	109	5.4	1.5	49
With skin, fried	1	162	9.6	2.7	60
Skin removed, fried	1	113	5.7	1.6	53
Turkey					
Breast:					
With skin, roasted	4 oz.	212	8.3	2.4	83
Skin removed, roasted	4 oz.	152	0.8	0.3	73
Leg:					
With skin, roasted	1	418	13.3	4.1	171
Skin removed, roasted	1	355	8.5	2.8	170
MISCELLANEOUS					
Baking powder	1 tsp	3	tr	tr	0
Baking soda	1 tsp	0	0.0	0.0	0
Chocolate, baking-type	1 oz.	139	14.6	8.7	tr
Chocolate powder drink mix, sugar sweetened	1 Tb	83	0.6	0.0	0
Chocolate syrup (Bosco-tm)	1 Tb	50	0.1	0.0	0
Cocoa, unswtn	⅓ cup	115	3.6	3.0	0
Cocoa mix (Hershey)	1 oz.	115	2.2	1.0	0
Cream of coconut	1 Tb	36	3.4	3.0	0
Flour, all-purpose	1 Tb	25	0.1	0.0	0
Honey, plain	1 Tb	61	0.0	0.0	0
Jam or jelly	1 Tb	55	0.1	0.0	0
Ketchup	1 Tb	16	0.1	0.0	0
Molasses	1 Tb	46	0.0	0.0	0
Mustard, yellow	1 Tb	11	0.7	n/a	0
Olives:					
Black	2 lg	37	4.0	0.5	0
Green	2 med	15	1.6	0.2	0
Ovaltine, choc. powder	¾ oz.	77	0.6	0.4	0
Pickle relish, sweet	1 Tb	21	0.1	tr	0
Pickles:					
Dill	1 lg	11	0.2	tr	0
Sweet	1 lg	146	0.4	0.2	0
Shake and Bake (General Foods)	¼ pkt	69	2.6	1.4	tr
Sugar:					
Brown	1 Tb	52	0.0	0.0	0
White, granular	1 Tb	46	0.0	0.0	0
White, powdered	1 Tb	42	0.0	0.0	0

Food	Portion	Total cal.	Total fat (gm)	Sat. fat (gm)	Chol. (mg)
Strawberry Quik	1 Tb	90	0.0	0.0	0
Syrup, pancake	1 Tb	50	0.0	0.0	0
Tapioca	1 Tb	32	tr	0.0	0
Tartar sauce	1 Tb	70	7.9	1.3	5
Vinegar, cider or distilled	1 Tb	2	0.0	0.0	0

NUTS AND SEEDS

NUTS

Food	Portion	Total cal.	Total fat (gm)	Sat. fat (gm)	Chol. (mg)
Almonds, dried	1 oz.	167	14.8	1.4	0
Almond butter	1 Tb	101	9.5	0.9	0
Brazil nuts, dried	1 oz.	186	18.8	4.6	0
Cashews, dry roasted	1 oz.	163	13.2	2.6	0
Chestnuts, roasted	1 oz.	70	0.6	0.1	0
Coconut, fresh	2″ × 2″ pc	159	15.1	13.4	0
Coconut, dried, flaked, sweetened	½ cup	170	12.2	10.8	0
Filberts or hazelnuts, dried	1 oz.	179	17.8	1.3	0
Macadamia nuts, dried	1 oz.	199	20.9	3.1	0
Macadamia nuts, oil roasted	1 oz.	204	21.7	3.3	0
Peanuts, dry roasted	1 oz.	161	14.0	1.9	0
Peanuts, oil roasted	1 oz.	165	14.0	1.9	0
Peanut butter	1 Tb	95	8.2	1.4	0
Pecans, dried	1 oz.	190	19.2	1.5	0
Pistachio nuts, dry roasted	1 oz.	172	15.0	1.9	0
Soybean kernels, roasted	1 oz.	129	6.8	0.9	0
Walnuts, black, dried	1 oz.	172	16.1	1.0	0
Walnuts, English, dried	1 oz.	182	17.6	1.6	0

SEEDS

Food	Portion	Total cal.	Total fat (gm)	Sat. fat (gm)	Chol. (mg)
Pumpkin seed kernels, dry roasted	1 oz.	148	12.0	2.3	0
Sesame seed kernels, dried	1 Tb	47	4.4	0.6	0
Sesame seed paste (Tahini)	1 Tb	89	8.1	1.1	0
Sunflower seed kernels, dry roasted	1 oz.	165	14.1	1.5	0
Sunflower seed kernels, oil roasted	1 oz.	175	16.3	1.7	0
Sunflower seed butter	1 Tb	93	7.6	0.8	0

PASTA
See Combination Foods; Grain Products

Food	Portion	Total cal.	Total fat (gm)	Sat. fat (gm)	Chol. (mg)
PIZZA					
See Combination Foods; Fast Foods					
POULTRY					
See Meat, Fish, and Poultry					
SALAD DRESSINGS					
See Fats and Oils					
SAUSAGES AND LUNCHEON MEATS					
Barbecue loaf, beef and pork	1 oz.	49	2.5	0.9	11
Bologna, beef	1 oz.	89	8.0	3.3	16
Bologna, beef and pork	1 oz.	89	8.0	3.0	16
Bologna, turkey	1 oz.	57	4.3	0.8	28
Chicken roll	1 oz.	45	2.9	0.6	14
Corned beef brisket	1 oz.	71	5.4	1.8	28
Corned beef loaf	1 oz.	46	1.9	0.8	12
Frankfurter, beef	1	145	13.2	5.4	22
Frankfurter, beef and pork	1	144	13.1	4.8	22
Frankfurter, chicken	1	116	8.8	2.5	45
Frankfurter, turkey	1	102	8.0	2.2	48
Ham, chopped	1 oz.	48	3.6	1.2	11
Ham, extra-lean (5% fat)	1 oz.	37	1.4	0.5	13
Ham, regular (11% fat)	1 oz.	52	3.0	1.0	15
Honey loaf, beef and pork	1 oz.	36	1.3	0.4	10
Italian sausage, cooked	1 oz.	92	7.3	2.6	11
Kielbasa, pork and beef	1 oz.	88	7.7	2.8	19
Lebanon bologna, beef	1 oz.	64	4.2	1.8	19
Liverwurst, pork	1 oz.	93	8.1	3.0	45
Luncheon loaf, beef and pork	1 oz.	100	9.1	3.3	15
Olive loaf, pork	1 oz.	67	4.7	1.7	11
Pastrami, beef	1 oz.	99	8.3	3.0	26
Pepperoni, beef and pork	1 oz.	139	12.2	4.5	12
Polish sausage, pork	1 oz.	92	8.1	2.9	20
Pork sausage, patty, cooked	1 oz.	100	8.4	2.9	22
Pork sausage, link, cooked	1 link	48	4.1	1.4	11
Salami, cooked-type, beef and pork	1 oz.	71	5.7	2.3	18
Salami, cooked-type, turkey	1 oz.	56	3.9	0.9	23
Salami, dry or hard, pork	1 oz.	115	9.4	3.3	22
Turkey breast	1 oz.	31	0.5	0.1	12

Food	Portion	Total cal.	Total fat (gm)	Sat. fat (gm)	Chol. (mg)
Turkey ham	1 oz.	37	1.4	0.5	16
Turkey pastrami	1 oz.	40	1.8	0.5	20
Turkey roll, light and dark meat	1 oz.	42	2.0	0.6	16
Turkey roll, light meat	1 oz.	42	2.1	0.6	12

SOUPS, SAUCES, AND GRAVIES
Whole milk is assumed for soups and sauces prepared with milk.

SOUPS

Food	Portion	Total cal.	Total fat (gm)	Sat. fat (gm)	Chol. (mg)
Bean with bacon, cnd, water prep	1 cup	173	5.9	1.5	3
Bean with ham, chunky, cnd	1 cup	231	8.5	3.3	22
Beef broth or bouillon	1 cup	16	0.5	0.3	tr
Beef noodle, cnd, water prep	1 cup	84	3.1	1.2	5
Chicken broth	1 cup	39	1.4	0.4	1
Chicken, chunky, cnd	1 cup	178	6.6	2.0	30
Chicken noodle, cnd, water prep	1 cup	75	2.5	0.7	7
Chicken noodle, dried, water prep	1 cup	53	1.2	0.3	3
Chili beef, cnd, water prep	1 cup	169	6.6	3.3	12
Clam chowder, Manhattan, cnd	1 cup	78	2.3	0.4	2
Clam chowder, New England, milk prep	1 cup	163	6.6	3.0	22
Crab/vegetable	1 cup	76	1.5	0.4	10
Cream of celery, cnd, condensed	1 cup	180	11.2	2.8	28
Cream of celery, cnd, water prep	1 cup	90	5.6	1.4	15
Cream of chicken, cnd, condensed	1 cup	233	14.7	4.2	20
Cream of chicken, cnd, water prep	1 cup	116	7.4	2.1	10
Cream of mushroom, cnd, condensed	1 cup	257	19.0	5.2	3
Cream of mushroom, cnd, water prep	1 cup	129	9.0	2.4	2
Gazpacho	1 cup	57	2.2	0.3	0
Lentil with ham, cnd	1 cup	140	2.8	1.1	7
Minestrone, cnd	1 cup	83	2.5	0.5	2
Onion, cnd	1 cup	57	1.7	0.3	0
Onion, dry powder	1 pkt	115	2.3	0.5	2

Food	Portion	Total cal.	Total fat (gm)	Sat. fat (gm)	Chol. (mg)
Onion, dried, water added	1 cup	28	0.6	0.1	0
Oyster stew, milk prep	1 cup	134	7.9	5.1	32
Pea, cnd, water prep	1 cup	164	2.9	1.4	0
Pea with ham, chunky	1 cup	184	3.9	1.6	7
Split pea with ham, cnd, water prep	1 cup	189	4.4	1.8	8
Tomato, cnd, water prep	1 cup	86	1.9	0.4	0
Turkey noodle, cnd, water prep	1 cup	69	2.0	0.6	5
Turkey vegetable	1 cup	74	3.0	0.9	2
Vegetable, vegetarian, cnd	1 cup	72	1.9	0.3	0
Vegetable beef, cnd	1 cup	79	1.9	0.9	5
Vegetable beef, dried, water prep	1 cup	53	1.1	0.6	1

SAUCES

Commercial, Ready-to-Serve

Barbecue sauce	1 cup	188	4.5	0.7	0
Soy sauce	1 cup	11	0.0	0.0	0
Teriyaki sauce	1 cup	15	0.0	0.0	0

Dried, Powdered Mixes

Cheese, milk prep	1 cup	307	17.1	9.3	53
Hollandaise, butter prep	1 cup	237	19.7	11.6	51
Mushroom, milk prep	1 cup	228	10.3	5.4	34
Stroganoff, milk prep	1 cup	271	10.7	6.8	38
Sweet and sour, water prep	1 cup	294	0.1	0.0	0
Teriyaki, water prep	1 cup	131	0.9	0.1	0
White, milk prep	1 cup	241	13.5	6.4	34

GRAVIES

Canned, Ready-to-Serve

Au jus	1 cup	38	0.5	0.2	1
Beef	1 cup	124	5.5	2.8	7
Chicken	1 cup	189	13.6	3.4	5
Mushroom	1 cup	120	6.5	1.0	0
Turkey	1 cup	122	5.0	1.5	5

Dried, Powdered Mixes

Au jus, water prep	1 cup	19	0.8	0.4	1
Brown, water prep	1 cup	9	0.2	0.1	0
Chicken, water prep	1 cup	83	1.9	0.5	3
Mushroom, water prep	1 cup	70	0.9	0.5	1
Onion, water prep	1 cup	80	0.7	0.5	1
Pork, water prep	1 cup	76	1.9	0.8	3
Turkey, water prep	1 cup	87	1.9	0.6	3

Food	Portion	Total cal.	Total fat (gm)	Sat. fat (gm)	Chol. (mg)
SOY PROTEIN PRODUCTS					
Bac-O-Bits (General Mills)	1 Tb	33	1.3	0.2	0
Beef-style roll, frz (Worthington)	2.5 oz.	140	9.0	n/a	0
Beef-style roll, frz, smoked (Worthington)	2.5 oz.	170	10.0	n/a	0
Beef-style slices, frz, smoked (Worthington)	6 sl	130	7.0	n/a	0
Big Franks, can (Loma Linda)	1	95	4.6	0.6	0
Bologna, frz (Loma Linda)	2 sl	140	8.0	1.0	0
Bolona, frz (Worthington)	2 sl	70	3.0	0.4	0
Breakfast Links (Morningstar Farms)	5	190	13.3	3.3	0
Breakfast Patties (Morningstar Farms)	2	224	14.9	3.4	0
Breakfast Strips (Morningstar Farms)	3	92	8.5	1.2	0
Chicken, fried, frz (Loma Linda)	1 pc	140	10.0	n/a	0
Country Crisps Nuggets (Morningstar Farms)	3 oz.	280	19.0	3.0	0
Cutlets, cnd (Worthington)	1½ sl	100	2.0	n/a	0
Fillets, frz (Worthington)	2 pcs	180	10.0	n/a	0
Fri Chik, cnd (Worthington)	2 pcs	190	16.0	n/a	0
Granburger, dry (Worthington)	6 Tbs	110	1.0	0.2	0
Griddle steaks, frz (Loma Linda)	1 steak	160	11.0	n/a	0
Grillers (Morningstar Farms)	1 patty	184	11.6	n/a	0
Linketts, cnd (Loma Linda)	2	140	4.4	n/a	0
Little Links, cnd (Loma Linda)	2	85	4.6	n/a	0
Miso, fermented soybean	3.5 oz.	171	4.6	n/a	0
Natto, fermented soybean	3.5 oz.	167	7.4	n/a	0
Ocean Fillet, frz (Loma Linda)	1	180	11.0	n/a	0
Prime Stakes, cnd (Worthington)	1 pc	160	11.0	n/a	0
Prosage Links, frz (Worthington)	3	210	17.0	n/a	0
Redi-burger, cnd (Loma Linda)	½" sl	120	4.7	n/a	0
Salami, meatless, frz (Worthington)	2 sl	100	6.0	n/a	0

Food	Portion	Total cal.	Total fat (gm)	Sat. fat (gm)	Chol. (mg)
Savory Dinner Loaf, cnd (Loma Linda)	1 sl	140	9.7	n/a	0
Sizzle Burger, frz (Loma Linda)	1	190	11.0	n/a	0
Sizzle Frank, frz (Loma Linda)	2	160	13.0	n/a	0
Skallops, cnd (Worthington)	½ cup	70	2.0	n/a	0
Soybean milk	1 cup	87	4.0	0.6	0
Soybean milk powder	1 oz.	120	5.7	0.8	0
Soymeat, beef, cnd (Worthington)	2 sl	110	7.0	n/a	0
Soymeat, chicken, cnd (Worthington)	2 sl	130	10.0	n/a	0
Stakelets, frz (Worthington)	1 pc	150	9.0	n/a	0
Tofu, soybean curd	3.5 oz.	72	4.2	0.6	0
Tuno-Roll, frz (Worthington)	2 oz.	90	7.0	n/a	0
Turkey-like Slices, cnd (Worthington)	2½ sl	150	11.0	n/a	0
Veelet Parmesano, frz (Worthington)	7 oz.	340	21.0	n/a	0
Veg Steaks, cnd (Worthington)	2½ pcs	100	2.0	n/a	0
Vege-Burger, cnd (Loma Linda)	½ cup	110	1.0	n/a	0
Vegelona, cnd (Loma Linda)	½" slice	95	1.3	n/a	0
Vegetarian Burger, cnd (Worthington)	½ cup	160	6.0	0.8	0
Wham, cnd (Worthington)	3 sl	130	8.0	n/a	0

SUGAR AND SWEET FOODS
See Miscellaneous

VEGETABLES
See also Juices, Fruit and Vegetable; Legumes

Food	Portion	Total cal.	Total fat (gm)	Sat. fat (gm)	Chol. (mg)
Alfalfa sprouts, raw	3.5 oz.	41	0.6	0.1	0
Artichoke, cooked	1 lg	44	0.2	tr	0
Asparagus, cooked	⅔ cup	20	0.2	tr	0
Avocado, raw, California	1 med	306	30.0	4.5	0
Avocado, raw, Florida	1 med	339	27.0	5.3	0
Bamboo shoots, cnd	1 cup	21	0.1	tr	0

Food	Portion	Total cal.	Total fat (gm)	Sat. fat (gm)	Chol. (mg)
Bean sprouts, Mung, cnd	1 cup	23	0.1	tr	0
Beets, cooked	½ cup	27	0.1	tr	0
Broccoli, cooked	½ cup	27	0.3	tr	0
Brussels sprouts, cooked	6–8 med	36	0.4	0.1	0
Cabbage, cooked	½ cup	18	0.2	tr	0
Cabbage, raw, shredded	1 cup	24	0.2	tr	0
Carrot, raw	1 lg	42	0.2	tr	0
Carrot, cooked	⅔ cup	31	0.2	tr	0
Cauliflower, raw	1 cup pcs	27	0.2	tr	0
Cauliflower, cooked	1 cup	25	0.2	tr	0
Celery, raw, diced	1 cup	17	0.1	tr	0
Corn, white, frz	½ cup	88	0.9	0.2	0
Corn, yellow, ear, cooked	4″ ear	100	1.0	0.2	0
Corn, yellow, frz	½ cup	88	0.7	0.1	0
Cucumber, w/skin	½ med	8	0.1	tr	0
Cucumber, w/o skin	½ med	7	0.1	tr	0
Eggplant, cooked	½ cup	19	0.2	tr	0
Greens:					
Beet greens, cooked	½ cup	18	0.2	tr	0
Chard, cooked	½ cup	16	0.2	tr	0
Collards, cooked	½ cup	29	0.6	0.1	0
Dandelion, cooked	½ cup	33	0.6	0.1	0
Kale, frz	½ cup	28	0.5	0.1	0
Mustard, cooked	½ cup	23	0.4	tr	0
Spinach, raw	3.5 oz.	26	0.3	tr	0
Spinach, cooked	½ cup	21	0.5	0.1	0
Turnip, cooked	⅔ cup	20	0.2	tr	0
Green beans, frz	⅔ cup	29	0.2	tr	0
Hominy, cnd	1 cup	140	1.0	0.1	0
Kohlrabi, cooked	⅔ cup	24	0.1	tr	0
Lettuce, raw, avg all varieties	3.5 oz.	14	0.2	tr	0
Lima beans, baby-type, frz	½ cup	128	0.5	0.1	0
Mushrooms, raw	10 sm	28	0.5	0.1	0
Mushrooms, cnd	⅓ cup	17	0.2	tr	0
Okra, frz	½ cup	26	0.2	tr	0
Onion, raw	1 med	38	0.1	tr	0
Onion, cooked	½ cup	29	0.1	tr	0
Parsnips, cooked	½ cup	66	0.5	0.1	0
Peas, green, frz	⅗ cup	81	0.5	0.1	0
Pepper, sweet, raw	1 lg	22	0.2	tr	0
Potato:					
Baked	1 med	95	0.1	tr	0
Boiled, w/skin	1 med	76	0.1	tr	0

Food	Portion	Total cal.	Total fat (gm)	Sat. fat (gm)	Chol. (mg)
Boiled, w/o skin	1 med	65	0.1	tr	0
French fried, home, w/liquid oil	¾ cup	138	5.5	0.8	0
Mashed, w/milk and margarine	½ cup	94	4.3	1.1	2
Salad, home, w/mayonnaise	1 cup	363	23.0	3.6	20
Pumpkin, cnd	½ cup	35	0.3	0.2	0
Radish, raw	10 sm	17	0.1	tr	0
Sauerkraut, cnd	⅔ cup	21	0.2	tr	0
Snow peas, frz	6 oz.	90	0.3	0.1	0
Squash, acorn, baked	½ med	86	0.2	tr	0
Squash, butternut, boiled, mashed	1 cup	100	0.2	tr	0
Squash, yellow/summer, boiled	½ cup	14	0.1	tr	0
Succotash, frz	½ cup	94	0.8	0.1	0
Sweet potato, baked	1 sm	141	0.5	0.1	0
Sweet potato, boiled, peeled	1 lg	172	1.3	0.2	0
Sweet potato, candied, cnd	1 sm	114	0.2	tr	0
Tomato, raw	1 med	33	0.3	tr	0
Tomato, cnd	½ cup	25	0.3	tr	0
Tomato paste, cnd	1 cup	215	1.0	0.1	0
Tomato sauce, cnd	½ cup	38	0.4	tr	0
Turnip, cooked	⅔ cup	23	0.2	tr	0
Water chestnuts, cnd	16 med	80	0.2	tr	0
Zucchini	½ cup	16	0.1	tr	0

Quick and Easy Recipes Low in Fat and Cholesterol

Most of the recipes in this Appendix were provided by my patients and friends and have been tested by them. Half a dozen recipes for oat bran dishes come from the Quaker Oats Company. Each recipe has been analyzed by Katie Hannah and Katherine Boyd, R.D., M.S., using the Nutritionist III software package (N-Squared Computing, © 1986), for calories, total fat, saturated fat, cholesterol, carbohydrate, and protein. These figures can help you keep tabs on what you are eating.

When an oil is indicated, canola oil was chosen for analysis; oils low in saturated fat (less than two grams per tablespoon) as listed on p. 308 can be substituted if desired. For analysis, a corn oil tub margarine was chosen. When the type of fish is unspecified in a recipe, haddock was used in the analysis.

The recipes are organized into the following groups. Within each group, the recipes are listed alphabetically.

Breads, muffins, and breakfast ideas	Rice and vegetables
Desserts	Salads
Entrées	Soups

Breads, Muffins, and Breakfast Ideas

Always Ready Bran Muffins

3 cups wheat bran cereal (All-Bran extra fiber)	½ cup margarine
1 cup boiling water	2 egg whites
1 cup sugar	2½ cups flour
	2½ teaspoons baking soda

1   teaspoon salt   1   teaspoon cinnamon
½   teaspoon nutmeg   1   pint buttermilk

Instructions

Preheat oven to 400 degrees. Put 1 cup bran in small bowl. Add boiling water, stir, and let stand. In large bowl, cream sugar and margarine. Beat egg whites slightly and add to mixture. Add combined flour, baking soda, salt, and spices. Stir until mixed. Add the softened bran, remaining bran, and buttermilk. Mix well. Store in tightly covered container; refrigerate minimum of 12 hours. (Will keep up to 6 weeks.)

Line muffin tins with paper baking cups, fill ⅔ full. Bake 18 minutes. (After baking, may dip top of muffin in melted margarine, then in sugar-cinnamon mixture.)

number of servings: 30   *serving size: 1 muffin*

Content per Serving

total fat ...... 3.4 gm   cholesterol ..... 1 mg   carbohydrate ... 21 gm
saturated fat .. 0.6 gm   calories 112   protein .... 3 gm

This recipe was submitted by Kay Baker.

Apple Cinnamon Muffins

2   cups oat bran cereal   2   egg whites
¼   cup brown sugar   2   tablespoons vegetable oil
1¼ teaspoons cinnamon   1   medium apple, chopped
1   tablespoon baking powder   ¼   cup chopped walnuts
½   cup skim milk   ¼   cup raisins
¾   cup frozen apple juice
    concentrate

Instructions

Preheat oven to 425 degrees. In a medium bowl, mix dry ingredients. In a large bowl, mix milk, apple juice concentrate, egg whites, and oil. Add the dry ingredients, mixing well. Fold in apple, walnuts, and raisins.

Line 12 muffin tins with paper baking cups. Fill cups ⅔ full. Bake 17 minutes. Store muffins in airtight container to retain moisture.

no. of servings: 12   *serving size: 1 muffin*

Content per Serving

total fat ...... 5.0 gm   cholesterol ..... 0 mg   carbohydrate ... 26 gm
saturated fat .. 0.4 gm   calories 164   protein .... 5 gm

This recipe was submitted by David Riter.

Apple Oatmeal Bars

½   cup all-purpose flour   ¼   cup oat bran
¼   cup whole wheat flour   ½   teaspoon baking soda

⅓ cup brown sugar
½ cup margarine
1 cup rolled oats

2 tablespoons margarine
2½ cups apple slices
½ cup sugar

Instructions

In a large bowl, combine all-purpose flour, whole wheat flour, oat bran, baking soda, and brown sugar. Add margarine and oats, and cream until crumbly. Spread half of mixture in greased 7 × 10-inch pan. Arrange apple slices over it. Dot margarine on apples. Sprinkle sugar on top. Cover with remaining mixture. Bake 40 minutes. Cut into 2 × 2-inch squares while warm.

no. of servings: 16   *serving size: one square*

Content per Serving

total fat ...... 7.6 gm
saturated fat .. 1.3 gm

cholesterol .....0 mg
calories 154

carbohydrate ...21 gm
protein ....2 gm

This recipe was submitted by Mrs. Kenneth Campbell.

Apple Raisin Coffee Cake

½ cup margarine
1½ cups sugar
½ cup Egg Beaters (equivalent to
   2 eggs)
1 teaspoon vanilla
1½ cups flour

1 teaspoon cinnamon
⅛ teaspoon cloves
1 teaspoon nutmeg
4½ teaspoons baking powder
½ cup raisins
3 apples, chopped

Instructions

Preheat oven to 350 degrees. In a large bowl, cream sugar and margarine. Add egg substitute and vanilla. Beat well. Add combined flour, spices, and baking powder. Mix well. Fold in raisins and apples. Pour into 9 × 9-inch pan sprayed with vegetable oil spray. Bake 55 minutes.

no. of servings: 9   *serving size: one 3 × 3-inch piece*

Content per Serving

total fat ..... 12.7 gm
saturated fat .. 2.4 gm

cholesterol .....0 mg
calories 364

carbohydrate ...63 gm
protein ....4 gm

This recipe was submitted by Leah Hertz.

Apricot Oat Bread

½ cup uncooked oats
1 cup whole wheat flour (or ½
   cup whole wheat flour and ½
   cup oat flour)
½ cup diced dried apricots
¼ cup wheat germ

¼ cup pecans
2 teaspoons baking powder
1 teaspoon ground cinnamon
½ teaspoon baking soda
½ teaspoon salt
¾ cup skim milk

½ cup honey   ¾ teaspoon vanilla extract
¼ cup vegetable oil   ¼ cup Egg Beaters

Instructions

Preheat oven to 350 degrees. Spray 8½ × 4½-inch loaf pan with vegetable oil spray. In large bowl mix oats and next 8 ingredients. In small bowl mix milk and next 4 ingredients. Stir the two mixtures together in the large bowl. Pour batter into pan. Bake 45 minutes. Cool pan. Remove from pan and cool completely on rack.

   no. of servings: 12   *serving size: one ¾-inch slice*

Content per Serving

total fat ...... 6.8 gm   cholesterol .....0 mg   carbohydrate ...27 gm
saturated fat .. 0.5 gm   calories 176   protein .... 4 gm

---

Blueberry Muffins

1 cup oatmeal, uncooked   1 cup skim milk
¼ cup firmly packed brown sugar   ¼ cup Egg Beaters (equivalent to
1 tablespoon baking powder   1 egg)
½ teaspoon salt   3 tablespoons vegetable oil
½ teaspoon cinnamon   1 cup fresh or frozen blueberries

Instructions

Preheat oven to 425 degrees. In a large bowl, combine dry ingredients. Add milk, egg substitute, and oil. Stir until dry ingredients are moistened. Fold in blueberries. Spray 12 medium muffin tins with vegetable oil spray or line with paper baking cups. Fill muffin cups ⅔ full. Bake 25 to 30 minutes.

   no. of servings: 12   *serving size: 1 muffin*

Content per Serving

total fat ...... 4.2 gm   cholesterol .....0 mg   carbohydrate ...12 gm
saturated fat .. 0.4 gm   calories 94   protein .... 2 gm

---

Breakfast Waffle

¼ cup oat bran   ⅓ cup skim milk
¼ cup fat-free pancake mix   1 egg white
¼ teaspoon baking powder   dash vanilla

Instructions

Mix dry ingredients. Add milk and vanilla (if mix is stiff, add one more tablespoon milk). Fold whipped egg white. Heat waffle maker, sprayed lightly with vegetable oil spray. Pour batter into waffle maker and bake until golden brown.

no. of servings: 1

Content per Serving

total fat ...... 2.8 gm	cholesterol ..... 1 mg	carbohydrate ... 47 gm
saturated fat .. 0.5 gm	calories 283	protein .... 17 gm

This recipe was submitted by Judith Katz.

Cottage Cheese Muffins

¼ cup melted margarine
3 to 4 tablespoons sugar
6 egg whites
1 cup all-purpose flour

2 teaspoons baking poweder
12 ounces low-fat cottage cheese
(Light 'n Lively 1% milkfat)

Instructions

Melt margarine and add to sugar in mixer. In another bowl, beat egg whites until stiff. Add ⅓ of beaten egg whites to margarine-sugar mixture. To this add flour and baking powder, mixing until smooth. Fold in remainder of egg whites and cottage cheese.

Fill individual lined muffin pans ⅔ full with batter. Bake 15 to 20 minutes at 400 degrees until golden brown.

no. of servings: 12   *serving size: 1 muffin*

Content per Serving

total fat ...... 4.1 gm	cholesterol ..... 1 mg	carbohydrate ... 12 gm
saturated fat .. 0.8 gm	calories 111	protein .... 6 gm

This recipe was submitted by Stephanie Attman.

French Toast

1 cup skim milk
1 cup Egg Beaters (equivalent to 4 eggs)
½ teaspoon salt

½ teaspoon almond flavoring
2 tablespoons sugar
8 slices whole wheat bread
1 tablespoon margarine

Instructions

In a shallow bowl, combine first 5 ingredients. Beat until well-blended. Melt margarine in a skillet. Soak slices of bread in the mixture. Fry bread slices, turning after about 1 minute.

no. of servings: 4   *serving size: 2 slices*

Content per Serving

total fat ...... 5.4 gm	cholesterol ..... 1 mg	carbohydrate ... 35 gm
saturated fat .. 0.8 gm	calories 238	protein .... 14 gm

This recipe was submitted by Jane Anderson.

Fruity Nut Bread

1 cup all-purpose flour	2 egg whites
½ cup whole wheat flour	½ cup oat bran
½ cup sugar	¼ cup nuts
1½ teaspoons baking powder	½ cup dates
½ teaspoon baking soda	½ cup pineapple
¾ cup orange juice	½ cup raisins
2 tablespoons margarine	1½ cups blueberries, chopped

Instructions

Preheat oven to 350 degrees. In a large bowl, combine flour, sugar, baking powder, and baking soda. Stir in orange juice, margarine, and egg whites. Mix well. Fold in remaining ingredients. Put into greased 9 × 5-inch loaf pan. Bake for 55 minutes until toothpick inserted in center comes out clean. Cool for 15 minutes before removing from pan.

no. of servings: 18   *serving size: one ½-inch slice*

Content per Serving

total fat ...... 2.6 gm	cholesterol .....0 mg	carbohydrate ...25 gm
saturated fat .. 0.3 gm	calories 128	protein .... 3 gm

This recipe was submitted by Mrs. Kenneth Campbell.

Ippy's Staff of Life Bread

1¾ cups skim milk	⅓ cup bran
4 tablespoons margarine	3 tablespoons wheat germ
⅔ cup honey	3¾ to 4¼ cups all-purpose flour
1½ teaspoons salt	¼ cup white sugar
½ cup rolled oats	¼ cup dark brown sugar
1 package yeast	1 teaspoon cinnamon

Instructions

Heat milk and margarine. As it warms, add honey and salt. When it boils, remove from heat and stir in rolled oats. Let cool 1½ hours. Pour into mixing bowl. Stir in yeast, bran, and wheat germ. Add flour, small amounts at a time. Turn onto floured board and knead 8–10 minutes or until resilient. Add flour if needed. Place in greased bowl. Cover and let rise until doubled. Mix sugars and cinnamon.

When bread has doubled in size, punch down and place on a lightly floured board. Form into a flat oval. Sprinkle with half of cinnamon sugar mixture. Roll oval up tightly. Flatten into oval again by punching. Sprinkle on remaining cinnamon sugar and roll up perpendicular to first roll. Place loaf in greased 9 × 5-inch bread pan, lightly covered. Let rise 1 hour.

Preheat oven to 350 degrees. Bake loaf 25 minutes, then cover loaf securely with foil. Bake 30 minutes more. Remove from oven, cool in pan 15 minutes. Remove from pan and cool thoroughly before slicing. Delicious toasted.

no. of servings: 18   *serving size: one ½-inch slice*

Content per Serving

total fat ...... 3.1 gm	cholesterol ..... 0 mg	carbohydrate ... 34 gm
saturated fat .. 0.6 gm	calories 179	protein .... 4 gm

Submitted by Janet Johansen. Source: Baltimore Sun.

Michele's Pancakes

3 tablespoons squeeze margarine
2 tablespoons sugar
¼ cup Egg Beaters
1¼ cups flour

3 teaspoons baking powder
1 cup skim milk
1 teaspoon vanilla

Instructions

Mix first 6 ingredients with an electric beater. Add vanilla and mix well. Cook in skillet sprayed with vegetable oil spray.

no. of servings: 6   *serving size: two 4" pancakes*

Content per Serving

total fat ...... 5.9 gm	cholesterol ..... 1 mg	carbohydrate ... 24 gm
saturated fat .. 1.1 gm	calories 172	protein .... 5 gm

This recipe was submitted by Bonnie Stafford.

Oat Bran Muffins

2 cups Quaker Oat Bran Cereal
¼ cup firmly packed brown sugar
2 teaspoons baking powder
½ teaspoon salt (optional)

1 cup skim milk or 2% low-fat milk
2 egg whites, slightly beaten
¼ cup honey or molasses
2 tablespoons vegetable oil

Instructions

Heat oven to 425 degrees. Line 12 medium muffin cups with paper baking cups, or spray bottoms only with vegetable oil cooking spray. Combine dry ingredients. Add milk, egg whites, honey, and oil; mix just until dry ingredients are moistened. Fill prepared muffin cups almost full; bake 15–17 minutes or until golden brown.

number of servings: 12   *serving size: 1 muffin*

Content per Serving

total fat ...... 3.3 gm	cholesterol ... 0.3 mg	carbohydrate ....19 gm
saturated fat .. 0.3 gm	calories 122	protein .... 4 gm

This recipe is from the Quaker Oats Company.

Omelet

3 egg whites	1 two-cubic-inch block Kraft
2 teaspoons dried minced onion	Golden Image cheese, sliced

Instructions

Beat egg whites with onion. Pour into 8-inch Teflon pan sprayed with vegetable oil spray. Slice cheese into 3 pieces and place of top of eggs. Cook slowly. When mixture begins to set, fold one half over the other. Serve immediately.

no. of servings: 1

Content per Serving

total fat ..... 10.6 gm	cholesterol ..... 6 mg	carbohydrate .... 1 gm
saturated fat .. 2.4 gm	calories 179	protein .... 18 gm

This recipe was submitted by Bernard Swerbilow.

Strawberry Pecan Bread

½ cup vegetable oil	1 teaspoon baking soda
1 cup sugar	1 teaspoon baking powder
2 egg whites	½ teaspoon salt
1 cup mashed strawberries	½ teaspoon vanilla
2 cups all-purpose flour	¼ cup chopped pecans

Instructions

Beat oil and sugar. Add egg whites and mashed strawberries; beat well. Sift dry ingredients; add to strawberry mixture with vanilla. Mix well and stir in nuts.

Preheat oven to 350 degrees. Pour into 9 × 5-inch loaf pan sprayed with vegetable oil spray. Cool well and store overnight before slicing.

no. of servings: 16   *serving size: one ½-inch slice*

Content per Serving

total fat ...... 8.2 gm	cholesterol ..... 0 mg	carbohydrate ... 24 gm
saturated fat .. 0.6 gm	calories 176	protein .... 2 gm

This recipe was submitted by Santa Krieger.

Whole Wheat Bread

2 cups skim milk	2 tablespoons dry yeast
3 tablespoons vegetable oil	⅓ cup warm water
1 tablespoon salt	5½ cups whole wheat flour
½ cup honey	

Instructions

Heat milk to simmering. Stir in oil, salt, and honey; cool to lukewarm. Dissolve yeast in warm water. Add to cooled milk. With electric mixer at low speed, beat in 3 cups flour; beat for 8 minutes. Add 2 cups flour and mix well. Turn out on floured board (this is where the additional ½ cup flour is used for the several kneadings) and knead until dough is smooth and elastic.

Place in oiled bowl, cover and set in warm place to rise until doubled in bulk (at least 1 hour). Punch down, knead lightly, and return to bowl to rise again. When double in bulk, punch down and form into two loaves. Place in 2 lightly greased loaf pans. Cover, let rise.

When double, uncover and bake at 375 degrees for 40 minutes. Remove from pans and cool on rack.

no. of servings: 2 loaves, 18 slices each   *serving size: 1 slice*

Content per Serving

total fat ...... 1.5 gm	cholesterol ..... 0 mg	carbohydrate ... 17 gm
saturated fat .. 0.2 gm	calories 91	protein .... 3 gm

This recipe was submitted by Margaret Rose.

Desserts

Applesauce Cake

1 1-pound can applesauce	1 teaspoon cinnamon
½ cup margarine	½ teaspoon ground cloves
2 teaspoons baking soda	1 cup raisins
1½ cups sugar	1 tablespoon flour
2½ cups flour	

Instructions

Preheat oven to 350 degrees. Heat applesauce. Add margarine, baking soda, and sugar. Mix well. In another bowl sift flour and spices together. Add to the applesauce mixture and mix. Sprinkle raisins with flour and stir into mixture.

Bake in greased and floured tube pan 40 to 50 minutes, or put in lightly greased microwave-safe pan and cook at 100 percent power for 8 minutes, turning ¼ turn at 2-minute intervals.

no. of servings: 10   *serving size: ¹⁄₁₀ of cake*

Content per Serving

total fat ...... 9.4 gm	cholesterol ..... 0 mg	carbohydrate ... 71 gm
saturated fat .. 1.6 gm	calories 371	protein .... 4 gm

This recipe was submitted by Janet Johansen.

Banana Walnut Cake

⅔ cup mashed bananas (mash
   ripe banana with a fork)
⅓ cup margarine
6 large egg whites
¾ cup water

2 cups unbleached white flour
2 teaspoons baking powder
1 teaspoon baking soda
1 teaspoon cinnamon
½ cup walnuts
½ cup raisins

Instructions

Preheat oven to 350 degrees. In a mixing bowl, beat together mashed bananas and margarine until creamy. Add egg whites and water. Beat well. Stir in flour, baking powder, baking soda, and cinnamon. Beat until smooth. Add walnuts and raisins.

Spoon batter into a 9 × 13-inch baking pan, sprayed with vegetable oil spray. Bake 20 minutes or until a knife inserted comes out clean. Cool and cut into 3 × 3-inch squares.

no. of servings: 12   *serving size: 1 square*

Content per Serving

total fat ...... 7.5 gm   cholesterol ..... 0 mg   carbohydrate ... 24 gm
saturated fat .. 1.0 gm   calories 178   protein .... 5 gm

This recipe was submitted by Frieda Miller.

Cocoa Cupcakes

1½ cups flour
1 cup sugar
1 teaspoon baking soda
4 tablespoons cocoa

3 tablespoons vegetable oil
1 teaspoon vanilla
1 tablespoon vinegar
1 cup cold water

Instructions

Preheat oven to 350 degrees. In a medium bowl, combine flour, sugar, and baking soda. In a large bowl, combine cocoa, oil, vinegar, and vanilla, mixing well. Add dry ingredients to cocoa mixture. Add water in several additions. Mix well. Pour into muffin tins lined with wax paper. Bake 25 to 30 minutes.

no. of servings: 12   *serving size: 1 cupcake*

Content per Serving

total fat ...... 3.8 gm   cholesterol ..... 0 mg   carbohydrate ... 27 gm
saturated fat .. 0.4 gm   calories 148   protein .... 2 gm

This recipe was submitted by Judith Katz.

Crunchy Pie Crust

Bottom crust:
- ½ cup all-purpose flour
- ¼ cup whole wheat flour
- ¼ cup oat bran
- ⅓ cup vegetable oil
- ¼ cup skim milk
- ¼ cup rolled oats

Top crust:
- ⅓ cup flour
- ¼ cup brown sugar
- ¼ cup rolled oats
- 3 tablespoons margarine

Instructions

Bottom crust: In a large bowl, combine all ingredients. Mix well. Press onto bottom and sides of 9-inch pie pan.

Top crust: Combine flour, brown sugar, and oats. Cut in softened margarine until it resembles fine crumbs. Sprinkle over pie filling.

no. of servings: 8   serving size: ⅛ of pie

Content per Serving (crust only)

total fat ..... 13.5 gm	cholesterol ..... 0 mg	carbohydrate ... 24 gm
saturated fat .. 1.4 gm	calories 229	protein .... 3 gm

Note: This crust should be filled with a low-fat pie filling. For example, pudding mix made with skim milk; or, for a fruit filling, ¼ cup melted grape jelly and 1 pint whole fresh strawberries.

This recipe was submitted by Mrs. Kenneth Campbell.

Deep Dish Brownie

- ¾ cup melted margarine
- 1½ cups sugar
- 1½ teaspoons vanilla flavoring
- ¾ cup unsifted all-purpose flour
- ½ cup Hershey's cocoa
- ½ teaspoon baking powder
- ½ teaspoon salt
- 6 egg whites

Instructions

Preheat oven to 350 degrees. In a large bowl, combine margarine, sugar, and vanilla. In another bowl, combine flour, baking powder, and salt. Add to margarine mixture. Mix well. Beat egg whites until stiff; fold into mixture until well blended.

Spread into 8 × 8-inch baking pan sprayed with vegetable oil spray. Bake for 40 to 45 minutes or until brownie begins to pull away from edge of pan. Cool and cut into 2 × 2-inch squares.

no. of servings: 16   serving size: 1 brownie

Content per Serving

total fat ..... 10.8 gm	cholesterol ..... 0 mg	carbohydrate ... 28 gm
saturated fat .. 3.0 gm	calories 230	protein .... 6 gm

This recipe was submitted by Stephanie Attman.

Frozen Fruit Dessert

1 6-ounce can frozen orange
  juice
1 6-ounce can frozen lemonade
20 ounces frozen strawberries

5–6 bananas, sliced
1 12-ounce can pineapple
  chunks

Instructions

Mix all ingredients and freeze in a large container. When ready to serve, thaw until slushy. Good alone or with plain cake.

no. of servings: 10   *serving size: 1 cup*

Content per Serving

total fat ...... 0.5 gm   cholesterol ..... 0 mg   carbohydrate ... 51 gm
saturated fat .. 0.1 gm   calories 198   protein .... 2 gm

This recipe was submitted by Robin Stowell.

Ginger Cookies

¾ cup sugar
1 cup margarine
3 egg whites
½ cup molasses
½ teaspoon baking soda
1 teaspoon baking powder

1 teaspoon ginger (or less,
  according to taste)
1 cup whole wheat flour
1½ cups all-purpose flour
¾ cup oat bran
1 cup raisins

Instructions

Preheat oven to 325 degrees. In a large bowl, cream sugar, margarine, and egg whites. Add molasses, baking soda, baking powder, and ginger. Mix well. Stir in flour and oat bran. Fold in raisins. Drop by spoonfuls onto greased 11 × 15-inch cookie sheet with sides. Pat down to cover entire pan. Bake 25 to 30 minutes. Cut into squares and cool in pan.

no. of servings: about 40   *serving size: one 2 × 2-inch cookie*

Content per Serving

total fat ...... 4.7 gm   cholesterol ..... 0 mg   carbohydrate ... 15 gm
saturated fat .. 0.8 gm   calories 108   protein .... 2 gm

This recipe was submitted by Mrs. Kenneth Campbell. Source: Houghton Heritage Cookbook.

Honey Cake

4 egg whites
½ cup sugar
½ cup vegetable oil
½ cup honey

½ cup strong tea
1½ cups flour
¾ teaspoon baking powder
½ teaspoon baking soda

½ teaspoon nutmeg   ½ teaspoon cinnamon
½ teaspoon ground cloves   ¼ cup slivered almonds

Instructions

Preheat oven to 350 degrees. Beat egg whites. Add sugar, oil, honey, and tea, mixing well. In another bowl, combine flour, baking powder, baking soda, nutmeg, cloves, and cinnamon. Stir in the flour and spice mixture in several additions. Pour mixture into a 9 × 5-inch loaf pan lined with wax paper. Sprinkle with almonds. Bake for 50 to 55 minutes. (Bake at 325 degrees for 55 to 60 minutes if using a glass pan.)

no. of servings: 18   serving size: one ½-inch slice

Content per Serving

total fat ...... 6.9 gm	cholesterol ..... 0 mg	carbohydrate ... 19 gm
saturated fat .. 0.5 gm	calories 142	protein .... 2 gm

This recipe was submitted by Linda Finifter.

Lebkuchen

⅔ cup margarine   2½ cups all-purpose flour
1½ cups brown sugar   1 teaspoon cinnamon
½ cup Egg Beaters (equivalent to   1 teaspoon cloves
   2 eggs)   1 teaspoon allspice
1 tablespoon lemon juice   1 teaspoon baking soda
1 tablespoon lemon rind   1 cup dried fruit, chopped
4 tablespoons water   1 cup chopped nuts

Instructions

Preheat oven to 350 degrees. In a large bowl, combine margarine, sugar, Egg Beaters, lemon juice, lemon rind, and water. In another bowl, combine flour, spices, and baking soda. Stir in the flour and spice mixture in several additions. Mix well. Stir in fruit and nuts.

Bake for 20 minutes in a 10½ × 15-inch pan. Cut into squares immediately. Do not remove from pan until cool.

no. of servings: 50   serving size: one 2 × 2½-inch piece

Content per Serving

total fat ...... 3.9 gm	cholesterol ..... 0 mg	carbohydrate ... 14 gm
saturated fat .. 0.5 gm	calories 95	protein .... 2 gm

This recipe was submitted by Leah Hertz.

Low-Fat Banana Shake

½ banana   ½ cup vanilla ice milk (4.3% fat)
½ to ⅓ cup skim milk   1 tablespoon oat bran

Instructions

Blend all ingredients in a blender at high speed. Serve immediately.

no. of servings: 1   *serving size: one 12-ounce shake*

Content per Serving

total fat ...... 3.7 gm	cholesterol .... 11 mg	carbohydrates .. 38 gm
saturated fat .. 2.1 gm	calories 210	protein .... 9 gm

This recipe was submitted by Carol McCarthy.

Low-Fat Chocolate Shake

1 package Alba-77 Chocolate   ½ cup skim milk
   Shake Mix   ½ cup vanilla ice milk (4.3% fat)

Instructions

Blend all ingredients in a blender at high speed. Serve immediately.

no. of servings: 1   *serving size: one 12-ounce shake*

Content per Serving

total fat .... 4 gm	cholesterol .... 11 mg	carbohydrate ... 32 gm
saturated fat .... 2 gm	calories 205	protein .... 13 gm

This recipe was submitted by Judy Falcon.

Pie Pastry

2 cups all-purpose flour   ⅓ cup oil
1¼ teaspoons salt   3 tablespoons cold skim milk

Instructions

Preheat oven to 425 degrees. In a large bowl, sift flour and salt together. Mix oil with milk, and pour at once into the flour. Stir with a fork until well blended, adding more liquid if necessary to make the dough hold together. Divide into 2 portions. Refrigerate a few minutes to make dough easier to work.

Flatten one ball of dough slightly and place on a sheet of wax paper or cellophane wrap. Put another sheet over top, and roll out quickly. Do not roll too thin. Remove top sheet and turn over dough into pie plate. Remove second sheet and lift crust around the edge so it settles into the plate. Trim and flute the edge with a fork or your fingers. Crust may be refrigerated.

no. of servings: 8   *serving size: ⅛ pie*

Content per Serving (pastry only)

total fat ...... 8.8 gm	cholesterol ..... 0 mg	carbohydrate ... 24 gm
saturated fat .. 0.6 gm	calories 193	protein .... 3 gm

Note: For examples of low-fat pie filling, see recipe for *Crunchy Pie Crust.*

This recipe was submitted by Sondra Hinckley. Source: The American Heart Association Cookbook, *1975.*

Pineapple Cake

1 20-ounce can crushed pineapple with juice	½ cup Egg Beaters
2 cups sugar	2 tablespoons baking soda
2 cups flour	½ cup nuts

Instructions

Preheat oven to 350 degrees. In a large bowl, combine first 5 ingredients. Mix well, fold in nuts. Pour into 10 × 10-inch sheet cake pan. Bake 45 minutes.

no. of servings: 16   *serving size: one 2½ × 2½-inch piece*

Content per Serving

total fat ...... 2.4 gm	cholesterol .....0 mg	carbohydrate ...38 gm
saturated fat .. 0.7 gm	calories 182	protein .... 3 gm

This recipe was submitted by Mary Kloss.

Sorbet

¼ cup low-fat yogurt	1 to 3 teaspoons sugar
2 egg whites	3 cups frozen fruit, cut in chunks
1 to 2 teaspoons lemon or lime juice	

Instructions

Place yogurt, egg whites, juice, and sugar in food processor; blend briefly. With processor running, gradually add frozen fruit until sorbet is formed (2–3 minutes).

no. of servings: 6   *serving size: 1 cup*

Content per Serving

total fat ...... 0.5 gm	cholesterol ..... 1 mg	carbohydrate ... 11 gm
saturated fat .. 0.1 gm	calories 50	protein .... 2 gm

This recipe was submitted by Anna Hare.

Strawberries and "Cream"

1 pint fresh strawberries, washed, hulled, and sliced	1 8-ounce carton nonfat plain yogurt
	1 teaspoon vanilla flavoring

Instructions

In a large bowl, combine all ingredients. Chill 1 to 2 hours, to allow juice from strawberries to mix with yogurt.

no. of servings: 6   *serving size: about ¾ cup*

Content per Serving

total fat ...... 0.2 gm   cholesterol ..... 1 mg   carbohydrate .... 6 gm
saturated fat .. 0.1 gm   calories 36   protein .... 2 gm

This recipe was submitted by Myrna Brams.

Vanilla Ice Cream

1 cup Egg Beaters (equivalent to   3 tablespoons flour
   4 eggs)   5 cups skim milk, scalded
¾ cup sugar or 15 packets Equal   1 tablespoon vanilla

Instructions

Mix Egg Beaters, sugar, and flour. Add milk. Cook over medium heat until slightly thickened (consistency of soft custard). Cool and flavor with vanilla. Freeze in ½-gallon hand crank or electric ice cream freezer.

   no. of servings: 12   *serving size: 1 cup*

Content per Serving

total fat ...... 0.2 gm   cholesterol ..... 2 mg   carbohydrate ... 19 gm
saturated fat .. 0.1 gm   calories 98   protein .... 6 gm

This recipe was submitted by J. Galen Metzger.

Wacky Cake

1½ cups flour   5 tablespoons vegetable oil
 1 cup sugar   1 tablespoon vinegar
 3 rounded teaspoons   1 teaspoon vanilla
   unsweetened cocoa 1 cup cold water
 1 teaspoon baking soda

Instructions

Preheat oven to 350 degrees. Mix dry ingredients together in ungreased 9 × 9-inch pan. Add liquid ingredients. Stir thoroughly. Bake 30–35 minutes.

   no. of servings: 9   *serving size: one 3 × 3-inch piece*

Content per Serving

total fat ...... 8.1 gm   cholesterol ..... 0 mg   carbohydrate ... 37 gm
saturated fat .. 0.8 gm   calories 231   protein .... 3 gm

This recipe was submitted by Mrs. Max Moore.

Walnut Pie

 5 egg whites   ¾ teaspoon vanilla
1½ cups sugar   1 cup finely chopped walnuts
 ¾ teaspoon baking powder   2 tablespoons margarine
 1 cup Saltine cracker crumbs

Instructions
Beat egg whites until stiff. Add sugar, baking powder, cracker crumbs, and vanilla. Mix well. Fold in walnuts. Grease pie plate with margarine. Pour mixture into pie plate and bake for 30 minutes at 350 degrees, until top splits. Cool and cover with wax paper.

no. of servings: 10 slices   *serving size: ¹⁄₁₀ of pie*

Content per Serving

total fat ..... 10.3 gm	cholesterol ..... 3 mg	carbohydrate ... 38 gm
saturated fat .. 1.2 gm	calories 260	protein .... 6 gm

This recipe was submitted by Donna Askin.

Entrées

Baked Fish Fillet

1 fish fillet (4 ounces)	½ teaspoon dried dill weed
1 lemon	2 tablespoons onion, minced
1 teaspoon margarine	

Instructions
Preheat oven to 350 degrees. Place fillet in baking pan sprayed with vegetable oil spray. Squeeze juice of lemon over fish. Rub fish with margarine and sprinkle with dill and chopped onions. Bake 15 minutes or until fish flakes easily with a fork.

no. of servings: 1

Content per Serving

total fat ...... 4.7 gm	cholesterol .... 63 mg	carbohydrate .... 7 gm
saturated fat .. 0.8 gm	calories 156	protein .... 22 gm

---

Baked Fish Provençal

4 white fish fillets (about 1 pound)	¼ cup shredded part-skim mozzarella cheese
¾ cup water	2 tablespoons grated parmesan cheese
½ cup dry white wine	
½ cup Quaker Oat Bran cereal, uncooked	2 tablespoons chopped fresh parsley or 1 tablespoon dry parsley flakes
1 large tomato, chopped	

Instructions

Preheat oven to 425 degrees. Place fish in 11¾ × 7½-inch baking dish. In medium saucepan, combine water, wine, and cereal. Cook over medium heat 3 to 4 minutes or until thickened. Add tomato. Pour over fish. Sprinkle with cheese and parsley. Bake 20 minutes or until fish flakes easily with a fork.

no. of servings: 4   *serving size: 1 fillet*

Content per Serving

total fat ...... 3.5 gm   cholesterol .... 69 mg   carbohydrates ... 7 gm
saturated fat .. 1.6 gm   calories 174   protein .... 26 gm

This recipe comes from the Quaker Oats Company.

Broiled Hawaiian Fish Fillets

⅓ cup soy sauce
1 tablespoon firmly packed brown sugar
2 tablespoons vegetable oil
1 tablespoon cider vinegar

½ teaspoon ground ginger
1 clove garlic, crushed
4 white fish fillets (about 1½ pounds)
1 tablespoon minced fresh parsley

Instructions

In a small bowl, combine soy sauce, brown sugar, oil, vinegar, ginger, and garlic. Place fish fillets in shallow pan. Pour sauce over fish and marinate 20 minutes. Reserve sauce.

Arrange fish fillets in shallow baking pan. Broil 5 inches from heat for 4 minutes. Turn, baste with sauce, and broil 4 minutes more. Sprinkle with parsley and serve immediately.

no. of servings: 4   *serving size: 1 fillet*

Content per Serving

total fat ...... 8.0 gm   cholesterol .... 94 mg   carbohydrate .... 6 gm
saturated fat .. 0.7 gm   calories 233   protein .... 33 gm

This recipe was submitted by Janet Johansen. Source: Cook's Corner, Baltimore Sun.

Chicken Fried Rice

1 cup cooked, skinned, diced chicken
1 tablespoon soy sauce

¼ cup vegetable oil
1 cup uncooked rice
2 cups chicken bouillon

Instructions

Toss chicken with soy sauce. Set aside. Heat oil in large skillet. Add rice and fry over medium heat, stirring constantly until rice is browned. Add chicken bouillon and chicken mixture. Cover and simmer 15 minutes or until liquid is absorbed.

(May add any of the following: diced onions, celery, broccoli, carrots, or pea pods. Simmer and stir another 5 minutes.)

   no. of servings: 4   *serving size: about 1 cup*

Content per Serving

total fat ..... 15.8 gm   cholesterol ....31 mg   carbohydrate ...38 gm
saturated fat .. 1.5 gm   calories 372   protein ....17 gm

This recipe was submitted by Barbara Alexander.

Chicken Nuggets

1½ pounds boneless, skinless   dash McCormick Lemon and
   chicken breasts, cubed   Pepper
¼ cup flour   3 tablespoons vegetable oil

Instructions

Roll chicken in flour and sprinkle with McCormick Lemon and Pepper. Fry in skillet in oil until brown.

   no. of servings: 5   *serving size:1 cup*

Content per Serving

total fat ..... 11.8 gm   cholesterol ....85 mg   carbohydrate .... 4 gm
saturated fat .. 1.5 gm   calories 260   protein ....32 gm

Chicken Tetrazzini

1 cup onion, chopped   dash pepper
½ cup green pepper, chopped   1 chicken bouillon cube
¼ cup celery, chopped   2 cups diced, cooked chicken
¼ cup margarine   2 cups cooked spaghetti
¼ cup fine, dry, seasoned bread   1½ cups cooked French green
   crumbs   beans
¼ cup grated parmesan cheese   1 2½-ounce jar whole button
¼ cup unsifted flour   mushrooms, drained
dash salt   1 tablespoon diced pimiento

Instructions

Preheat oven to 400 degrees. In a large skillet, sauté onion, green pepper, and celery in 2 tablespoons margarine, until tender. Remove vegetables, blend bread crumbs and cheese into margarine in saucepan, then remove from saucepan and set aside. Melt remaining margarine in skillet. Blend in flour, salt, and pepper. Gradually stir in skim milk. Add bouillon cube and sautéed vegetables. Cook over medium heat, stirring until mixture comes to a boil. Stir in cooked chicken, spaghetti, green beans, and pimiento. Pour into 2-quart casserole. Sprinkle with reserved cheese and bread crumbs mixture. Bake 30 minutes.

no. of servings: 6   *serving size:* ⅙ *of casserole*

Content per Serving

total fat ..... 11.5 gm   cholesterol ....46 mg   carbohydrate ... 32 gm
saturated fat .. 2.8 gm   calories 332   protein .... 25 gm

This recipe was submitted by Elena Harman. Source: Sensible Eating Can Be Fun, presented by the makers of Fleischmann's Margarine and Egg Beaters Low-Cholesterol Egg Substitute.

Chicken with Peppers in Peking Sauce

4½ ounces boneless, skinless   1 teaspoon cornstarch
    chicken breast meat cut in   1 ounce water
    strips   1 medium green pepper, cut in
 1 tablespoon soy sauce   strips
 1 teaspoon gin   ½ large onion, cut in strips
 1 tablespoon Hoi Lein sauce   6 ounces water

Instructions

Marinate chicken in mixture of soy sauce and gin for 30 minutes. Combine Hoi Lein sauce, cornstarch, and 1 ounce water; reserve. In wok, bring 6 ounces water to boil and add chicken, pepper, and onion. Cover and cook for 3 minutes. Add reserved Hoi Lein sauce. Cook and stir until sauce is thickened and all ingredients are well glazed with the sauce.

no. of servings: 1

Content per Serving

total fat ...... 3.9 gm   cholesterol ....82 mg   carbohydrate ... 14 gm
saturated fat .. 1.1 gm   calories 247   protein .... 35 gm

Source: The Low Calorie Chinese Gourmet Cookbook, *James Leang.*

Crab and Vegetables

 1 16-ounce package of mixed   4 tablespoons Kikkoman Lite
    vegetables (broccoli, carrots,   Soy Sauce (or any soy sauce)
    and water chestnuts)   ½ teaspoon garlic powder
 8 imitation crabmeat sticks, cut   ¼ teaspoon pepper
    in bite-sized pieces   ¼ cup white wine

Instructions

Defrost and cook vegetables according to package instruction, using a covered saucepan. Add crab pieces when vegetables are almost finished. Add spices and wine and stir occasionally until vegetables are cooked to desired softness.

no. of servings: 3   *serving size: about* 1½ *cups*

Content per Serving

total fat ...... 9.7 gm   cholesterol ....42 mg   carbohydrate ...15 gm
saturated fat .. 0.1 gm   calories 140   protein ....18 gm

This recipe was submitted by Nathan Kantor.

Eggplant Parmesan

1 medium eggplant (about 1 pound)
2 medium tomatoes, chopped
1 6-ounce can low-sodium vegetable juice (⅔ cup)
½ cup Quaker Oat Bran cereal, uncooked
¼ teaspoon oregano leaves, crushed
2 cloves garlic, minced
½ cup part-skim mozzarella cheese, shredded
2 tablespoons parmesan cheese

Instructions

Preheat oven to 350 degrees. Peel eggplant, cut into ½-inch slices. Layer in 1½-quart casserole dish sprayed with vegetable oil spray. Top with tomatoes. In a small bowl, combine remaining ingredients except cheese. Spread over vegetables. Sprinkle evenly with mozzarella cheese, then parmesan cheese. Bake 35 to 40 minutes.

no. of servings: 4   *serving size: 1 cup*

Content per Serving

total fat ...... 4.5 gm   cholesterol ....11 mg   carbohydrate ...20 gm
saturated fat .. 2.2 gm   calories 148   protein ....9 gm

This recipe comes from the Quaker Oats Company.

Fish and Vegetables

2 tablespoons vegetable oil
½ cup chopped onion
⅔ cup celery, cut in 1-inch matchsticks
⅔ cup carrots, cut in 1-inch matchsticks
⅔ cup zucchini, cut in 1-inch matchsticks
3 cups diced tomatoes
1 cup water
1 teaspoon basil leaves, crushed
½ teaspoon garlic powder
½ teaspoon salt
dash pepper
4 fish fillets (4 ounces each)

Instructions

In large skillet, heat oil and sauté onion for 2 minutes. Add celery, carrots, and zucchini, and sauté 1 minute. Add tomatoes, water, basil, garlic powder, salt, and pepper. Simmer 2 minutes more. Arrange fish fillets on top of vegetables. Cover and simmer 3 minutes.

no. of servings: 4   *serving size: 1 fillet and 1 cup vegetables*

Content per Serving

total fat ...... 7.7 gm	cholesterol .... 63 mg	carbohydrate .... 6 gm
saturated fat .. 0.6 gm	calories 184	protein .... 22 gm

This recipe was submitted by Stella Figinski.

Grilled Tuna Steak with Dill Sauce

DILL SAUCE

2 tablespoons nonfat plain
    yogurt
1 tablespoon light mayonnaise

dash tabasco sauce
¼ teaspoon dill weed

Instructions
  Combine all ingredients and refrigerate.

no. of servings: 2   *serving size: 1½ tablespoons*

Content per Serving

total fat ...... 2.0 gm	cholesterol ..... 3 mg	carbohydrate .... 2 gm
saturated fat .. 0.0 gm	calories 28	protein .... 1 gm

GRILLED TUNA STEAK

¼ cup diet Italian dressing

2 tuna steaks (about 4 ounces
    each)

Instructions
  Place salad dressing in a bowl and dip the raw tuna steaks in it. Turn to coat entire steak with dressing. Place tuna steaks under a hot broiler, allowing 2 minutes per side. Remove from broiler and place in a microwave-type dish. Cover with plastic wrap and cook in microwave on high level 4 to 5 minutes.

no. of servings: 2   *serving size: 1 steak*

Content per Serving

total fat ...... 4.6 gm	cholesterol .... 32 mg	carbohydrate .... 1 gm
saturated fat .. 0.4 gm	calories 141	protein .... 24 gm

This recipe was submitted by Roger Hartmuller III.

Healthy Coq au Vin

2½ pounds boneless, skinless
    chicken breast, diced
2 tablespoons onions, chopped
2 tablespoons vegetable oil
8 small onions
4 carrots, chopped
3 stalks celery, chopped

4 potatoes, quartered
1 clove garlic
1 3-ounce can mushrooms
3 to 4 sprigs parsley
¼ teaspoon thyme
2 cups red burgundy wine
1 tablespoon cornstarch

Instructions

Preheat oven to 350 degrees. In a large skillet, brown chicken and chopped onions in oil. Add whole onions, carrots, celery, potatoes, and garlic. Cook 3 minutes. Add mushrooms, parsley, and thyme. Arrange in a 2-quart casserole dish. Add wine. Cover and cook 2 hours; stir occasionally. Thicken with cornstarch and water at end of 2 hours.

no. of servings: 6   serving size: 1/6 of recipe

Content per Serving

total fat ..... 10.3 gm	cholesterol ...126 mg	carbohydrate ...29 gm
saturated fat .. 1.9 gm	calories 413	protein ....49 gm

This recipe was submitted by Sarah Nesbitt.

Lemon Herb Chicken

1 pound chicken breasts, boned, skinned, and chopped
2 tablespoons flour
¼ tablespoon salt
dash pepper

2 tablespoons margarine
½ cup chicken broth
1 tablespoon lemon juice
¼ teaspoon basil leaves, crushed

Instructions

Toss chicken pieces around in a plastic bag containing flour, salt, and pepper. In a skillet, brown chicken in margarine. Add all remaining ingredients. Cover and simmer 10 minutes or until tender. Serve with brown rice and mushrooms.

no. of servings: 4   serving size: about ⅔ cup

Content per Serving

total fat ...... 9.0 gm	cholesterol ....73 mg	carbohydrate .... 3 gm
saturated fat .. 1.9 gm	calories 212	protein ....28 gm

This recipe was submitted by Donna Askin.

Meatless Bean and Corn Stew

1 8-ounce box frozen cooked squash (butternut)
2 16-ounce cans plain pinto beans (pink)
1 16-ounce can corn

1 medium onion, chopped
2 cloves garlic, chopped
1 teaspoon cumin
Tabasco or cayenne to taste
dash salt (optional)

Instructions

Thaw the squash. Drain liquid from pinto beans and rinse: pour into saucepan and add the can of corn without draining liquid. Add the onions and garlic. Cook about 10 minutes. Add the squash and the spices. Cook 20 minutes at low temperature until onions are soft, stirring often. Add water if needed.

no. of servings: 8   *serving size: 1 cup*

Content per Serving

total fat ...... 1.0 gm   cholesterol .....0 mg   carbohydrate ...47 gm
saturated fat .. 0.1 gm   calories 234   protein .... 12 gm

This recipe was submitted by Silvia and Simon Grinspun.

Pasta and Cottage Cheese

1 cup shell or rotini pasta, raw   ½ cup low-fat cottage cheese
(or ½ cup elbow macaroni)   (1% fat)

Instructions

Cook pasta following directions on box. Combine cooked pasta with cottage cheese and stir gently.

no. of servings: 1

Content per Serving

total fat ...... 3.1 gm   cholesterol .....5 mg   carbohydrate ...81 gm
saturated fat .. 0.7 gm   calories 462   protein .... 28 gm

This recipe was submitted by Judith Katz.

Pasta with Cottage Cheese and Spinach Sauce

1 pound penne or other short   4 tablespoons margarine
  tubular macaroni   2 or 3 pinches salt
2 10-ounce packages of frozen   1 cup low-fat cottage cheese (1%
  leaf spinach, thawed   fat)

Instructions

Cook pasta following directions on box, and drain. Sauté spinach in skillet in melted margarine and salt for 2 minutes. Pour over pasta. Mix in the cottage cheese. Serve at once.

no. of servings: 6   *serving size: 2 cups*

Content per Serving

total fat ...... 9.4 gm   cholesterol .....2 mg   carbohydrate ...58 gm
saturated fat .. 1.6 gm   calories 374   protein .... 17 gm

Pita Pizza

1 large pita   ½ red pepper, chopped
5 tablespoons tomato sauce   dash basil
½ green pepper, chopped   1 onion, chopped

optional: 1 plum tomato, sliced   1 tablespoon grated parmesan
    thin   cheese

Instructions

Toast pita in toaster oven at low heat. Put warm pita on aluminum foil.
Spread tomato sauce on pita. Place vegetables on top. Top with some additional sauce, basil, and grated cheese. Bake in toaster oven on high temperature for 4 minutes.

number of servings: 1

Content per Serving

total fat ...... 3.6 gm	cholesterol ..... 5 mg	carbohydrate ... 50 gm
saturated fat .. 1.3 gm	calories 272	protein .... 12 gm

This recipe was submitted by Sandra Margulies.

Rice Balls

    1 pound lean ground beef   1 medium onion, chopped
      (10% fat)   ½ teaspoon salt
    ½ cup white rice, uncooked   ½ teaspoon pepper
    1 green pepper, chopped   1 quart canned tomatoes, diced

Instructions

Preheat oven to 350 degrees. Combine all ingredients except tomatoes and
shape into balls. Put in dutch oven. Pour tomatoes over top, cover. Bake 2
hours. If too dry, add tomato sauce for more juice.

no. of servings: 4   *serving size: ¼ of recipe*

Content per Serving

total fat ..... 14.8 gm	cholesterol ....71 mg	carbohydrate ... 32 gm
saturated fat .. 5.6 gm	calories 362	protein .... 26 gm

This recipe was submitted by Mary Van Horn.

Roast Chicken with Rice and Mushroom Stuffing

    1 cup uncooked rice   dash curry powder
    ¼ teaspoon poultry seasoning   1 5-pound roasting chicken
    ¼ cup margarine   ¼ teaspoon basil leaves, crushed
    ¼ cup green pepper, diced   dash pepper
    ½ cup onion, diced   ½ teaspoon thyme
    ½ cup celery, diced   ¼ teaspoon paprika
    1 4-ounce jar sliced mushrooms

Instructions

Preheat oven to 325 degrees. Prepare rice following directions on box, substituting poultry seasoning for salt. Set aside. In a skillet, melt margarine.

Sauté green pepper, onion, celery, and mushrooms. Sprinkle with curry powder. Combine and mix with rice.

Sprinkle inside of roasting chicken with basil. Fill chicken cavity with rice mixture. Rub chicken with small amount of margarine. Sprinkle with pepper, thyme, and paprika. Bake 1 hour and 40 minutes (or 20 minutes per pound). Carve, remove skin, and serve.

no. of servings: 8   *serving size: about 5 ounces*
chicken and ⅔ cup stuffing

Content per Serving

total fat ..... 10.9 gm	cholesterol ... 120 mg	carbohydrate ... 21 gm
saturated fat .. 2.4 gm	calories 377	protein .... 46 gm

This recipe was submitted by Margaret Filliaux.

Sante Fe Chicken

1 pound chicken breasts, boned and skinned	1 clove garlic, minced
¼ cup orange juice	½ teaspoon cinnamon
2 tablespoons dry white wine	¼ teaspoon chili powder
1 tablespoon honey	dash ground red pepper

Instructions

Preheat oven to 375 degrees. In a shallow baking pan, arrange chicken in a single layer. In a small bowl, combine remaining ingredients. Pour over chicken. Cover and refrigerate 1 hour. Bake chicken, uncovered, about 45 minutes. Baste occasionally.

no. of servings: 4   *serving size: ¼ of recipe*

Content per Serving

total fat ...... 3.0 gm	cholesterol .... 69 mg	carbohydrate .... 7 gm
saturated fat .. 0.8 gm	calories 163	protein .... 26 gm

This recipe was submitted by Myrna Brams.

Shrimp and Vegetable Pasta

1 small head broccoli, in flowerets	1 medium zucchini, sliced thin
1 large carrot, sliced thin	1 medium onion, chopped
3 cloves garlic	¾ pound cooked small shrimp
2 tablespoons margarine	8 ounces linguine, raw
	½ cup grated parmesan cheese

Instructions

Steam broccoli and carrots until crisp-tender. Set aside. Sauté garlic in margarine. Add zucchini and onions; sauté 2–3 minutes. Add shrimp; heat through. Boil linguine in water just until al dente (8–9 minutes). Serve vegetable mixture over linguine. Top with cheese.

no. of servings: 4   *serving size: 1 cup*

Content per Serving

total fat ..... 11.9 gm	cholesterol ...138 mg	carbohydrate ...47 gm
saturated fat .. 3.7 gm	calories 429	protein ....35 gm

This recipe was submitted by Anna Hare.

Spaghetti with Turkey Tomato Sauce

2 cups onion, chopped	2 cups water
dash garlic powder	1 bay leaf
1 pound ground turkey	dash salt and pepper
3 tablespoons oil	½ teaspoon oregano
3½ cups canned tomatoes	½ teaspoon basil
2 6-ounce cans tomato paste	15 ounces spaghetti
1 12-ounce can tomato sauce	

Instructions

In skillet, sauté onion, garlic powder, and turkey in oil until brown. Add remaining ingredients (except spaghetti) and simmer for 2 hours or until thick. Remove bay leaf. Serve over cooked spaghetti.

no. of servings: 10   *serving size: 1 cup spaghetti with*
                                       ¹⁄₁₀ of sauce

Content per Serving

total fat ...... 7.2 gm	cholesterol ....26 mg	carbohydrate ...49 gm
saturated fat .. 0.9 gm	calories 330	protein ....19 gm

This recipe was submitted by Debbie Keitt.

Spinach Cheese Pie

1 package chopped frozen spinach, cooked and well drained*	1 pound low-fat cottage cheese (1% fat)
¾ cup Egg Beaters (equivalent to 3 eggs)	4 ounces shredded low-fat cheese or tofu
	¼ cup minced onion
	dash nutmeg

*may use broccoli or zucchini

Instructions

Preheat oven to 375 degrees. In a bowl, combine all ingredients. Mix gently. Transfer to 9-inch pie plate. Bake 1 hour or until browned on top and knife inserted in center comes out clean.

no. of servings: 6   *serving size: ¹⁄₆ of pie*

Content per Serving

total fat ...... 4.0 gm	cholesterol ....14 mg	carbohydrate ....7 gm
saturated fat .. 2.4 gm	calories 137	protein .... 19 gm

This recipe was submitted by Myrna Brams.

Stir Fry Chicken

2 pounds boneless, skinless
chicken breast, cut in thin
strips
1 to 2 cloves garlic
2 tablespoons vegetable oil

½ cup each chopped onion,
carrots, broccoli, and cabbage
¼ cup chicken broth
2 to 3 tablespoons soy sauce

Instructions

In a large Teflon fry pan, sauté chicken and garlic in oil. Add onion, carrots, broccoli, cabbage, chicken broth, and soy sauce. Cover and cook until vegetables are tender-crisp, stirring occasionally.

no. of servings: 6   *serving size: 1 cup*

Content per Serving

total fat ...... 8.7 gm	cholesterol ....97 mg	carbohydrate ....4 gm
saturated fat .. 1.5 gm	calories 250	protein .... 37 gm

This recipe was submitted by Ruth Lovell.

Sweet and Sour Mini Kabobs

1 20-ounce can pineapple
chunks in heavy syrup,
drained (reserve syrup)
1 pound chicken breasts, boned,
skinned, and cut into 1-inch
pieces

2 medium green peppers, cut
into 1-inch chunks
1 envelope tomato-onion soup
mix
¼ cup water
2 tablespoons vinegar

Instructions

Preheat oven to 350 degrees. On wooden toothpicks, alternately thread pineapple, chicken, and green pepper. Place kabobs in shallow baking pan and bake 20 minutes or until chicken is tender.

Meanwhile, in medium saucepan, blend tomato-onion soup mix, reserved syrup, water, and vinegar. Bring to a boil, then simmer, stirring constantly, until sauce is thickened (about 5 minutes). Serve with kabobs.

no. of servings: 48 kabobs   *serving size: 1 kabob*

Content per Serving

total fat ...... 0.3 gm	cholesterol .....6 mg	carbohydrate ....2 gm
saturated fat .. 0.1 gm	calories 21	protein .... 2 gm

This recipe was submitted by Carol Hodrick.

Sweet and Sour Turkey Meatballs

2 egg whites
1¼ pounds ground turkey
3 tablespoons fine, dry bread crumbs
1 teaspoon onion powder
1 tablespoon vegetable oil
1 16-ounce can crushed pineapple

¼ cup firmly packed brown sugar
¼ cup vinegar
2 tablespoons low-sodium soy sauce
1 large green pepper, cut into ¼-inch strips
2 tablespoons cornstarch
2 tablespoons water

Instructions

In a large bowl, beat egg whites slightly. Add turkey, bread crumbs, and onion powder. Mix well. Form into 24 meatballs. Heat oil in large skillet. Cook meatballs in skillet over medium-high heat until brown. Drain oil.

Drain pineapple, reserving juice. Set aside pineapple. Add enough water to reserved juice to make 1 cup liquid. In a bowl, combine juice/water mixture, brown sugar, vinegar, and soy sauce. Mix and pour over meatballs in skillet.

Heat to boiling. Reduce heat, cover, and simmer 20 minutes, stirring occasionally. Stir in pineapple and green peppers. Cover and simmer 10 minutes. In a cup, mix cornstarch and water. Stir into skillet. Simmer 5 minutes more, stirring constantly until sauce is thickened and clear. Serve over rice.

no. of servings: 6   serving size: 4 meatballs and
                                           ⅙ of sauce

Content per Serving

total fat ...... 6.1 gm	cholesterol ....54 mg	carbohydrate ...26 gm
saturated fat .. 1.3 gm	calories 250	protein ....23 gm

This recipe was submitted by Elena Harman. Source: The Turkey Store Cookbook.

Sweet and Sour Vegetables with Tofu

1 pound tofu cakes
6 tablespoons distilled white vinegar
¼ cup firmly backed brown sugar or honey
¼ cup tomato paste or catsup
3 tablespoons tamari soy sauce
1½ teaspoons fresh ginger root, grated
3 tablespoons vegetable oil
3 cups onions, thinly sliced
2 medium carrots, peeled and diagonally sliced ¼ inch thick

1 tablespoon fresh ginger root, grated
½ pound green beans, cut in 3-inch pieces
1 large sweet red or green pepper, sliced lengthwise
4 cups mushrooms, sliced
4 cups thinly sliced zucchini rounds (1¼ pounds)
¾ cup fresh or drained canned pineapple chunks

1 tablespoon cornstarch
dissolved in ½ cup pineapple
juice, vegetable stock, or water

2 green onions, thinly sliced

Instructions

Prepare tofu (see note below). In a small bowl, stir together vinegar, brown sugar, tomato paste, soy sauce, and ginger root. Set aside. Heat oil in wok. Add onion and stir-fry over medium-high heat until translucent. Add carrots and ginger root and continue cooking, stirring, for 3 to 4 minutes. Add green beans and cook 2 minutes longer. Add peppers and cook 2 more minutes. Stir in mushrooms and zucchini.

Reduce heat to medium-low. Cover wok and cook, stirring occasionally, until vegetables are tender-crisp, about 7 minutes. Stir in pineapple chunks, tofu, tomato paste mixture, and dissolved cornstarch. Bring to boiling. Lower heat and simmer, stirring gently, for 3 to 4 minutes or until thickened slightly. Top with sliced green onions. This recipe is good served over rice or noodles.

Note: To press tofu, place cakes between 2 flat plates or baking sheets. Weight top with bowl of water, stack of plates, or heavy can. The sides of the cakes of tofu should bulge a little, but not split. Let stand for at least 30 minutes; remove cakes and discard water.

no. of servings: 6   *serving size: ⅙ of recipe*

Content per Serving

total fat ..... 11.0 gm	cholesterol ..... 0 gm	carbohydrate ... 39 gm
saturated fat .. 0.6 gm	calories 275	protein .... 11 gm

This recipe was submitted by Carol Hodrick. Source: Family Circle.

Tamari-Ginger Fish

½ cup tamari
½ cup water
1 tablespoon dry sherry
1 tablespoon grated fresh ginger
½ cup scallions, minced

1 small clove garlic, crushed
2 teaspoons sesame oil
2 teaspoons dark vinegar
2 teaspoons sugar
1 white fish fillet (4 ounces)

Instructions

Preheat oven to 350 degrees. Combine all ingredients in shallow dish. Marinate fish several hours. Bake 10–20 minutes until fish flakes easily with a fork.

no. of servings: 1

Content per Serving

total fat ..... 10.4 gm	cholesterol ..... 63 gm	carbohydrate ... 27 gm
saturated fat .. 1.5 gm	calories 329	protein .... 34 gm

This recipe was submitted by Donna Askin.

Tofu-Vegetable Quiche

1 unbaked 9-inch pastry shell
1 pound soft tofu
¾ cup Egg Beaters
1 teaspoon seasoned salt
¼ teaspoon ground nutmeg
⅛ teaspoon pepper

1 10-ounce package frozen chopped broccoli or spinach
1 medium onion, minced
1 cup shredded part-skim mozzarella cheese (4 ounces)

Instructions

Preheat oven to 450 degrees. Bake pastry shell 10 minutes. Reduce oven temperature to 350 degrees. Put tofu, Egg Beaters, seasoned salt, nutmeg, and pepper in food processor or blender and process until smooth (if using blender, add tofu a quarter at a time, blending after each addition).

Steam frozen vegetables just until thawed. Drain well. Add to tofu mixture with onion and mix well. Stir in ½ cup cheese. Turn into pie shell and sprinkle with remaining ½ cup cheese. Bake 45 minutes or until firm.

no. of servings: 8　　　　　*serving size: ⅛ of quiche*

Content per Serving

total fat . . . . . 10.9 gm	cholesterol . . . . . 8 mg	carbohydrate . . . 14 gm
saturated fat . . 3.0 gm	calories 202	protein . . . . 13 gm

This recipe was submitted by Cecelia Justin. Source: Woman's Day.

Turkey Chili

1 pound ground turkey
1 onion, chopped
1 16-ounce can whole tomatoes
2 to 4 tablespoons chili powder
1 teaspoon sugar

1 16-ounce can kidney beans, drained
½ teaspoon ground pepper
½ teaspoon red pepper sauce (*optional*)

Instructions

Brown ground turkey and onion in large skillet sprayed with vegetable oil spray. Drain. Add remaining ingredients. Simmer about 45 minutes, stirring often.

no. of servings: 5　　　　　*serving size: ⅕ of chili*

Content per Serving

total fat . . . . . . 3.9 gm	cholesterol . . . . 52 mg	carbohydrate . . . 17 gm
saturated fat . . 1.2 gm	calories 202	protein . . . . 25 gm

This recipe was submitted by Shana Hughes.

Turkey Loaf with Cranberry-Orange Sauce

TURKEY LOAF

1½ pounds uncooked ground turkey

1¼ cups Quaker Oat Bran cereal, uncooked

½ cup onion, minced

¼ cup Egg Beaters (equivalent to 1 egg)

1 teaspoon poultry seasoning

Instructions

Preheat oven to 350 degrees. In a large bowl, combine all ingredients. Mix well. Pat into 9 × 5-inch loaf pan sprayed with vegetable oil spray. Bake 50 to 55 minutes. Let stand 5 minutes before slicing. Serve with cranberry-orange sauce (see below).

no. of servings: 8   *serving size: one 1⅛-inch slice*

Content per Serving

total fat ...... 4.2 gm   cholesterol ....49 mg   carbohydrate .... 9 gm

saturated fat .. 1.2 gm   calories 170   protein ....23 gm

CRANBERRY-ORANGE SAUCE

2 cups fresh or frozen cranberries (½ pound)

1¼ cups orange juice

1 tablespoon Quaker Oat Bran cereal, uncooked

1 teaspoon sugar

Instructions

In medium saucepan, combine all ingredients. Bring to a boil over medium heat. Boil 6–7 minutes or until cranberries pop and sauce is thickened. Chill.

no. of servings: 8   *serving size: 2⅔ tablespoons*

Content per Serving

total fat ...... 0.1 gm   cholesterol .....0 mg   carbohydrate .... 8 gm

saturated fat .. 0.0 gm   calories 33   protein .... 1 gm

This recipe comes from the Quaker Oats Company.

Rice and Vegetables

Carrot Bake

1 pound carrots, shredded

¾ cup Quaker Oat Bran cereal, uncooked

¼ cup egg substitute (equivalent to 1 egg)

¼ cup water

2 tablespoons snipped fresh or
frozen chives

2 tablespoons chopped nuts
⅛ teaspoon nutmeg

Instructions

Preheat oven to 350 degrees. In large bowl, combine all ingredients. Pour into 1-quart casserole or baking dish sprayed with vegetable oil spray. Bake 40 minutes.

no. of servings: 8   *serving size: ½ cup*

Content per Serving

total fat ...... 1.8 gm	cholesterol ..... 0 mg	carbohydrate ... 11 gm
saturated fat .. 0.2 gm	calories 70	protein .... 4 gm

This recipe comes from the Quaker Oats Company.

Nutted Wild Rice

1 cup wild rice
5½ cups water
¼ cup pecan halves
1 cup yellow raisins
1 grated orange rind
¼ cup chopped mint

4 green onions, diced
2 tablespoons vegetable oil
⅓ cup fresh orange juice
1½ teaspoons salt
dash pepper

Instructions

Wash rice thoroughly. Place rice and water in medium saucepan. Bring to boil and simmer uncovered for 45 minutes. Rice should not be too soft. Drain and transfer rice to bowl. Add remaining ingredients and toss gently. Let stand for 2 hours. Serve at room temperature.

number of servings: 6   *serving size: about ⅔ cup*

Content per Serving

total fat ...... 7.9 gm	cholesterol ..... 0 mg	carbohydrate ... 47 gm
saturated fat .. 0.6 gm	calories 263	protein .... 3 gm

Potato Skins

4 large (preferably long) potatoes
1 tablespoon vegetable oil

salt, pepper, paprika to taste

Instructions

Preheat oven to 450 degrees. Scrub potatoes. Cut them lengthwise into 6 wedges (like pickle spears). Dry the cut sides; put them in a large bowl and toss with oil and seasonings. Spread on baking sheet and bake for 20–30 minutes.

no. of servings: 4   *serving size: 1 potato*

Content per Serving

total fat ...... 3.6 gm	cholesterol .....o mg	carbohydrate ...51 gm
saturated fat .. 0.3 gm	calories 251	protein .... 5 gm

This recipe was submitted by Judith Katz. Source: Eater's Choice, Ron and Nancy Goor.

Pickled Beets

1 1-pound can sliced beets	1 teaspoon whole cloves
½ cup vinegar	1 stick cinnamon
½ cup sugar	1 small bay leaf
¼ teaspoon salt	

Instructions
Drain beets. Mix vinegar, sugar, salt, cloves, cinnamon, and bay leaf, and heat to dissolve sugar. Add beets to the liquid. Heat to just boiling and re-move from heat. Refrigerate. Serve chilled.

no. of servings: 5   *serving size: ½ cup*

Content per Serving

total fat ...... 0.4 gm	cholesterol .....o mg	carbohydrate ...27 gm
saturated fat .. 0.1 gm	calories 105	protein .... 1 gm

This recipe was submitted by Janet Johansen.

Sherried Mushrooms

12 ounces raw mushrooms, sliced	½ average raw onion, sliced
½ cup cooking sherry	

Instructions
In a nonstick fry pan, combine cooking sherry, onion, and mushrooms. Cover and cook on medium heat for 5–8 minutes. Serve as a side dish with lean meat or chicken.

no. of servings: 4   *serving size: ¾ cup*

Content per Serving

total fat ...... 0.5 gm	cholesterol .....o mg	carbohydrate .... 7 gm
saturated fat .. 0.1 gm	calories 43	protein .... 2 gm

This recipe was submitted by Roger Hartmuller III.

Spicy Brown Rice

2 cups defatted chicken broth	3 to 4 shakes Tabasco sauce
1 cup brown rice	1 teaspoon lemon juice
1 to 2 bay leaves	1 tomato, peeled and chopped

Instructions

In a pot bring chicken broth to a boil. Add all ingredients except tomato. Lower heat and simmer approximately 45 to 60 minutes or until chicken broth is absorbed. Remove from heat. Stir in tomato and re-cover. Let cool slightly and serve.

no. of servings: 6   *serving size: ½ cup*

Content per Serving

total fat ...... 1.1 gm	cholesterol ..... 0 mg	carbohydrate ...26 gm
saturated fat .. 0.1 gm	calories 134	protein .... 4 gm

---

Spinach Sauté

2 10-ounce packages frozen chopped spinach	⅓ cup Quaker Oat Bran cereal, uncooked
1 tablespoon margarine	¼ teaspoon salt
2 cloves garlic	¼ teaspoon nutmeg
½ cup skim milk	⅛ teaspoon lemon pepper

Instructions

Thaw spinach, reserving liquid. In medium saucepan, melt margarine. Sauté garlic 1 to 2 minutes. Add milk and oat bran cereal; stir 1 to 2 minutes or until thickened. Add spinach, reserved liquid, salt, nutmeg, and lemon pepper. Simmer about 10 minutes or until heated through.

no. of servings: 6   *serving size: ½ cup*

Content per Serving

total fat ...... 2.4 gm	cholesterol ..... 0 mg	carbohydrate .... 9 gm
saturated fat .. 0.4 gm	calories 69	protein .... 5 gm

This recipe comes from the Quaker Oats Company.

Stuffed Tomato Halves

1 medium green pepper, chopped (about ¾ cup)	¼ to ½ teaspoon basil leaves, crushed
4 large tomatoes (about 2 pounds)	¼ to ½ teaspoon oregano leaves, crushed
3 to 4 green onions, sliced	2 tablespoons chopped fresh parsley or 1 tablespoon dried parsley flakes
⅓ cup Quaker Oat Bran cereal, uncooked	
¼ cup Egg Beaters (equivalent to 1 egg)	

Instructions

Preheat oven to 350 degrees. In a small saucepan, simmer green pepper in a small amount of water 2 to 3 minutes. Drain and reserve. Slice each tomato in half crosswise. Scoop out pulp; drain tomato halves upside down.

Chop pulp; place in large bowl. Add green pepper and remaining ingredients except parsley. Place tomato halves cut side up in 13½ × 8¾-inch baking dish. Fill each half with about ⅓ cup stuffing mixture. Sprinkle parsley over top. Bake 30 minutes.

no. of servings: 8   *serving size: 1 tomato half*

Content per Serving

total fat ...... 0.4 gm   cholesterol .....0 mg   carbohydrate .... 6 gm
saturated fat .. 0.1 gm   calories 34   protein .... 2 gm

This recipe comes from the Quaker Oats Company.

Zucchini Casserole

3 cups shredded zucchini
1 tablespoon vegetable oil
½ cup chopped onion
1¼ cups Quaker Oat Bran cereal, uncooked
½ cup shredded part-skim mozzarella cheese
¼ cup Egg Beaters (equivalent to 1 egg)
½ teaspoon basil or oregano leaves, crushed
½ teaspoon salt
⅛ teaspoon pepper
⅓ cup tomato sauce

Instructions

Preheat oven to 375 degrees. Squeeze zucchini between paper towels to remove excess moisture. In a small skillet, heat oil; sauté onion until tender. Transfer to a large bowl. Add zucchini and remaining ingredients except tomato sauce. Mix well. Pour into 8 × 8-inch baking dish sprayed with vegetable oil spray. Spread tomato sauce evenly over top. Bake 30 minutes.

no. of servings: 8   *serving size: ⅓ cup*

Content per Serving

total fat ...... 3.3 gm   cholesterol .....2 mg   carbohydrate ... 11 gm
saturated fat .. 0.6 gm   calories 91   protein .... 5 gm

This recipe comes from the Quaker Oats Company.

Salads

Broccoli Salad

Salad:

- 1 bunch broccoli, broken into bite-sized pieces
- 1 to 2 cups bean sprouts
- 1 tin water chestnuts, drained
- 1 cup mushrooms, sliced

Dressing:

- ¼ cup soy sauce
- ¼ cup vegetable oil
- 1 teaspoon sesame seeds
- 2 tablespoons honey
- 1 pinch ginger

Instructions

In a bowl, combine broccoli, sprouts, water chestnuts, and mushrooms. In small bowl, combine and mix all ingredients for dressing. Pour dressing over vegetables and marinate overnight.

no. of servings: 8   *serving size: ⅛ of recipe*

Content per Serving

total fat ...... 7.3 gm	cholesterol ..... 0 mg	carbohydrate ... 11 gm
saturated fat .. 0.5 gm	calories 116	protein .... 4 gm

This recipe was submitted by Sherie and Sam Libber.

Cold Pasta Salad Vinaigrette

- ½ pound pasta (use medium shells, rotini, or fusili or other similar-sized pasta)
- 2 to 3 cups broccoli, flowers and stems, sliced (or combination of broccoli and cauliflower)
- ½ cup celery, sliced
- 1 cup mushrooms, sliced
- ½ cup matchstick carrots
- 1 cup onions, coarsely sliced
- 1 cup green peppers, sliced
- ½ cup peeled seeded cucumbers, sliced
- ½ cup seeded tomatoes, sliced
- ½ cup chickpeas, cooked
- ¼ cup Greek olives
- 3 to 4 tablespoons oil
- 3 to 4 tablespoons balsamic vinegar (or red wine vinegar)
- salt, pepper, and herbs to taste

Instructions

Cook pasta, toss with 1 teaspoon vegetable oil. In a steamer, steam broccoli, celery, mushrooms, carrots, onions, and peppers for 3–5 minutes until tender-crisp. (Steam the vegetables separately, for more control over the "crunch.") Toss all the ingredients together gently; add salt and pepper to taste. Herbs that go well are basil and oregano. Refrigerate 1 hour and serve.

no. of servings: 12   *serving size: 1 cup*

Content per Serving

total fat ...... 4.4 gm	cholesterol .....0 mg	carbohydrate ... 18 gm
saturated fat .. 0.3 gm	calories 118	protein .... 4 gm

This recipe was submitted by Judith Katz.

Corn Salad

2 16-ounce cans of corn (white, yellow, or shoestring), drained
6 hard-boiled eggs without the yolks, chopped

4 to 6 spring onions, chopped
2 tablespoons light mayonnaise
juice of 1 lemon

Instructions
Mix all ingredients together. Chill.

no. of servings: 6   *serving size: 1 cup*

Content per Serving

total fat ...... 2.5 gm	cholesterol .....2 mg	carbohydrate ... 22 gm
saturated fat .. 0.2 gm	calories 122	protein .... 6 gm

This recipe was submitted by Silvia and Simon Grinspun.

Cranberry Salad

1 3-ounce package Raspberry Jello
⅛ teaspoon salt
⅛ teaspoon cinnamon
dash of powdered cloves
¾ cup boiling water

1 8-ounce can whole cranberry sauce
1 tablespoon grated orange rind
1 medium-tart apple, finely chopped
⅓ cup walnuts, chopped

Instructions
Dissolve Jello, salt, cinnamon, and cloves in boiling water. Add cranberry sauce and orange rind. Chill until thickened. Fold in apple and nuts. Pour into 3-cup mold. Refrigerate 3 hours until firm.

no. of servings: 5   *serving size: ⅔ cup*

Content per Serving

total fat ...... 5.0 gm	cholesterol .....0 mg	carbohydrate ... 68 gm
saturated fat .. 0.3 gm	calories 311	protein .... 4 gm

This recipe was submitted by Mollie Tussing.

Cucumber-Radish Salad

½ cup nonfat plain yogurt
2 tablespoons vegetable oil

2 tablespoons fresh parsley, chopped

1 tablespoon white wine vinegar
½ teaspoon dry mustard
2 cups cucumber, thinly sliced

1 cup radishes, thinly sliced
¼ cup green onions, thinly sliced

Instructions

In a bowl, stir together first 5 ingredients. Add vegetables, toss to coat.

no. of servings: 6   *serving size: ½ cup*

Content per Serving

total fat ...... 4.7 gm
saturated fat .. 0.3 gm

cholesterol ..... 0 mg
calories 61

carbohydrate .... 4 gm
protein .... 1 gm

Curry Chicken Salad

1½ cups baked, skinned, boned
   chicken breast, cubed
½ cup celery, diced
2 apples, diced

1½ cups cooked white rice,
   chilled
2½ tablespoons light mayonnaise
2 tablespoons curry powder (or
   more to taste)

Instructions

Mix all ingredients together. Chill and serve on lettuce.

no. of servings: 8   *serving size: ⅔ cup*

Content per Serving

total fat ...... 2.3 gm
saturated fat .. 0.3 gm

cholesterol .... 24 mg
calories 121

carbohydrate ... 16 gm
protein .... 9 gm

This recipe was submitted by Bonnie Stafford.

Fruit Ambrosia

2 cups cantaloupe balls
1 cup blueberries

2 cups honeydew balls
2 12-ounce cans Diet 7-Up

Instructions

Layer cantaloupe balls, blueberries, and honeydew balls in a transparent
bowl. Pour chilled Diet 7-Up over fruit. Serve immediately.

no. of servings: 5   *serving size: about 1 cup*

Content per Serving

total fat ...... 0.4 gm
saturated fat .. 0.0 gm

cholesterol ..... 0 mg
calories 63

carbohydrate ... 16 gm
protein .... 1 gm

This recipe comes from the Diet Center Program, *by Sybil Ferguson (New York: Simon and
Schuster, 1986).*

Fruit Slaw

3 cups shredded cabbage
1 orange, peeled and sectioned
1 cup halved seedless red grapes
½ cup celery, sliced

1 8-ounce carton low-fat orange yogurt
1 small apple, chopped

Instructions
In a large salad bowl, combine cabbage, orange sections, grapes, and celery. In another bowl stir together yogurt and apple. Spread dressing over cabbage mixture. Cover and chill. Just before serving, toss gently. Serve on cabbage-lined plates.

no. of servings: 10   *serving size: about ½ cup*

Content per Serving

total fat ...... 0.5 gm	cholesterol ..... 1 mg	carbohydrate ... 12 gm
saturated fat .. 0.2 gm	calories 56	protein .... 2 gm

This recipe was submitted by Elena Harman. Source: Better Homes and Gardens.

Pea Salad

1 large can peas
¼ cup onions, diced
½ cup celery, diced
1 cup iceberg lettuce, sliced

6 stuffed olives, diced
1 tablespoon vinegar
5 teaspoons light mayonnaise

Instructions
In a medium bowl, blend all ingredients. Refrigerate.

no. of servings: 4   *serving size: ¼ of recipe*

Content per Serving

total fat ...... 2.9 gm	cholesterol ..... 2 mg	carbohydrate ... 16 gm
saturated fat .. 0.2 gm	calories 110	protein .... 5 gm

This recipe was submitted by Ruby Huebner.

Sweet 'n Sour Cabbage Salad

3 cups shredded cabbage (red or green)
½ cup water
2 apples, diced
1 tablespoon caraway seeds
½ cup light or dark raisins

1 teaspoon dill
2 tablespoons white vinegar
1 tablespoon Dijon mustard
1½ teaspoons sugar
½ teaspoon Tabasco
⅛ teaspoon salt

Instructions
Microwave cabbage and water on high for 7 minutes. Drain. Mix rest of ingredients and add to cabbage. Microwave 2–3 minutes until apples are crisp-tender. May be served warm or cold.

no. of servings: 4   *serving size: 1 cup*

Content per Serving

total fat ...... 0.7 gm   cholesterol ..... 0 mg   carbohydrate ... 31 gm
saturated fat .. 0.0 gm   calories 121   protein .... 2 gm

This recipe was submitted by Dorothy Lane.

Tabouli

4 ounces bulgur wheat
⅔ cup water
½ cup lemon juice
4 medium tomatoes, chopped
1 cup green onions, diced
1 cup green peppers, chopped
½ cup snipped parsley

2 tablespoons vegetable oil
1 teaspoon salt
1 teaspoon mint flakes
¼ teaspoon cumin
¼ teaspoon coriander
⅛ teaspoon pepper

Instructions

In a large bowl, combine bulgur wheat, water, and lemon juice. Cover and refrigerate 1 hour, until all liquid is absorbed. Add remaining ingredients and mix. Serve on lettuce leaf.

no. of servings: 4   *serving size: about 1 cup*

Content per Serving

total fat ...... 7.8 gm   cholesterol ..... 0 mg   carbohydrate ... 37 gm
saturated fat .. 0.5 gm   calories 224   protein .... 5 gm

This recipe was submitted by Donna Askin.

Soups

Creamy Squash Soup

2 cups potatoes, peeled and
  chopped
2 cups acorn squash, peeled and
  chopped
½ cup onion, chopped
1½ teaspoons snipped fresh
  marjoram, or ½ teaspoon dried
  marjoram, crushed

¾ teaspoon instant chicken
  bouillon granules
1 clove garlic, minced
1 cup water
⅛ teaspoon pepper
2 cups skim milk

Instructions

In a large saucepan, combine potatoes, squash, onion, marjoram, bouillon, garlic, water, and pepper. Bring to boiling. Reduce heat, cover, and simmer 20 minutes or until vegetables are tender.

Transfer about half of the vegetable mixture into a blender or food processor. Process until smooth. Repeat with second half of vegetable mixture. Return mixture to saucepan. Stir in milk. Heat thoroughly but do not boil.

no. of servings: 10   *serving size: about 1 cup*

Content per Serving

total fat ...... 0.2 gm	cholesterol ..... 1 mg	carbohydrate ... 15 gm
saturated fat .. 0.1 gm	calories 67	protein .... 3 gm

This recipe was submitted by Elena Harman.

Fish Chowder

2 large onions, coarsely chopped
2 green peppers, coarsely chopped
2 red peppers, coarsely chopped
8 ounces mushrooms, sliced
1½ cups carrots, diced
2 cups potatoes, diced
1 cup frozen or fresh cut corn
1 tablespoon vegetable oil
1 large bay leaf
2 cups chicken broth
1½ tablespoons vegetable oil
3 tablespoons flour
2 cups skim milk
2 cups any firm white fish, diced
1 cup tomatoes, chopped
4 to 6 cups water
optional: salt, pepper, nutmeg, Greek seasoning to taste

Instructions

Sauté/steam all the vegetables in 1 tablespoon oil; add the bay leaf. When onions are translucent, add broth. Make white sauce with 1½ tablespoons oil, flour, and milk. Add white sauce to vegetables in pot. Add cooked fish and tomatoes. Add water until soup is consistency of chowder. Season to taste.

no. of servings: 18   *serving size: 1 cup*

Content per Serving

total fat ...... 2.5 gm	cholesterol .... 12 mg	carbohydrate ... 11 gm
saturated fat .. 0.3 gm	calories 93	protein .... 7 gm

This recipe was submitted by Judith Katz.

Golden Harvest Soup

2 cups chicken broth, fat-free
2 cups cauliflower, chopped
1 cup carrots, chopped
½ cup onions, chopped
1 cup skim milk
¼ teaspoon nutmeg
dash pepper

Instructions

In a large pot, combine broth, cauliflower, carrots, and onions. Bring to a boil. Reduce heat and simmer 7 to 10 minutes, until vegetables are tender. Puree in a blender or food processor. Add milk and heat thoroughly, but do not boil. Stir in nutmeg and pepper.

no. of servings: 6   *serving size: about 1 cup*

Content per Serving

total fat ...... 0.7 gm	cholesterol ..... 1 mg	carbohydrate .... 8 gm
saturated fat .. 0.2 gm	calories 53	protein .... 4 gm

This recipe was submitted by Myrna Brams.

Grandma Anne's Vegetable Soup

1 large onion	dashes pepper, salt, dried dill
3 celery stalks	weed
3 carrots	1 tube of Goodman's Vegetable
¼ cup vegetable oil	Soup Mix with Mushrooms,
1 12-ounce can tomatoes	excluding flavor packet
3 quarts water	½ of 10-ounce bag of frozen
	mixed vegetables

Instructions

Chop onion in food processor. Slice celery and carrots in processor. Sauté onion and celery in oil until translucent. Add carrots and tomatoes. In a large pot, combine sautéed vegetables with 3 quarts of water. Add salt, pepper, and dill. Add tube of soup mix. Simmer for at least 2 hours. Add frozen vegetables 15 minutes before finishing.

no. of servings: 16   *serving size: 1 cup*

Content per Serving

total fat ...... 3.5 gm	cholesterol ..... 0 mg	carbohydrate .... 3 gm
saturated fat .. 0.2 gm	calories 52	protein .... 0.7 gm

This recipe was submitted by Donna Askin.

Hearty Pea Soup

2 tablespoons vegetable oil	2 teaspoons salt
1 onion, diced	dash pepper
1 bay leaf	1 carrot, chopped
1 teaspoon celery seed	3 stalks celery, diced
1 cup green split peas	½ cup snipped parsley
¼ cup barley	1 potato, diced
½ cup lima beans, dried	½ teaspoon basil
2 quarts water	½ teaspoon thyme

Instructions

Heat oil in saucepan. Add onion, bay leaf, and celery seed. Sauté 3 minutes. Stir in peas, barley, and lima beans. Transfer mixture into a large pot. Add 2 quarts water and bring to a boil. Cook on low heat partially covered for 1½ hours. Add salt, pepper, vegetables, and herbs. Simmer another 30 to 40 minutes on low heat.

no. of servings: 8   *serving size: 1 cup*

Content per Serving

total fat ...... 3.9 gm	cholesterol ..... 0 mg	carbohydrate ... 24 gm
saturated fat .. 0.3 gm	calories 150	protein .... 6 gm

This recipe was submitted by Gloria Katzenberg.

Lentil No-Fat Soup

1 cup dry lentils (prewashed)	1 cup carrots, diced
4 cups water	¼ teaspoon garlic powder
1 cup celery, diced	¼ teaspoon dried dill
1 medium onion, diced	salt and pepper to taste

Instructions

Combine ingredients in a large pot. Simmer for 1½ to 2 hours. May be frozen.

no. of servings: 4   *serving size: about 1½ cups*

Content per Serving

total fat ...... 0.2 gm	cholesterol ..... 0 mg	carbohydrate ... 30 gm
saturated fat .... 0 gm	calories 158	protein .... 11 gm

This recipe was submitted by Dorothy E. Jenney.

Low-Cal Cabbage Soup

6 large onions, chopped	1 large head cabbage, shredded
2 large carrots, chopped	1 bunch celery, chopped
1 yellow squash, chopped	1 pack dry onion soup mix
2 tomatoes, chopped	

Instructions

Combine all ingredients in a large pot; fill with water until ingredients are covered. Boil for 10 minutes. Cover, lower heat, and simmer until vegetables are soft.

no. of servings: 20   *serving size: 1 cup*

Content per Serving

total fat ...... 0.3 gm	cholesterol ..... 0 mg	carbohydrate .... 7 gm
saturated fat .... 0 gm	calories 32	protein .... 1 gm

This recipe was submitted by Edward Toney.

Seafood Chowder

4 slices Morningstar Farms
Breakfast Strips (soybean
imitation bacon)
½ cup chopped onion
½ cup chopped celery
1 tablespoon vegetable oil
½ clove garlic
1 pint water
1 can tomatoes

¼ cup ketchup
1 teaspoon salt
½ tablespoon Worcestershire
sauce
dash Tabasco
⅛ teaspoon curry powder
½ pound scallops
½ pound shrimp
½ pound steakfish (hake)

Instructions

In a large skillet, brown imitation bacon. Brown onion and celery in oil.
Add all ingredients except seafood. Simmer until tomatoes are cooked. Add
seafood. Cook about 15 minutes more.

no. of servings: 4   *serving size: about 1½ cups*

Content per Serving

total fat ...... 9.8 gm
saturated fat .. 1.1 gm

cholesterol ...111 mg
calories 252

carbohydrate ... 10 gm
protein ....31 gm

This recipe was submitted by Janet Johansen.

Glossary

Aerobic exercise. Repetitive, rhythmic exercise that requires oxygen from the atmosphere for the muscles to continue to contract. Examples are brisk walking, running, swimming, cycling, rowing, jumping rope, and skating.

Anaerobic exercise. Quick, short-term exercise that does not require oxygen from the atmosphere to continue. Examples are sprinting, weight lifting, push-ups, sit-ups, hand grip, and isometrics.

Angina pectoris. Pressing or tightening pain in the middle of the chest due to a significant blockage in a coronary artery that deprives the heart muscle of needed oxygen. The pain is usually related to physical exertion and may also radiate up into the throat or jaw or down the left arm.

Angiography, *see* Coronary angiography

Angioplasty, *see* Coronary artery balloon angioplasty

ApoA1. The major apolipoprotein of HDL; it is necessary for the action of lecithin cholesterol acyl transferase (LCAT).

ApoB. A major apolipoprotein of VLDL, IDL, and LDL (*see* LDL apoB).

ApoC2. An apolipoprotein that is necessary for the action of lipoprotein lipase.

ApoE. A major apolipoprotein of VLDL; it is also found on chylomicron remnants and VLDL remnants, where it facilitates the uptake of these lipoproteins from blood into the liver.

Apolipoproteins (apoA1, apoB, apoC2, apoE, etc.). Special proteins in the blood that bind with lipids such as cholesterol and triglyceride, forming a complex called lipoproteins.

Arachidonic acid. A polyunsaturated fat consisting of a chain of 20 carbons that has four areas of unsaturation (*see also* Omega-6 fatty acids).

Arcus, *see* Corneal arcus

Arrhythmia. Irregular heartbeats that can signal the presence of disease in the heart, including lack of oxygen due to coronary artery disease.

Arteriosclerosis. Literally means "hardening of the arteries." A broad term used to cover a variety of disease states (including atherosclerosis) that lead to abnormal thickening and hardening of the walls of arteries.

Atherosclerosis. A chronic disease process in which there is a gradual build-up of plaque on the inside walls of the arteries. Plaque consists of cholesterol, other lipids, fibrous material, and cellular debris.

Atromid-S®, *see* Clofibrate

Bile acid binding agent (bile acid sequestrant, bile acid resin drug). A drug used for patients with high blood LDL levels, consisting of a long chain (polymer) of organic molecules. The drug is not absorbed into blood, but binds bile acids in the intestine and prevents them from returning to the bloodstream. Instead, they are eliminated from the body in the stool.

Bran. The skin or husk of grains from wheat, rye, or oats, which can be separated from the flour by sifting.

Bypass, *see* Coronary artery bypass

Cardiac catheterization, *see* Coronary angiography

Cerebral vascular disease. A chronic disease process in which the arteries of the brain, called cerebral arteries, are gradually narrowed by atherosclerosis. This can lead to a stroke.

Cholesterol. A white, waxy substance that does not dissolve in water (*see* Lipid). Cholesterol is composed of 27 carbon atoms in the form of four "rings" with a tail. It is found only in animal cells, where it is used to make cell membranes and hormones.

Cholesteryl ester. That form of cholesterol in which a fatty acid is attached to its third carbon through a chemical bond called an ester bond (*see* Lipid). This is the storage form of cholesterol. It is found inside cells and also on the inside (or core) of the blood lipoproteins.

Cholestyramine. A bile acid binding agent that is used to lower blood LDL cholesterol (*see also* Bile acid binding agent). This drug comes in a powder form that must be mixed with liquid before drinking, or alternatively in the form of a "candy" bar.

Cholybar®. A new formulation of cholestyramine in the form of a flavored "candy" bar that can be eaten without mixing with liquid.

Chylomicron. A lipoprotein that transports dietary triglyceride and cholesterol from the intestine into the bloodstream. It is normally not present in blood after an overnight fast.

Chylomicron remnant. The breakdown product of chylomicron that results when triglyceride is broken down by lipoprotein lipase. This particle is relatively enriched in cholesterol and is rapidly removed from blood by the chylomicron remnant receptor in the liver.

Chylomicron remnant receptor. A protein on the surface of liver cells that recognizes apoE on the chylomicron remnant, leading to the removal of the lipoprotein from blood.

Clofibrate. A drug used to treat elevated blood VLDL and triglyceride levels. A derivative of fibric acid, this agent was found in the World Health Organization Trial to reduce the incidence of coronary heart disease, but it also increased death from non-cardiovascular diseases. Consequently, its use is limited to treatment of type 3 disease and very high blood triglyceride levels that do not respond to other lipid-lowering drugs.

Colestid®, *see* Colestipol

Colestipol. A bile acid binding agent that is used to treat patients with high blood LDL levels (*see* Bile acid binding agent). It is a powder which must be mixed with a liquid before drinking.

Corneal arcus. Deposit of cholesterol in the clear outer covering (cornea) of the eye that usually occurs in the shape of a half moon (arcus). Corneal arcus before the age of 55 usually indicates the presence of a blood lipid problem. Corneal arcus in the elderly (arcus senilis) or in blacks (arcus not so senilis) does not usually indicate a blood lipid problem.

Coronary angiography. A test used to determine whether there are significant blockages in the coronary arteries. A hollow plastic tube (catheter) is inserted in the large femoral artery in the groin. The catheter is threaded through the femoral artery, into the aorta, and up to the aortic valve, which separates the aorta from the main pumping part of the heart, the left ventricle. The catheter is placed in the openings of the coronary arteries (which begin just above the aortic valve), and a small amount of dye is injected. The appearance of the dye in the arteries is photographed using a special camera that enables the cardiologist to watch the heart on a television monitor. This test is also sometimes referred to as cardiac catheterization.

Coronary artery. An artery that supplies blood with its nutrients and oxygen to the heart muscle. There are three major coronary arteries: the right coronary artery, the left anterior descending coronary artery, and the left circumflex coronary artery.

Coronary artery balloon angioplasty. A procedure that does not require open heart surgery and that is used to treat blocked coronary arteries. A thin, flexible tube containing an uninflated balloon is inserted into the artery underneath the blockage, and the balloon is then inflated to "squash down" the blockage.

Coronary artery bypass. An open heart operation in which a blood vessel graft (the saphenous vein from the leg) is used to connect the aorta with a coronary artery at a point beyond its blockage with atherosclerosis. One or more vessel grafts may be used (e.g., triple vessel bypass for three blocked arteries). In patients in whom multiple distal blockages rule out the use of a bypass graft, an artery (the internal mammary from the chest) is implanted beyond the blocked coronary artery. In some cases, an implant may be combined with a bypass graft.

Coronary heart disease. Results from blockages of atherosclerosis in the arteries of the heart called the coronary arteries. This can lead to angina pectoris, heart attack, and sudden death. Coronary heart disease that develops before age 55 is called premature (or early) coronary heart disease.

DHA (docosahexaenoic acid). A polyunsaturated fatty acid enriched in fish oils that has a chain of 22 carbons and six areas of unsaturation. DHA is plentiful in the fats of the brain and may have a role in the normal development of the eye and the brain. (*See also* Omega-3 fatty acids.)

EKG (resting; stress exercise; stress thallium exercise). A recording or tracing that is used to detect electrical impulses as they travel through the various parts of the heart muscle. Electrodes are attached to the body to detect these impulses at rest (resting EKG), during exercise (stress exercise), or during exercise after the injection of a small amount of radioactive thallium (stress thallium exercise). An abnormal tracing results when the electrical impulses do not travel through the heart muscle properly, or when the thallium is not distributed evenly throughout the heart. Such results indicate that the heart muscle has been previously damaged, or that under the stress of exercise, sufficient blood is not reaching part of the heart muscle owing to a blockage in a coronary artery.

EPA (eicosapentaenoic acid). A polyunsaturated fatty acid enriched in fish oil that consists of a chain of twenty carbons and five areas of unsaturation. (See also Omega-3 fatty acids.)

Familial combined hyperlipidemia (FCH). An inherited disorder causing premature coronary heart disease in which affected relatives have either a high blood cholesterol level alone (type 2a lipoprotein pattern), a high blood triglyceride level alone (type 4 lipoprotein pattern), or an elevation in both cholesterol and triglyceride (type 2b lipoprotein pattern). FCH is due to the liver making too much VLDL (and therefore triglyceride, cholesterol, and apoB).

Familial hypercholesterolemia (FH). An inherited disorder producing premature coronary heart disease that is characterized by high levels of blood cholesterol and LDL cholesterol. FH is due to an inherited defect in the LDL receptor that prevents the removal of LDL from the blood at a normal rate. Persons with one faulty gene for the LDL receptor are called FH heterozygotes; those in whom both genes are faulty are called FH homozygotes.

Familial hypertriglyceridemia (FHT). An inherited disorder characterized by high VLDL and triglyceride levels. LDL cholesterol is normal; HDL cholesterol is often low. FHT is often associated with obesity, diabetes, and gout and therefore with some increased risk of coronary heart disease and peripheral vascular disease.

Fat, *see* Monounsaturated fat, Polyunsaturated fat, Saturated fat

Fatty acid. A member of the lipid family. A fatty acid is insoluble in water. It consists of a chain of carbon atoms whose length and degree of saturation can vary. A saturated fatty acid is one in which all the positions in the carbon chain are occupied (saturated) with hydrogen atoms. A mono-unsaturated fatty acid is one in which one position in the chain of carbons is unsaturated: that is, two adjacent carbons are each missing one hydrogen atom, producing what is referred to as a "double bond." A polyunsaturated fatty acid is one in which two or more positions in the carbon chain are unsaturated; thus two or more areas contain "double bonds" and are not saturated with hydrogen atoms.

Fatty streak. The early form of atherosclerosis, at which time cholesterol and other materials from the blood are deposited in the lining of the arteries but the buildup has not begun to narrow the opening of the artery.

FCH, *see* Familial combined hyperlipidemia

Fenofibrate. A drug used to lower blood VLDL and triglyceride levels; a derivative of fibric acid.

FHT, *see* Familial hypertriglyceridemia

Fiber (water-soluble, water-insoluble). Vegetable material that is resistant to digestion. Fiber may be water-insoluble, such as wheat bran, or water-soluble, such as oat brain, guar gum from legumes, and pectin from fruits.

Fibric acid derivative. A drug derived from the compound fibric acid that may help to lower blood VLDL and triglyceride levels (*see* Clofibrate, Fenofibrate, Gemfibrozil).

Fibrous plaque. An intermediate form of atherosclerosis in which cholesterol and other materials from the blood are starting to narrow the opening of the artery but a significant amount of blockage has not yet occurred.

Gemfibrozil. A drug used to lower blood VLDL and triglyceride levels; it also increases HDL cholesterol levels.

Gene. A unit of genetic material or DNA that is responsible for the production of a protein (including an enzyme) by the cell.

Guar gum. A water-soluble fiber found in legumes, particularly their seeds.

HDL, *see* High-density lipoprotein

Heart attack, *see* Myocardial infarction

Hepatic triglyceride lipase. A protein (enzyme) on the surface of liver cells that breaks down the triglyceride in the core of lipoproteins (such as intermediate-density lipoprotein, or IDL). A modified particle is produced.

Heterozygote. A term used to indicate that a person carries one faulty gene for an inherited condition and one normal gene.

High blood pressure, *see* Hypertension

High-density lipoprotein (HDL). A blood lipoprotein that carries about 20 to 25 percent of the cholesterol in blood. About 50 percent of HDL is protein, the major one being apoA1. HDL removes cholesterol from the surface of cells, esterifies it, and then transfers the cholesteryl ester to other lipoproteins for delivery to the liver for processing. HDL is sometimes referred to as the "good cholesterol" because high levels of HDL are associated with a lower risk of coronary heart disease and low levels with a higher risk.

HMG CoA reductase inhibitor. A class of drugs that blocks the manufacture of cholesterol by cells by inhibiting the action of an enzyme called HMG CoA reductase. These drugs reduce the amount of cholesterol inside cells, leading to an increase in the number of LDL receptors on the surface of cells and an increased removal of LDL from the blood.

Homozygote. A term used to indicate that a person carries two faulty genes for a specific trait (one from the father and one from the mother).

HyperapoB. A disorder associated with premature coronary heart disease and characterized by high blood levels of LDL apoB (*see* LDL apoB) but by normal or only moderately elevated levels of LDL cholesterol. The increased number of small, dense LDL particles in hyperapoB is due to the overproduction of VLDL in the liver, which leads to increased synthesis of its breakdown product, LDL.

Hypercholesterolemia. A high level of total cholesterol in the blood.

Hyperlipidemia. A high level of total cholesterol *and* triglyceride in the blood.

Hypertension. A condition in which the blood pressure is elevated, leading to increased chance of having a stroke and developing kidney disease. Hypertension is also called "high blood pressure."

Hypertriglyceridemia. A high level of triglyceride in the blood.

HypoHDL. A disorder associated with premature coronary heart disease in which the blood levels of HDL cholesterol are very low and the LDL cholesterol, LDL apoB, and triglyceride levels are normal.

Intermediate-density lipoprotein (IDL). A by-product of the breakdown of triglyceride in VLDL and VLDL remnants. IDL is relatively enriched in cholesterol. Some IDL is removed from the liver by the LDL (B, E) receptor; the rest is converted into LDL.

Ischemia. Lack of oxygen to cells, leading to injury and, if severe enough, to permanent damage or scarring of the tissue.

LCAT (Lecithin cholesterol acyl transferase). The enzyme that is responsible for converting cholesterol to cholesteryl ester by removing a fatty acid from lecithin and transferring it to cholesterol. This reaction occurs primarily in HDL. The cholesteryl ester is then transferred to other lipoproteins or can be taken up by the liver directly from HDL.

LDL, *see* Low-density lipoprotein

LDL apoB. The major apolipoprotein of LDL and the major carrier of cholesterol in the blood. It also is responsible for the recognition of LDL by the LDL receptor.

LDL (B, E) receptor. A protein on the surface of cells that (1) binds LDL apoB and allows the LDL to be taken into the cell and processed; and (2) binds apoE on VLDL remnants and IDL and facilitates their uptake into the liver from blood.

Lecithin. A phospholipid found in cell membranes and also lipoproteins (*see also* Lipid). Lecithin consists of a backbone called glycerol, to which are attached two fatty acids, and a chemical compound called phosphorylcholine.

Legumes. Vegetables, like beans, with pods that enclose seeds, and which contain the water-soluble fiber guar gum.

Linoleic acid. A polyunsaturated fatty acid enriched in many plant oils. It has a chain of eighteen carbons and two areas of unsaturation (*see* Omega-6 fatty acids).

Lipid. Any of various substances that are insoluble in water but will dissolve in solvents such as chloroform or ether. Examples of lipids are cholesterol, cholesteryl esters, triglyceride, phospholipids, and fatty acids.

Lipid profile. A blood test in which the blood levels of cholesterol, LDL cholesterol, HDL cholesterol, and triglyceride are measured.

Lipidil®, *see* Fenofibrate

Lipoprotein. A complex of proteins called apolipoproteins and lipids, such as cholesterol, cholesteryl esters, triglyceride, and phospholipids. Blood lipoproteins are responsible for transporting lipids between various organs of the body.

Lipoprotein lipase. An enzyme that is responsible for the breakdown of triglyceride in either chylomicrons or VLDL.

Lipoprotein pattern. Refers to a particular interpretation of a lipid profile in which the result is categorized according to which lipoprotein classes are elevated or depressed.

Lopid®, *see* Gemfibrozil

Lorelco®, *see* Probucol

Lovastatin. One of the HMG CoA reductase inhibitors. This drug lowers high levels of blood cholesterol and LDL cholesterol.

Low-density lipoprotein (LDL). The major carrier of cholesterol in blood. About 50 percent of LDL is cholesterol and cholesteryl ester; 25 percent is protein, mostly apoB. A high level of LDL promotes atherosclerosis and coronary heart disease.

Mevacor®, *see* Lovastatin

Monounsaturated fat. A clear, oily substance that is liquid at room temperature. Monounsaturated fats are rich in monounsaturated fatty acids; examples are olive oil, peanut oil, and canola oil (*see* Lipid).

Myocardial infarction. The muscle of the heart (myocardium) is deprived of oxygen, leading to death of the muscle cells (infarction). This process is often called a heart attack. It leaves a scar over the injured area.

Myristic acid. A saturated fatty acid that contains fourteen carbons in its chain. Foods high in myristic acid increase blood levels of cholesterol and LDL cholesterol.

Niacin. Another chemical name for nicotinic acid. However, this term is also used by nutritionists to refer to vitamin B_3, which contains two components, nicotinic acid and nicotinamide.

Nicotinamide. A derivative of nicotinic acid that is essential for many chemical reactions in the body but does not lower blood lipid levels.

Nicotinic acid. A component of vitamin B_3. When nicotinic acid is used in high doses, it becomes a drug that lowers high blood levels of cholesterol, triglyceride, and VLDL but raises HDL levels. Nicotinic acid decreases the production of VLDL (and therefore apoB, triglyceride, and cholesterol) in the liver.

Oat bran. A water-soluble fiber found in the husks of oats. Oat bran can lower the blood cholesterol level.

Oleic acid. A monounsaturated fatty acid that has a chain of eighteen carbons and contains one area of unsaturation between carbons 9 and 10. Olive oil, canola oil, and peanut oil are enriched in oleic acid.

Omega-3 fatty acids. A group of polyunsaturated fatty acids in which the last area of unsaturation occurs at the third position from the tail end (which contains the last, or omega, carbon) (see DHA, EPA).

Omega-6 fatty acids. A group of polyunsaturated fatty acids in which the last area of unsaturation occurs at the sixth position from the tail end (see Arachidonic acid, Linoleic acid).

P/S ratio. A term used to describe the amount of polyunsaturated fat (P) as compared to the amount of saturated fat (S) in a specific food or overall in the diet. The P/S ratio does not take monounsaturated fat into account. Generally, a diet with a low P/S ratio will increase blood cholesterol and a diet with a high P/S ratio will lower blood cholesterol.

Palmitic acid. A saturated fatty acid that has a chain of sixteen carbons and no areas of unsaturation. Foods high in palmitic acid increase blood levels of cholesterol and LDL cholesterol.

Pectin. A water-soluble fiber found in the skin and white rind of fruits. Pectin can lower blood cholesterol levels when ingested in large amounts.

Peripheral vascular disease. A chronic disease process in which the arteries of the legs are narrowed owing to atherosclerosis.

Phospholipids. A class of lipids usually containing a glycerol backbone, two fatty acids, and a third component in which a chemical compound is attached to the glycerol through its phosphorus component (see also Lecithin).

Plaque, see Atherosclerosis

Polyunsaturated fat. A clear, oily substance that is liquid at room temperature and whose main component is polyunsaturated fatty acids (see also Lipid). Examples of polyunsaturated fats are corn oil, safflower oil, and sunflower seed oil.

Probucol. A drug used to lower LDL levels in the blood. This drug is a chemical compound called butylphenol, which is soluble in lipids. When the drug is taken, it finds its way into the core of LDL and speeds the removal of LDL from blood. Probucol also decreases the production of HDL and thereby lowers the blood HDL cholesterol level.

Prostaglandin I$_2$. A product derived from arachidonic acid that dilates blood vessels and inhibits the clumping of platelets in blood. In this way, it helps to prevent the formation of blood clots in the arteries.

Prostaglandin I$_3$. A derivative of eicosapentaenoic acid (EPA). It dilates the blood vessels, inhibits clumping of platelets in blood, and thus helps to prevent the formation of blood clots in the arteries.

Questran®, *see* Cholestyramine

Saturated fat. A white, oily substance that is solid at room temperature and whose main component is saturated fatty acids. Saturated fats are the main component of the white marbling in meats, of the visible fat around meat, of butter and cheese, and of whole milk and ice cream. Saturated fats are also plentiful in coconut oil, palm kernel oil, and palm oil, three plant oils widely used in commercially processed foods.

Stearic acid. A saturated fatty acid that has a chain of eighteen carbons and no areas of unsaturation. Unlike palmitic acid, stearic acid does *not* increase blood cholesterol and LDL cholesterol levels and may have some lowering effect; it is the exception to the rule that saturated fatty acids raise blood cholesterol. This is probably because stearic acid is converted in the body into oleic acid, a monounsaturated fatty acid.

Step One diet. A diet recommended by the Adult Treatment Panel of the National Cholesterol Education Program, National Institutes of Health, in which less than 30 percent of the calories are from total fat, less than 10 percent from saturated fat, no more than 10 percent from polyunsaturated fat, and between 10 and 15 percent from monounsaturated fat. Cholesterol is limited to less than 300 mg per day. In this diet, 50–60 percent of the calories are from carbohydrate and 10–20 percent from protein.

Step Two diet. A stricter diet recommended by the Adult Treatment Panel of the National Cholesterol Education Program, National Institutes of Health, for lowering blood total and LDL cholesterol levels. Total fat is less than 30 percent of the calories, with less than 7 percent from saturated fat, no more than 10 percent from polyunsaturated fat, and 10–15 percent from monounsaturated fat. Cholesterol is restricted to less than 200 mg per day. As in the Step One diet, 50–60 percent of the calories are from carbohydrate and 10–20 percent from protein.

Stress test, *see* EKG

Thromboxane A$_2$. A product derived from arachidonic acid that causes blood vessels to become narrower and promotes clotting by causing platelets to clump in the blood.

Thromboxane A₃. A product derived from eicosapentaenoic acid (EPA) that is biologically inactive: that is, it does not cause blood vessels to narrow or platelets to clump.

Triglyceride. A member of the lipid class in which three fatty acids are attached to a glycerol backbone through a chemical bond called an ester bond. Triglyceride is obtained from the diet and is also made in the liver. Triglyceride is transported through blood on either chylomicrons or VLDL.

Type 3 disease. A disorder associated with premature coronary heart disease characterized by very high levels of blood cholesterol and triglyceride. These high levels are due to the inability of the body to process normally chylomicron remnants from the diet and VLDL remnants from the liver. ApoE, the apolipoprotein responsible for recognition of chylomicron remnants and VLDL remnants by the liver, is defective in patients with this condition. Patients with full-blown type 3 also overproduce VLDL in the liver.

Type 5 disease. A disorder in which cholesterol, and particularly triglyceride, are elevated because of an increased amount of both chylomicrons and VLDL in the blood. This can be due to one or both of two abnormalities: overproduction of VLDL by the liver, and/or slower hydrolysis of triglyceride in chylomicrons and VLDL. A major problem associated with type 5 disease is pancreatitis. Type 5 is often associated with obesity, diabetes, and low HDL cholesterol levels, and as such can also increase the risk of coronary heart disease and peripheral vascular disease.

Unsaturated fat. A clear, oily substance that is liquid at room temperature and in which monounsaturated and polyunsaturated fatty acids predominate (*see also* Lipid).

Very-low-density lipoprotein (VLDL). The major carrier of triglyceride in the blood of a fasting patient. VLDL is made primarily in the liver and contains about 65 percent of its weight as triglyceride. It also contains cholesterol and phospholipid. The major apolipoproteins of VLDL are apoE and apoB. As the triglyceride in VLDL is broken down by lipoprotein lipase, VLDL remnants and then IDL are produced. Some of these particles are taken up in the liver through apoE, but the rest are converted into cholesterol-rich LDL.

VLDL remnants. The breakdown products of VLDL. VLDL remnants contain triglyceride and relatively more cholesterol than VLDL. Some VLDL remnants may be taken up by the liver; the rest are converted into intermediate-density lipoprotein (IDL).

VO₂ max. The maximum rate of oxygen uptake, or the greatest amount of oxygen that can be taken up from the air during exercise. The higher the VO₂ max, the more work that can be performed.

Wheat bran. A water-insoluble fiber from the husks of wheat. Wheat bran does *not* lower blood cholesterol levels.

Xanthelasma. An orange, flat deposit of cholesterol on the eyelids or under the eyes, indicating that a blood lipid problem is probably present.

Xanthoma. A deposit of cholesterol and/or triglyceride in the skin or tendons of the body. Xanthomas occur in people with several different kinds of blood lipid problems.

General Index

Index of Recipes